The Science and Applications of 3D Bioprinting

The field of 3D bioprinting has witnessed significant growth over the past decade, with groundbreaking advances in the development of bioprinted tissues, organs, and implants. The use of 3D bioprinting has the potential to revolutionize regenerative medicine, drug development, and personalized healthcare. *The Science and Applications of 3D Bioprinting* provides an in-depth exploration of the science of 3D bioprinting, covering the latest advancements in materials, techniques, and applications, and serves as a comprehensive guide to this emerging field.

Features:

- Begins with a historical overview of bioprinting, followed by an exploration of the materials, bioinks, and CAD design used in bioprinting.
- Covers current bioprinting techniques, including bioprinting for regenerative medicine, drug development, and pharmaceutical testing.
- Includes numerous real-world case studies that highlight practical applications of 3D bioprinting, allowing readers to see how 3D bioprinting is being used in regenerative medicine, drug development, and pharmaceutical testing.
- Discusses the ethical and regulatory considerations associated with bioprinting.
- Provides insights into future directions and emerging trends.

This book is intended for scientists, researchers, students, and professionals interested in understanding the principles of 3D bioprinting, its applications, and the ethical considerations surrounding this exciting and rapidly advancing field.

Prof. Dr. Thiago Domingues Stocco is a Full Professor and researcher in Bioengineering at the Scientific and Technological Institute of Brasil University, where he leads the BioRegenera.Lab research group. His work focuses on advanced strategies in 3D bioprinting and biofabrication for the development of patient-specific regenerative implants, especially applied to the regeneration of tissues of the musculoskeletal system. He has also served as a Visiting Professor and postdoctoral researcher at Harvard Medical School. Dr. Stocco is an affiliate member of the Academy of Sciences of the State of São Paulo (ACIESP), a member of the editorial boards of scientific journals, and the author of multiple peer-reviewed publications in top-ranked outlets, contributing to the advancement of biofabrication and translational tissue engineering.

Dr. Shabir Hassan is an Assistant Professor of Biology in Khalifa University. Before joining Khalifa, he was an Early Career Investigator at Harvard Medical School, USA. His main focus of research has been devising *in vitro* platforms for diseases such as cancer and different tissues for drug discovery and drug delivery applications. Additionally, his interest revolves around 3D bioprinting of disease models to study genetic and rare diseases. He has published more than 75 research papers and has won many awards from the governments of India and Australia, Harvard Medical School, Swiss NSF, Yonsei University, and TERMIS. He was awarded the BRICS 2025 Award for Excellence in Research. Dr. Hassan serves as an Associate Editor for *Frontiers in Biomaterials Science.* He served as a Founding Associate Editor for *MIT Science Policy Review* in 2020. Additionally, he edits special issues for *Polymers, Frontiers in Pharmacology,* and many others.

Prof. Dr. Anderson de Oliveira Lobo is a Full Professor at the Center for Technology of the Federal University of Piauí. He is a CNPq Research Productivity Fellow Level A. He was an affiliated member of the Brazilian Academy of Sciences in the area of engineering from 2020 to 2025. He is a fellow of the international organizations: Core Academy – Biological Science and Engineering, Materials Tech, and the International Association of Advanced Materials. He is included among the top 2% of the most influential scientists in the world since 2021 in the area of Biomedical Engineering/Bioengineering. He possesses didactic-scientific experience in the area of Materials and Biomedical Engineering. He works directly on the development of biomimetic and bioinspired biomaterials applied to tissue engineering and nanomedicine. He has supervised more than 120 postgraduate and undergraduate students across various projects in this subfield. He has more than 200 indexed articles in journals with a selective editorial policy, over 5,600 citations, and an H-index of 41. Dr. Lobo serves as an Associate Editor-in-Chief for the *International Journal of Nanomedicine.* He serves as an ad hoc advisor for several international journals and Brazilian and international grant agencies. He also has edited several special issues for scientific journals, including the *International Journal of Bioprinting* and many others.

Emerging Materials and Technologies

Series Editor: Boris I. Kharissov

The *Emerging Materials and Technologies* series is devoted to highlighting publications centered on emerging advanced materials and novel technologies. Attention is paid to those newly discovered or applied materials with potential to solve pressing societal problems and improve quality of life, corresponding to environmental protection, medicine, communications, energy, transportation, advanced manufacturing, and related areas.

The series takes into account that, under present strong demands for energy, material, and cost savings, as well as heavy contamination problems and worldwide pandemic conditions, the area of emerging materials and related scalable technologies is a highly interdisciplinary field, with the need for researchers, professionals, and academics across the spectrum of engineering and technological disciplines. The main objective of this book series is to attract more attention to these materials and technologies and invite conversation among the international R&D community.

Emerging Materials for Biofuel Developments
Edited by Selvakumar Periyasamy, Eduardo Alberto López-Maldonado, and R. Balachandran

Nanostructured Materials for Energy Applications
Edited by Abdullah M. Al-Enizi, Mohd Ubaidullah, Mohd Shkir, and Abhay Kumar Singh

Boron Nitride Nanostructures
Applications in Energy and Healthcare
Indranil Lahiri, Amrita De Adhikari, Souvik Ghosh, Rita Joshi, Satish Jaiswal, and Debrupa Lahiri

Smart Polymers
An Emerging Vista for Nanotheranostics
Dipankar Chattopadhyay, Adrija Ghosh, Jonathan Tersur Orasugh, and Suprakas Sinha Ray

Lightweight Materials for Electric Vehicles
Sustainable Materials, Production Process, and Modeling Techniques
Edited by R. Suresh, C. Durga Prasad, Satish Kumar, Bharath K.N., and Ajith G. Joshi

Graphitic Carbon Nitrides
Michio Inagaki, Masahiro Toyoda, and Yasushi Soneda

The Science and Applications of 3D Bioprinting
Edited by Thiago Domingues Stocco and Anderson de Oliveira Lobo

For more information about this series, please visit www.routledge.com/Emerging-Materials-and-Technologies/book-series/CRCEMT

The Science and Applications of 3D Bioprinting

Edited by

Thiago Domingues Stocco, Shabir Hassan, and Anderson de Oliveira Lobo

CRC Press
Taylor & Francis Group
Boca Raton London New York

CRC Press is an imprint of the
Taylor & Francis Group, an **informa** business

Designed cover image: © 2026 Shutterstock

First edition published 2026
by CRC Press
2385 NW Executive Center Drive, Suite 320, Boca Raton FL 33431

and by CRC Press
4 Park Square, Milton Park, Abingdon, Oxon, OX14 4RN

CRC Press is an imprint of Taylor & Francis Group, LLC

ISBN: 978-1-032-63814-0 (hbk)
ISBN: 978-1-032-63815-7 (pbk)
ISBN: 978-1-032-63816-4 (ebk)

DOI: 10.1201/9781032638164

Typeset in Times
by codeMantra

Contents

Preface

Three-dimensional bioprinting has progressed from a formative concept to a structured scientific and technological field with growing impact across bioengineering and the life sciences. This book was developed to provide a coherent route through that landscape. It connects foundational ideas, enabling methods, and current applications in a sequence that mirrors how researchers, students, and practitioners typically encounter and integrate the subject. Our aim is to offer a clear, balanced, and authoritative overview that helps readers understand what the field is, why it matters, and how its core components relate to one another.

The volume opens with a concise historical perspective that establishes how bioprinting emerged and matured. It then examines bioinks and materials, recognizing that the selection, formulation, and characterization of these systems underlie the performance of printed constructs. Building on that foundation, the book addresses the translation from digital design to fabrication through computer-aided design workflows that prepare geometries and toolpaths for biological manufacturing.

Subsequent chapters survey current techniques and tools used in bioprinting, presenting the principal strategies and platforms that define practice today. The discussion then turns to information technology as it relates to bioprinting, including software frameworks and computational workflows that support design, process control, and data handling. With this infrastructure in place, the book advances to applications in regenerative medicine, outlining representative uses and considerations that guide the deployment of bioprinting in tissue engineering contexts.

The next section focuses on engineering scaled-up tissues via bioprinting, addressing design and fabrication considerations that arise when moving from small constructs to larger systems. The book then explores how bioprinting interfaces with organ-on-chip technology, highlighting the conceptual and practical connections between these platforms. A dedicated chapter compiles in vivo studies of bioprinted tissues and organs, providing an integrated view of approaches and outcomes reported to date.

The closing chapter looks ahead to bioprinting horizons, identifying emerging trends and future directions that may influence research and translation in the coming years. Throughout, the emphasis remains on clarity, rigor, and relevance to both established investigators and those entering the field. By organizing the topics in a linear progression from history to future directions, this book offers a structured reference that can be read end-to-end or consulted selectively according to the need.

We hope this work serves as a dependable guide for learning, research, and development in 3D bioprinting. It reflects the collective effort of authors and reviewers who brought together diverse expertise to produce a resource that is both accessible and comprehensive within its defined scope.

Contributors

Samile Bezerra de Aguiar
São Carlos Institute of Chemistry (IQSC – USP)
São Carlos, Brazil

Mohammed Aldhuhoori
Department of Biological Sciences
College of Medicine and Health Sciences, Khalifa University
Abu Dhabi, United Arab Emirates

Shahd Alshehhi
Department of Biological Sciences
College of Medicine and Health Sciences, Khalifa University
Abu Dhabi, United Arab Emirates

Paulo Henrique Junqueira Amorim
Renato Archer Information Technology Center
Campinas, Brazil

Renan Nascimento Araújo
São Carlos Institute of Chemistry (IQSC – USP)
São Carlos, Brazil

Maria Eduarda de Almeida Astolfo
São Carlos Institute of Chemistry (IQSC – USP)
São Carlos, Brazil

Huseyin Avci
Cellular Therapy and Stem Cell Production Application and Research Centre
ESTEM, Eskisehir Osmangazi University
Eskisehir, Türkiye
and
Department of Metallurgical and Materials Engineering
Eskisehir Osmangazi University
Eskisehir, Türkiye
and
Translational Medicine Research and Clinical Center (TATUM)
Eskisehir Osmangazi University
Eskisehir, Türkiye

Fawzi Banat
Chemical and Petroleum Engineering
Khalifa University
Abu Dhabi, United Arab Emirates
and
Food Security and Technology Center
Khalifa University
Abu Dhabi, United Arab Emirates

Judy Bassaleh
Department of Biological Sciences
College of Medicine and Health Sciences, Khalifa University
Abu Dhabi, United Arab Emirates

Kaoutar Chattahy
Trinity Centre for Biomedical Engineering
Trinity College Dublin
Dublin, Ireland

Gabriela Morais da Costa
Federal University of ABC
São Bernardo do Campo, Brazil
and
Quantis Biotechnology
São Paulo, Brazil

Chuyue Cui
School of Health Sciences and Biomedical Engineering
Hebei University of Technology
Tianjin, China

Shadab Dabagh
Institute of Applied Physics "Nello Carrara"
National Research Council of Italy (CNR)
Sesto Fiorentino, Italy

Janaina de Andréa Dernowsek
3D Biofabrication Training and Innovation Center, BioEdTech
São Paulo, Brazil
and
Quantis Biotechnology
São Paulo, Brazil

Aliakbar Ebrahimi
Department of Biomedical Engineering
Ankara Yildirim Beyazit University
Ankara, Türkiye
and
Cellular Therapy and Stem Cell Production Application and Research Centre
ESTEM, Eskisehir Osmangazi University
Eskisehir, Türkiye

Jiaxuan Fan
Department of Orthopaedics
Orthopaedic Research Institute, West China Hospital, Sichuan University
Chengdu, China

Thais Amaral França
Federal University of ABC
São Bernardo do Campo, Brazil
and
Quantis Biotechnology
São Paulo, Brazil

Hamed Ghorbanpoor
Cellular Therapy and Stem Cell Production Application and Research Centre, ESTEM
Eskisehir Osmangazi University
Eskisehir, Türkiye

Marcília Valéria Guimarães
Renato Archer Information Technology Center
Campinas, Brazil

Somayeh Asadi Haris
Department of Chemistry, Faculty of Science
Eskisehir Osmangazi University
Eskisehir, Türkiye

Shabir Hassan
Department of Biological Sciences
College of Medicine and Health Sciences, Khalifa University
Abu Dhabi, United Arab Emirates
and
Center for Biotechnology
Khalifa University
Abu Dhabi, United Arab Emirates

Paula Midori Kaneko
Renato Archer Information Technology Center
Campinas, Brazil

Aliaa S. Karam
Trinity Centre for Biomedical Engineering
Trinity College Dublin
Dublin, Ireland

Gabriela S. Kronemberger
Trinity Centre for Biomedical Engineering
Trinity College Dublin
Dublin, Ireland

Anderson Oliveira Lobo
Interdisciplinary Laboratory for Advanced Materials, Materials Science & Engineering Graduate Program
Federal University of Piauí
Teresina, Brazil

Zeyu Luo
Department of Orthopaedics
Orthopaedic Research Institute, West China Hospital, Sichuan University
Chengdu, China

Leonardo Mendes Ribeiro Machado
Renato Archer Information Technology Center
Campinas, Brazil

Bianca Chieregato Maniglia
São Carlos Institute of Chemistry (IQSC – USP)
São Carlos, Brazil

Juliano Marcello
Post-Graduation Program in Biotechnology
University of Araraquara
Araraquara, Brazil

Pamela Ferreira do Nascimento
Quantis Biotechnology
São Paulo, Brazil

Pedro Yoshito Noritomi
Renato Archer Information Technology Center
Campinas, Brazil

Ayça Bal Öztürk
Department of Analytical Chemistry
Faculty of Pharmacy
Istinye University
Istanbul, Türkiye
and
Department of Stem Cell and Tissue Engineering
Institute of Health Sciences
Istinye University
Istanbul, Türkiye
and
Department of Biomedical Engineering
Faculty of Engineering & Natural Sciences
Istinye University
Istanbul, Türkiye
and
Stem Cell and Tissue Engineering Application and Research Center (ISUKOK)
Istinye University
Istanbul, Türkiye

Kamilla da Costa Pantoja
Quantis Biotechnology
São Paulo, Brazil

Rodrigo Alvarenga Rezende
Post-Graduation Program in Biotechnology
University of Araraquara
Araraquara, Brazil

Arthur Schimith
Post-Graduation Program in Biotechnology
University of Araraquara
Araraquara, Brazil

Claudia Larissa Viana da Silva
Quantis Biotechnology
São Paulo, Brazil

Luciano Paulino Silva
Embrapa Genetic Resources and Biotechnology
Brasilia, Brazil

Hemant Singh
Department of Biological Sciences
College of Medicine and Health Sciences
Khalifa University
Abu Dhabi, United Arab Emirates
and
Center for Biotechnology
Khalifa University
Abu Dhabi, United Arab Emirates
and
Chemical and Petroleum Engineering
Khalifa University
Abu Dhabi, United Arab Emirates
and
Food Security and Technology Center
Khalifa University
Abu Dhabi, United Arab Emirates

Francesca D. Spagnuolo
Trinity Centre for Biomedical Engineering
Trinity College Dublin
Dublin, Ireland

Thiago Domingues Stocco
BioRegenera.Lab, Bioengineering Program
Scientific and Technological Institute, Brasil University
São Paulo, Brazil

Ergün Alperay Tarım
Department of Mechanical Engineering and Applied Mechanics
University of Pennsylvania
Philadelphia, Pennsylvania

Larissa Tessaro
São Carlos Institute of Chemistry (IQSC – USP)
São Carlos, Brazil

Muath Tuffaha
Department of Biological Sciences
College of Medicine and Health Sciences, Khalifa University
Abu Dhabi, United Arab Emirates

Gabriela Mendes da Rocha Vaz
Institute of Biological Sciences
University of Brasilia
Brasilia, Brazil

Rukshana Veettil
Department of Biological Sciences
College of Medicine and Health Sciences, Khalifa University
Abu Dhabi, United Arab Emirates

Thomas J. Webster
School of Health Sciences and Biomedical Engineering
Hebei University of Technology
Tianjin, China
and
Division of Pre-college and Undergraduate Studies
Brown University
Providence, Rhode Island
and
School of Engineering
Saveetha University
Chennai, India

1 From Concept to Reality
A Brief History of Bioprinting

Thiago Domingues Stocco
and Anderson Oliveira Lobo

1.1 INTRODUCTION

The emergence of three-dimensional (3D) bioprinting represents not a singular invention, but the remarkable culmination of two parallel, yet initially distinct, scientific revolutions of the late 20th century: additive manufacturing (AM) and tissue engineering (TE). 3D bioprinting is an advanced AM approach that utilizes living cells, biomaterials (collectively termed "bioinks"), and biological molecules to fabricate bioengineered constructs that mimic the architecture and function of native tissues and organs [1] (Figure 1.1). Its history is a compelling story of convergence, where an industrial drive for rapid prototyping fortuitously provided the tools to address the profound clinical challenges of organ shortage and tissue repair, needs that were simultaneously giving rise to the field of TE.

The central promise of TE, to restore, maintain, or improve tissue function, was historically limited by the challenge of fabricating constructs with the requisite structural complexity and cellular organization of native tissues [2]. Traditional methods often involved the manual seeding of cells onto preformed scaffolds, a

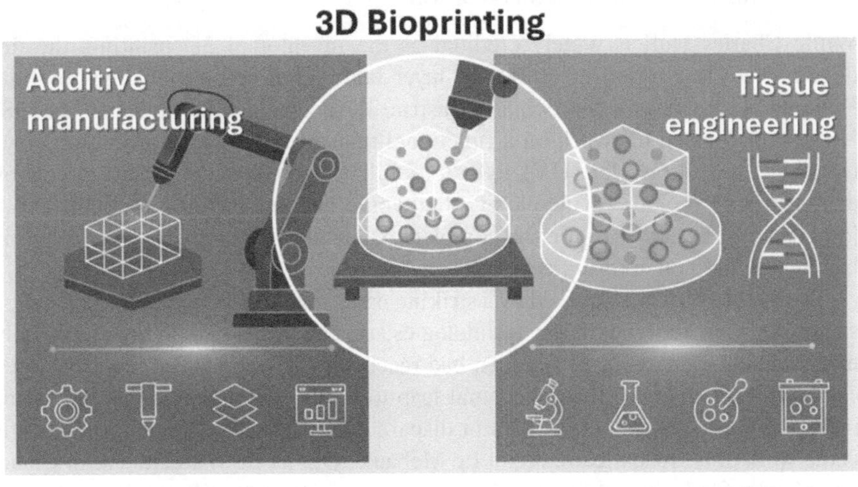

FIGURE 1.1 Historical convergence: from additive manufacturing and tissue engineering to bioprinting.

DOI: 10.1201/9781032638164-1

process that offered limited control over cell distribution and architectural fidelity [3]. Concurrently, the world of manufacturing was being transformed by AM, or 3D printing, a technology that enabled the layer-by-layer fabrication of complex, inert objects directly from a digital blueprint [4]. The true genesis of bioprinting occurred at the intersection of these two fields: the moment researchers realized that the precision and automation of AM could be harnessed to pattern not just plastics and metals, but the very building blocks of life.

This chapter traces the historical confluence of these disciplines, highlighting the key conceptual leaps, technological breakthroughs, and pioneering figures that transformed a speculative idea into a tangible and rapidly evolving scientific discipline. It will chronicle the journey from the first 3D-printed plastic part to the first deposition of living cells, and from the foundational principles of TE to the ambitious era of biofabrication, setting the stage for the detailed scientific and application-focused discussions that follow in this book.

1.2 THE DAWN OF ADDITIVE MANUFACTURING: FROM PROTOTYPING TO PRINTING OBJECTS

The technological bedrock of bioprinting is AM, a process born not from biomedical ambition but from industrial necessity. Its initial purpose was to accelerate product development cycles by rapidly creating inert plastic prototypes, a process that came to be known as "rapid prototyping" [5]. This industrial origin was a critical, if unintentional, prerequisite for the later development of bioprinting; it ensured that by the time biologists began to consider the possibility of printing cells, a robust, precise, and commercially available hardware platform already existed.

1.2.1 The Conceptual Origins: Hideo Kodama and Early Photopolymerization

While Charles Hull is widely credited as the inventor of 3D printing, the first documented description of a layer-by-layer fabrication process belongs to Hideo Kodama of the Nagoya Municipal Industrial Research Institute in Japan. In 1981, Kodama published his work on a functional photopolymer rapid prototyping system that used ultraviolet (UV) light to solidify photosensitive resin, effectively demonstrating the core principle of what would become stereolithography (SLA) [6]. However, he failed to file the complete patent application before the deadline, leaving the field open for others.

The history of AM is marked by a striking pattern of near-simultaneous invention, suggesting that the underlying technologies; accessible lasers, photocurable polymers, and computer control systems; had reached a critical level of maturity in the early 1980s. This made the conceptual leap to layer-by-layer fabrication an almost inevitable next step for researchers in disparate locations. Further evidence of this is the work of a French team, Alain Le Méhauté, Olivier de Witte, and Jean Claude André, who filed a patent for a SLA process on July 16, 1984 [7], a full three weeks before Hull's application. In a telling historical footnote, their corporate sponsors abandoned the patent, seeing little commercial potential in the technology, a powerful illustration of the difficulty in recognizing the value of disruptive innovations at their inception.

1.2.2 The Invention of SLA: Charles Hull and the Birth of an Industry

The individual who successfully translated the concept of layer-by-layer fabrication into a commercial reality was American engineer Charles "Chuck" Hull. In 1983, while working for a company that used UV lamps to cure protective coatings on tabletops, Hull independently conceived of a method to build 3D objects from liquid photopolymer. That year, he produced the world's first 3D-printed part [8].

On August 8, 1984, Hull filed his groundbreaking patent, US4575330A, for an "Apparatus for production of three-dimensional objects by stereolithography," which was granted on March 11, 1986 [9]. In this patent, Hull coined the term *stereolithography* (from the Greek *stereo* for solid and *lithography* for writing) and defined it as a method for making solid objects by successively "printing" thin layers of a UV-curable material one on top of the other. The process involved focusing a beam of UV light onto the surface of a vat of liquid photopolymer. Guided by a computer, the beam would trace the cross-section of an object, causing the resin to solidify, or cure. A platform would then lower the object slightly into the vat, and the process would repeat for the next layer.

Recognizing the immense potential of his invention for rapid prototyping, Hull cofounded 3D Systems in 1986, the world's first 3D printing company. In 1987, 3D Systems commercialized the first 3D printer, the SLA-1, marking the true birth of the AM industry. Crucially, alongside the hardware, Hull's team also developed the SLA file format, a standard for translating computer-aided design (CAD) data into instructions for the printer. This software innovation was a foundational contribution that created the digital workflow essential for all subsequent 3D printing technologies [10].

1.2.3 Diversification of Technologies: The Emergence of Selective Laser Sintering (SLS) and Fused Deposition Modeling (FDM)

Following the invention of SLA, the late 1980s and early 1990s saw the development of other key AM technologies that would later be adapted for biomedical applications. In 1986, Carl Deckard, at the University of Texas at Austin, filed a patent for Selective Laser Sintering, a process that uses a laser to fuse powdered materials, such as plastic, ceramic, or metal, layer by layer [11]. The ability to print with metals was a significant advancement. Shortly thereafter, in 1989, Scott Crump developed FDM, a technique that extrudes a filament of molten thermoplastic material to build an object [12]. FDM technology would eventually become the basis for the widespread and affordable "desktop 3D printers" that brought AM to a much broader audience. Together, these technologies formed the robust industrial toolkit that biomedical pioneers would later repurpose for an entirely unforeseen application: the fabrication of living tissue.

1.3 THE GENESIS OF A NEW FIELD: THE PRINCIPLES OF TISSUE ENGINEERING

Running parallel to the advancements in manufacturing, a separate revolution was brewing in the fields of biology and medicine. Driven by the persistent clinical problem of organ failure and the severe shortage of donor organs, researchers began to explore the possibility of creating functional biological substitutes *de novo*. This endeavor would coalesce into the interdisciplinary field of TE.

1.3.1 Early Foundations: From Cell Culture to the First Engineered Tissues

The conceptual roots of TE can be traced to early 20th-century cell culture techniques, which first demonstrated that cells could be sustained and grown outside the body [2]. However, the first concerted efforts to fabricate tissues began in the 1970s. A landmark achievement occurred in the late 1970s and early 1980s through the work of John F. Burke at Massachusetts General Hospital and Ioannis V. Yannas at the Massachusetts Institute of Technology (MIT) [13]. They developed the first clinically successful tissue-engineered product: an artificial skin for treating severe burn patients. This "integumentary template" was composed of a porous, cross-linked scaffold made from collagen (a structural protein) and glycosaminoglycans (polysaccharides found in the extracellular matrix), which was then covered by a silicone layer to prevent dehydration. This bilayer scaffold guided the regeneration of a new dermal layer from the patient's own cells. This success provided the first definitive proof that an engineered biomaterial could be used to regenerate complex living tissue, laying a critical foundation for the entire field.

1.3.2 Langer and Vacanti: Defining the Field and the Scaffold-Cell-Signal Triad

The moment that truly defined and codified TE came from the seminal collaboration between Joseph P. Vacanti, a pediatric surgeon at Boston Children's Hospital, and Robert S. Langer, a chemical engineer at MIT [14]. Vacanti, confronted daily with the tragic shortage of organs for his young patients, sought out Langer, an expert in polymers, with an idea to move beyond simply seeding cells on existing matrices. Their goal was to prospectively design and fabricate synthetic, biodegradable polymer scaffolds that could actively orchestrate tissue formation. This partnership established an interdisciplinary imperative that became the bedrock of the field; the fusion of clinical need with engineering solutions was not just beneficial, but essential for progress.

In a foundational 1988 paper, they described their new approach, which they termed "chimeric neomorphogenesis" [15]. They detailed the harvesting of various cell types, seeding them onto scaffolds made of bioabsorbable polymers like polyglactin 910, and implanting these cell-polymer constructs into animals. The study demonstrated successful engraftment and the formation of new, vascularized tissue masses. This work represented a crucial conceptual leap, reframing the scaffold from a passive structural support into an active, instructive template. By engineering the scaffold's properties, such as porosity and degradation rate, one could program the delivery of architectural and temporal information to guide biological self-assembly. This idea of an information-rich matrix is the direct intellectual precursor to the digital blueprints used in bioprinting.

In 1993, Langer and Vacanti published a landmark review in *Science* that formally defined the burgeoning field. They described TE as "an interdisciplinary field that applies the principles of engineering and the life sciences toward the development of biological substitutes that restore, maintain, or improve tissue function" [2]. This paper articulated the foundational triad of TE: the synergistic interplay between (1) living cells, (2) a biomaterial scaffold to provide structural support and guidance, and (3) biochemical signals, such as growth factors, to direct cell behavior.

1.3.3 The "Vacanti Mouse": A Landmark in Public and Scientific Consciousness

While the scientific principles of TE were well established within the research community by the mid-1990s, the field was thrust into the global public consciousness in 1997 with the publication of the "Vacanti mouse" [16]. This now-iconic image showed a nude mouse with a structure shaped like a human ear growing on its back. The structure was created by seeding bovine chondrocytes into a biodegradable, ear-shaped polymer scaffold and implanting it under the mouse's skin. The image was both captivating and, for some, unsettling, but it powerfully communicated the futuristic promise of growing replacement body parts. It became a symbol of the field's potential and cemented the concept of TE in the minds of scientists and the public alike.

1.4 THE BIRTH OF BIOPRINTING

By the late 1990s, the two historical streams of AM and TE were mature, independent fields. AM had established a robust technological platform for creating complex, inert objects, while TE had established the biological principles for creating living tissues. The birth of bioprinting occurred at the confluence of these two streams, when pioneers began to integrate the precision of AM with the biological components of TE.

1.4.1 Early Medical Applications of 3D Printing: Anatomical Models and Scaffolds

The first foray of AM into the medical world was non-biological. Beginning in the 1990s, clinicians and researchers began using SLA to convert data from computed tomography and magnetic resonance imaging scans into highly accurate, patient-specific 3D anatomical models. These models were invaluable tools for surgical planning, allowing surgeons to visualize complex anatomies and rehearse procedures before entering the operating room [8].

The next logical step was to use 3D printing to fabricate the scaffolds central to TE. Instead of creating scaffolds by hand, researchers could now design them in CAD software with precise control over pore size, interconnectivity, and overall geometry, and then print them using biocompatible and biodegradable polymers. These 3D-printed scaffolds were then seeded with cells using traditional manual techniques [17]. This hybrid approach represented the first true integration of the two fields, but the fabrication of the scaffold and the addition of the biological components remained two separate, distinct steps.

1.4.2 The Leap to Living Matter: Modifying Printers for Cells

The radical conceptual breakthrough that defined the birth of bioprinting was the realization that the printer itself could be used to deposit not just the scaffold material, but the living cells as well, in a single, integrated process. This was a revolutionary idea, as the prevailing assumption was that the high temperatures and mechanical shear stresses inherent in printing processes would inevitably destroy delicate cell membranes. The pioneers of bioprinting were characterized by a "hacking" or "repurposing" ethos; they did not invent entirely new machines from scratch but instead ingeniously adapted existing, off-the-shelf technologies, demonstrating that cells were far more resilient than previously thought.

1.4.3 Foundational Bioprinting Modalities: A Technological Triad

In a remarkable period of innovation between 1999 and 2004, three foundational bioprinting technologies emerged almost simultaneously, each adapting a different existing printing method. These modalities did not arise as competitors, but rather as complementary solutions to different aspects of the biofabrication challenge, providing the nascent field with a versatile toolkit from its very inception.

1.4.3.1 Inkjet-Based Bioprinting: The Pioneering Work of Thomas Boland

The first and most accessible approach was based on standard desktop inkjet printing. In the early 2000s, a group led by Thomas Boland at Clemson University began experimenting with modifying commercial inkjet printers, such as those made by Hewlett-Packard and Lexmark [18,19]. They emptied standard ink cartridges and refilled them with biological materials, first printing proteins and then, crucially, suspensions of living cells. Their groundbreaking discovery was that cells could survive the thermal and mechanical stresses of the droplet ejection process, with post-printing high viability rates.

On September 17, 2003, Boland filed the first patent for the process of printing viable cells, a landmark event that can be considered the formal birth of the bioprinting field [20]. In seminal papers published in 2003, Boland's group, in collaboration with Vladimir Mironov's team, further described the use of thermosensitive gels as a substrate, which allowed for the printing of successive layers to build true 3D cellular constructs [21]. Inkjet bioprinting offered the advantages of high speed, low cost, and wide availability, making it a powerful tool for early exploration.

1.4.3.2 Microextrusion Printing: The Development of the 3D-Bioplotter by Landers et al.

Contemporaneously, a second major modality, microextrusion, was developed. In 2002, Rüdiger Landers and his team in Germany reported on a system that used pneumatic or mechanical (piston-driven) pressure to extrude a continuous filament of a viscous, such as a hydrogel [22]. This technology, which adapted principles from industrial robotic dispensing systems, was later commercialized as the "3D-Bioplotter." Unlike the discrete droplets of inkjet printing, the continuous filament deposition of microextrusion was particularly well-suited for creating larger, more mechanically robust scaffolds with high structural integrity, addressing a key challenge in engineering load-bearing tissues.

1.4.3.3 Laser-Assisted Bioprinting: From Laser-Guided Writing to High-Resolution Cell Deposition

The third foundational technology, laser-assisted bioprinting (LAB), emerged from a completely different technological domain: microelectronics. LAB is a nozzle-free technique based on a process called laser-induced forward transfer (LIFT), which was originally developed for the high-resolution patterning of metals [23]. The conceptual groundwork was laid in 1999 by David Odde and Michael Renn, who described using "laser-guided direct writing" to precisely position individual cells using optical forces [24].

The first direct application of LIFT for printing viable mammalian cells was demonstrated in 2004 by a group at the U.S. Naval Research Laboratory led by J.A. Barron [25]. In their process, a focused laser pulse is aimed at an energy-absorbing layer on a transparent ribbon coated with a bioink. The laser energy creates a high-pressure bubble that propels a precise droplet of the bioink onto a receiving substrate below. This method offered unparalleled advantages: the absence of a nozzle eliminated the risk of clogging, and it allowed for the printing of highly viscous bioinks with very high cell densities at micrometer-scale resolution, all while maintaining excellent cell viability. This precision was critical for attempts to replicate the intricate micro-architectures of native tissues.

1.5 THE ERA OF BIOFABRICATION: KEY MILESTONES AND EVOLVING PARADIGMS

With the three foundational printing modalities established, the field entered a new phase in the mid-2000s, moving beyond simple demonstrations of cell deposition toward the ambitious goal of biofabrication: the automated construction of functional, multicomponent living tissues.

1.5.1 Coining "Organ Printing" and the Scaffold-Free Approach

A profound conceptual shift occurred with the articulation of a new vision for the field, spearheaded by Vladimir Mironov, Gabor Forgacs, Thomas Boland, and their colleagues. In a seminal 2003 paper in *Trends in Biotechnology*, they coined the term "organ printing" and laid out a comprehensive roadmap for the automated, layer-by-layer robotic biofabrication of 3D organs [21]. Their framework encompassed three key stages: preprocessing (creating a digital blueprint of the organ), processing (the actual printing), and post-processing (maturation of the printed construct in a bioreactor).

Central to their vision was a move toward a scaffold-free bioprinting paradigm. This approach represented a significant intellectual departure from the traditional TE model. Instead of relying on a synthetic scaffold to dictate structure, this new method leveraged the innate biological capacity of cells for self-organization. Drawing inspiration from the principles of embryonic development, Mironov et al. proposed using multicellular aggregates, or "tissue spheroids," as the fundamental building blocks [26]. The underlying principle was that when these living spheroids are printed in close proximity, they naturally fuse, sort, and remodel (a process called tissue fusion) to form larger, more complex tissues, much like cells do during embryogenesis. This reframed the printer's role from creating a static house for cells to live in, to precisely placing "smart" biological units that would then build the house themselves. It was a paradigm shift from an engineering-led to a biology-led approach to biofabrication.

1.5.2 From Simple Tissues to Complex Architectures

The decade following the establishment of the core technologies saw a series of landmark achievements that demonstrated the growing power and versatility of bioprinting. These "firsts" served as critical proofs-of-concept, validating the potential of biofabrication to create increasingly complex tissues.

- **First Bioprinted Skin:** A team led by Lee et al. reported the fabrication of the first multilayered skin constructs, successfully printing layers containing both dermal fibroblasts and epidermal keratinocytes to mimic the bilayered structure of native skin [27]. This was a milestone in recreating complex, heterocellular tissues.
- **First Bioprinted Blood Vessels:** Researchers at University of Missouri demonstrated the printing of the first scaffold-free vascular tubes using the tissue spheroid approach. Creating perfusable vascular networks is considered one of the most critical challenges in engineering any large-scale organ, making this a pivotal achievement [28].
- **Bioprinted Cartilage:** Several groups reported success in printing stem cells and differentiating them into chondrocytes to form stable cartilage tissue, showcasing the potential for treating musculoskeletal injuries and diseases like osteoarthritis [29,30].
- **Other Milestones:** This period also saw progress in printing a variety of other tissue types, including early demonstrations of miniature kidney units [31], lab-grown bladders for implantation [32], and constructs of beating heart tissue [33].

1.5.3 Commercialization and Democratization of Bioprinting Technology

The maturation of bioprinting from an academic curiosity to a viable technology was cemented by its commercialization. The founding of Organovo in 2007, the first company dedicated to bioprinting, was a pivotal moment. In 2009, Organovo, in partnership with Invetech, launched the Novogen MMX, one of the first commercial bioprinters.

This commercialization drove a pragmatic bifurcation of the field's goals. While the long-term, publicly-facing vision remained the printing of transplantable organs, the immediate commercial viability was found in a different application: creating miniaturized human tissue models for *in vitro* research. In 2014, Organovo released the first commercially available bioprinted product: 3D human liver tissue models for pharmaceutical toxicology testing. This was a critical development, as it established bioprinting as a valuable research tool that could help make drug discovery cheaper and more effective long before it could become a mainstream clinical therapy. This strategy provided a sustainable business model and a vital revenue stream to fund further research and development toward the ultimate therapeutic goals [34].

In the following years, the rise of companies like Allevi and Cellink (now BICO) further accelerated the field by focusing on developing more affordable, accessible, and user-friendly bioprinters. This "democratization" of technology lowered the barrier to entry, enabling a much wider range of academic and industrial labs to adopt bioprinting and explore its applications, leading to an explosion of innovation that continues to this day.

1.6 CONCLUSIONS

The history of bioprinting is a testament to the power of interdisciplinary convergence. It is a story that begins in two disparate worlds: the industrial factory floor, with Chuck Hull's first rudimentary plastic prototype, and the advanced medical laboratory, with Langer and Vacanti's first engineered tissues. The journey from these independent origins to the sophisticated biofabrication platforms of today was driven by a series of crucial conceptual and technological shifts.

First was the resourceful adaptation of industrial hardware, where pioneers repurposed commercial inkjet, dispensing, and laser systems for the radical new task of patterning living cells. This was followed by the integration of TE principles, which provided the biological "software" (the cells, scaffolds, and signals) necessary to transform printed structures into living constructs. Finally, a paradigm shift toward a developmental biology–inspired approach, using self-assembling tissue spheroids as building blocks, opened a new frontier in scaffold-free biofabrication, bringing the field closer to mimicking the elegant processes of nature itself.

This historical journey has established a robust and versatile technological foundation. The early trifurcation into inkjet, extrusion, and laser-assisted modalities provided a complementary toolkit suitable for fabricating a wide array of tissues, while the pragmatic commercial focus on *in vitro* models has created a sustainable ecosystem for continued innovation. The story of bioprinting's past is the essential prologue to its future. The challenges that were identified and the foundations that were laid during these formative decades are the direct antecedents of the cutting-edge research and applications discussed in the subsequent chapters of this book. Having moved from concept to reality, the field now stands poised to address the next set of grand challenges (including full-scale vascularization, long-term function, and regulatory approval) on its path toward revolutionizing regenerative medicine, drug discovery, and our fundamental understanding of human biology.

REFERENCES

1. Briones Y, Pascua B, Tiangco N, Crisostomo I, Casiguran S, Remenyi R. Assessing the landscape of clinical and observational trials involving bioprinting: a scoping review. *3D Print Med* 11(1), 5 (2025).
2. Langer R, Vacanti JP. Tissue engineering. *Science* 260(5110), 920–926 (1993).
3. Ashammakhi N, GhavamiNejad A, Tutar R et al. Highlights on advancing frontiers in tissue engineering. *Tissue Eng Part B Rev* 28(3), 633–664 (2022).
4. Patel R, Desai C, Kushwah S, Mangrola MH. A review article on FDM process parameters in 3D printing for composite materials. *Mater Today Proc* 60, 2162–2166 (2022).
5. Coon C, Pretzel B, Lomax T, Strlič M. Preserving rapid prototypes: a review. *Herit Sci* 4(1), 40 (2016).
6. Kodama H. Automatic method for fabricating a three-dimensional plastic model with photo-hardening polymer. *Rev Sci Instrum* 52(11), 1770–1773 (1981).
7. Andre J-C, Le Mehaute A, De Witte O. FR2567668A1 (1984).
8. Whitaker M. The history of 3D printing in healthcare. *Bull R Coll Surg Engl* 96(7), 228–229 (2014).
9. Hull CW. US4575330A (1984).
10. Melchels FPW. Celebrating three decades of stereolithography. *Virtual Phys Prototyp* 7(3), 173–175 (2012).
11. Deckard CR. US4863538 A (1986).
12. Crump SS. US5121329 A (1989).
13. Burke JF, Yannas IV, Quinby WC, Bondoc CC, Jung WK. Successful use of a physiologically acceptable artificial skin in the treatment of extensive burn injury. *Ann Surg* 194(4), 413–428 (1981).
14. Vacanti CA. The history of tissue engineering. *J Cell Mol Med* 10(3), 569–576 (2006).
15. Vacanti JP, Morse MA, Saltzman WM, Domb AJ, Perez-Atayde A, Langer R. Selective cell transplantation using bioabsorbable artificial polymers as matrices. *J Pediatr Surg* 23(1), 3–9 (1988).
16. Cao Y, Vacanti JP, Paige KT, Upton J, Vacanti CA. Transplantation of chondrocytes utilizing a polymer-cell construct to produce tissue-engineered cartilage in the shape of a human ear. *Plast Reconstr Surg* 100(2), 297–302 (1997).
17. Derby B. Printing and prototyping of tissues and scaffolds. *Science* 338(6109), 921–926 (2012).
18. Xu T, Jin J, Gregory C, Hickman JJ, Boland T. Inkjet printing of viable mammalian cells. *Biomaterials* 26(1), 93–99 (2005).
19. Roth EA, Xu T, Das M, Gregory C, Hickman JJ, Boland T. Inkjet printing for high-throughput cell patterning. *Biomaterials* 25(17), 3707–3715 (2004).
20. Boland T, Wilson WC Jr, Xu T. US7051654B2 (2003).

21. Mironov V, Boland T, Trusk T, Forgacs G, Markwald RR. Organ printing: computer-aided jet-based 3D tissue engineering. *Trends Biotechnol* 21(4), 157–161 (2003).
22. Landers R, Hübner U, Schmelzeisen R, Mülhaupt R. Rapid prototyping of scaffolds derived from thermoreversible hydrogels and tailored for applications in tissue engineering. *Biomaterials* 23(23), 4437–4447 (2002).
23. Bohandy J, Kim BF, Adrian FJ. Metal deposition from a supported metal film using an excimer laser. *J Appl Phys* 60(4), 1538–1539 (1986).
24. Odde DJ, Renn MJ. Laser-guided direct writing for applications in biotechnology. *Trends Biotechnol* 17(10), 385–389 (1999).
25. Barron JA, Wu P, Ladouceur HD, Ringeisen BR. Biological laser printing: a novel technique for creating heterogeneous 3-dimensional cell patterns. *Biomed Microdevices* 6(2), 139–147 (2004).
26. Mironov V, Visconti RP, Kasyanov V, Forgacs G, Drake CJ, Markwald RR. Organ printing: tissue spheroids as building blocks. *Biomaterials* 30(12), 2164–2174 (2009).
27. Lee W, Debasitis JC, Lee VK et al. Multi-layered culture of human skin fibroblasts and keratinocytes through three-dimensional freeform fabrication. *Biomaterials* 30(8), 1587–1595 (2009).
28. Norotte C, Marga FS, Niklason LE, Forgacs G. Scaffold-free vascular tissue engineering using bioprinting. *Biomaterials* 30(30), 5910–5917 (2009).
29. Cohen DL, Malone E, Lipson H, Bonassar LJ. Direct freeform fabrication of seeded hydrogels in arbitrary geometries. *Tissue Eng* 12(5), 1325–1335 (2006).
30. Cui X, Breitenkamp K, Finn MG, Lotz M, D'Lima DD. Direct human cartilage repair using three-dimensional bioprinting technology. *Tissue Eng Part A* 18(11–12), 1304–1312 (2012).
31. Homan KA, Kolesky DB, Skylar-Scott MA et al. Bioprinting of 3D convoluted renal proximal tubules on perfusable chips. *Sci Rep* 6(1), 34845 (2016).
32. Atala A, Bauer SB, Soker S, Yoo JJ, Retik AB. Tissue-engineered autologous bladders for patients needing cystoplasty. *The Lancet* 367(9518), 1241–1246 (2006).
33. Gaetani R, Doevendans PA, Metz CHG et al. Cardiac tissue engineering using tissue printing technology and human cardiac progenitor cells. *Biomaterials* 33(6), 1782–1790 (2012).
34. Choudhury D, Anand S, Naing MW. The arrival of commercial bioprinters – towards 3D bioprinting revolution!. *Int J Bioprint* 4(2), 139 (2024).

2 Bioinks and Materials for 3D Bioprinting

Janaina de Andréa Dernowsek,
Claudia Larissa Viana da Silva,
Pamela Ferreira do Nascimento,
Thais Amaral França, Kamilla da Costa Pantoja,
and Gabriela Morais da Costa

2.1 INTRODUCTION

As 3D bioprinting (3DBP) techniques evolve, so does the very concept of bioink, directly shaping our understanding of the field. This interplay of concepts led to earlier classifications that grouped bioinks by their intended function: support, fugitive, structural, and functional bioinks [1]. Under this framework, terminology was justified by usage, and the material's type did not affect the bioink's definition.

However, in 2018, Groll proposed a new definition: *bioink is* "a formulation of cells suitable for processing by an automated biofabrication technology that may also contain biologically active components and biomaterials." Contemporary definitions emphasize that a bioink is characterized not by its function or application, but by the presence of viable cells. Regardless of their origin (animal, plant, fungal, or bacterial) or organization (as single cells, spheroids, organoids, microcarriers, or microtissues), if the cells are suitable for the bioprinting process, the material qualifies as a bioink [2].

Although cells are the key component, most 3DBP technologies require biomaterials that provide structural support and promote cell growth. According to Williams [3], biomaterials are "designed to take a form that, alone or as part of a complex system, is used to direct, by control of interactions with components of living systems, the course of any therapeutic or diagnostic procedure in human or veterinary medicine." It is important to note that the biomaterial's definition is based on its final application, regardless of its chemical composition. For this reason, it is essential to distinguish between bioinks and biomaterials. Biomaterials are classified based on their chemical nature: metals, polymers, ceramics, and composites [3]. Among these, polymers, particularly natural and synthetic hydrogels, are the most commonly used in 3DBP, due to their high water content, which mimics the living tissue environment and supports cell adhesion, proliferation, and differentiation [4].

Groll also defined "biomaterial ink" as printable materials free of living cells during fabrication, although cells may be seeded onto them afterward. Therefore, materials used for support, sacrificial purposes, bioactive dressings, bioengineered drugs,

 DOI: 10.1201/9781032638164-2

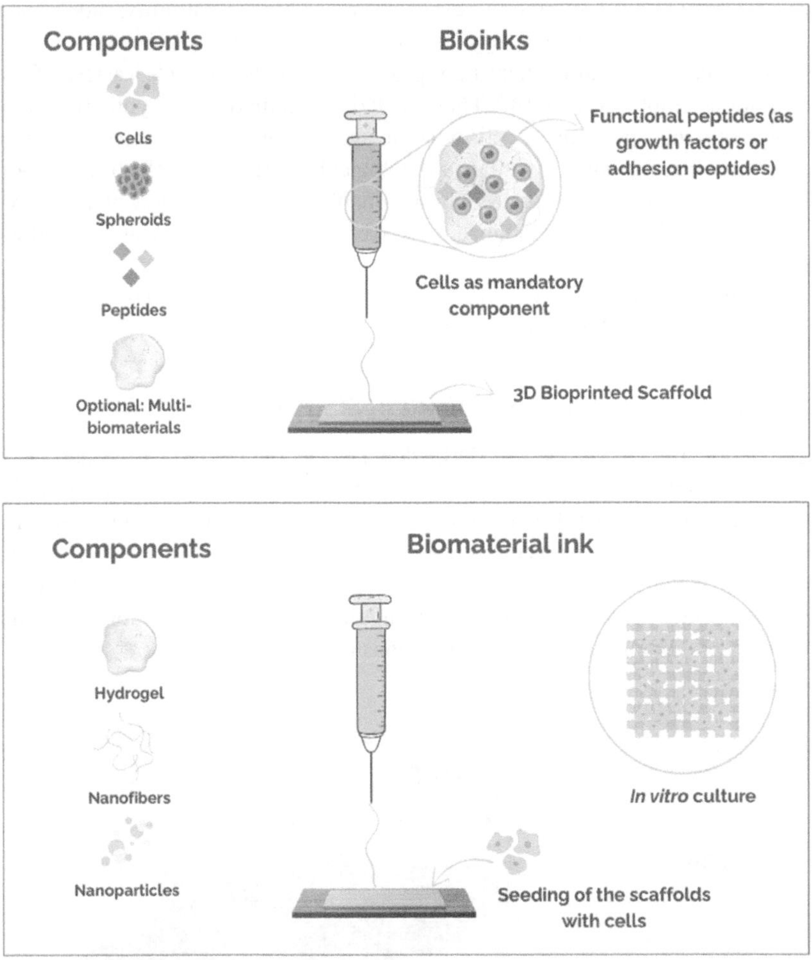

FIGURE 2.1 Comparison between bioinks and biomaterial inks. While bioinks contain cells as an obligatory component, in addition to spheroids, functional peptides, and, optionally, multiple biomaterials, biomaterial inks can have hydrogels, nanofibers, and nanoparticles as components and are subsequently seeded with cells after 3D printing of the scaffold.

or biodegradable implants do not qualify as bioinks if they lack cells at the time of printing, and thus do not constitute a 3DBP process [2]. As shown in Figure 2.1, bioinks differ from biomaterial inks primarily in that they incorporate cells directly into the printing process, whereas biomaterial inks are printed first and subsequently seeded with cells.

The conceptual complexity of bioinks reflects the multifaceted challenges involved in their development. Successful bioprinting depends on the properties of both bioinks and biomaterial inks, including their rheological, mechanical, and biological characteristics, in addition to the specific bioprinting technique employed. Currently, the development of bioinks represents one of the main challenges in the field, requiring careful attention to aspects such as biocompatibility, biodegradability, crosslinking methods, rheology, maturation, and sterility [1].

A brief search of major scientific repositories reveals the wide variety of bioink compositions employed in 3DBP. These include combinations of synthetic and natural polymers, incorporation of cell-inducing agents that stimulate biological activity, and the use of composites to enhance rheological properties. Such strategies aim to balance bioprintability with cell viability, enabling the fabrication of complex and high-resolution tissues. This balance is referred to as the "biofabrication window" or "bioprinting window" [5].

This chapter introduces core properties and material strategies for developing effective bioinks for 3DBP applications.

2.2 DESIRED PROPERTIES OF BIOINKS FOR 3D BIOPRINTING

The functionality of bioinks in 3DBP depends on their ability to simultaneously support bioprintability and biological performance (Figure 2.2). A successful bioink must ensure cell viability, allows for precise printing, and promotes integration with host tissues [4,5] This section reviews the key properties necessary to achieve these goals, including biocompatibility, biodegradability, bioprintability, rheological behavior, surface tension, mechanical strength, and oxygen permeability, for developing effective bioinks for 3DBP applications [2].

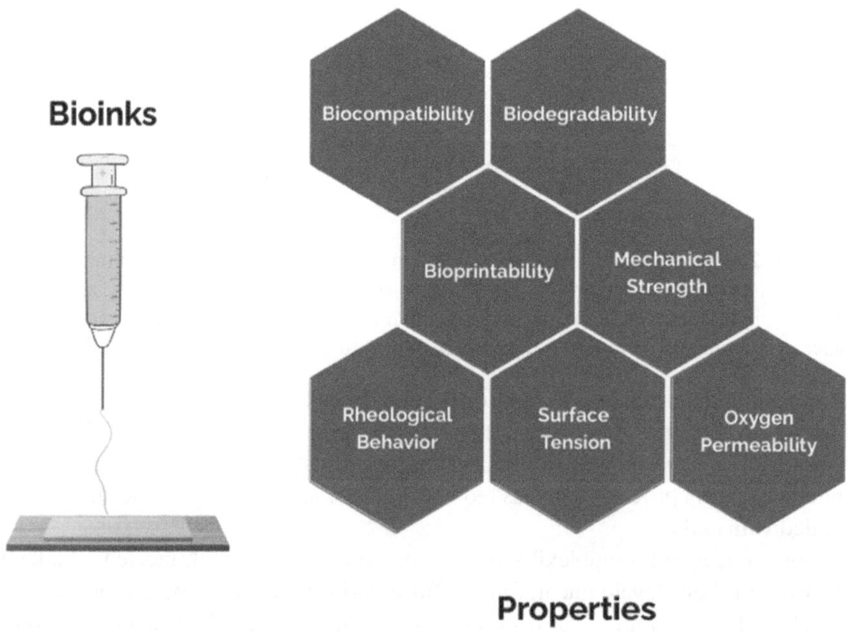

FIGURE 2.2 The functionality of bioinks in 3DBP enabling the creation of living, functional tissues.

2.2.1 Biocompatibility

Biocompatibility is a material's ability to perform its intended function without causing adverse effects, while actively supporting cellular activity. For bioinks, this means the material must be compatible with encapsulated cells and promote the health, viability, and proper function of the final printed tissue [1].

To ensure biocompatibility, bioinks are subject to an evaluation process that includes both *in vitro* and *in vivo* testing, as outlined by the ISO 10993 standards, which define a framework for the biological evaluation of medical devices and materials [6,7].

Biocompatibility is a dynamic, not a static, property. Its nature evolves over time, influenced by the material's composition, degradation profile, and surface characteristics, as well as the specific biological environment of the host tissue. Factors such as the release of degradation by-products, mechanical stress, or interactions with surrounding biological components can alter a bioink's compatibility. Consequently, bioinks must be engineered to maintain stable, nontoxic interactions throughout the entire tissue maturation process, either supporting long-term integration or undergoing controlled resorption, depending on the therapeutic goal [3,8,9].

In the field of 3DBP, achieving biocompatibility is a key requirement, demanding bioinks that are nontoxic, nonimmunogenic, and capable of seamless integration with the printed tissue. To meet these demands, researchers are leveraging advanced technologies. Transcriptomic profiling, *in silico* modeling, and AI-based predictions are now enabling more precise and predictive assessments of bioink–cell interactions. These tools are fundamental for designing next-generation bioinks with tailored biological responses, moving beyond traditional methods to optimize long-term tissue function and integration [10,11].

2.2.2 Biodegradability

Biodegradability refers to the capacity of a material to degrade into nontoxic by-products over time, usually through enzymatic or hydrolytic activity. In the context of bioinks, this property allows printed structures to gradually resorb while the native tissue regenerates, reducing the need for surgical removal and promoting natural integration [12,13].

Bioinks must exhibit controlled degradation rates that align with tissue maturation and maintain mechanical integrity during the early stages of regeneration [14]. Factors influencing degradation behavior include polymer composition, molecular weight, and the presence of hydrolysable bonds [15]. For instance, poly(lactic acid) (PLA), poly(glycolic acid), and poly(ε-caprolactone) (PCL) are widely used synthetic biodegradable polymers with varying degradation kinetics [16].

Natural biomaterials such as collagen, gelatin, and chitosan typically undergo enzymatic degradation, whereas synthetic counterparts often degrade primarily through hydrolysis. These degradation pathways influence not only material stability but also cell behavior and tissue remodeling. Advances in polymer chemistry now enable precise control of degradation rates through methods such as copolymerization, blending, and functional group modification [17–19].

Selecting biodegradable materials for bioinks requires balancing structural support with biocompatibility and degradation kinetics to avoid negative effects from by-products and ensure successful integration with host tissue [20].

2.2.3 Bioprintability

Bioprintability is the ability of a bioink to be printed in a precise and reproducible manner, maintaining shape fidelity during and after deposition. It depends on rheological properties, viscosity, surface tension, and crosslinking behavior, as well as printing parameters and technology [21,22].

Essential performance indicators include extrudability, filament fidelity, and structural integrity. Shear-thinning behavior is especially valuable, enabling better resolution while preserving cell viability, although a balance must be struck between viscosity and cell-friendly conditions [23,24].

Crosslinking and surface interactions also influence final structure accuracy. Rapid gelation prevents filament collapse, while wettability affects layer adhesion [25]. Besides that, bioprintability can be quantitatively evaluated using emerging methods such as printability factor assessments and computational modeling [26,27].

Ultimately, achieving optimal bioprintability requires a bioink formulation that meets two competing needs: the printing process and the biological environment. This involves designing a material that supports high print resolution and optimal cellular function, while adapting to the specific requirements of the selected bioprinting platform and the target tissue application [22,27].

2.2.4 Rheological Properties

Rheological properties define how bioinks flow and deform under applied forces, and arc fundamental for print fidelity, cell viability, and structural stability in 3DBP. These properties include viscosity, shear-thinning behavior, viscoelasticity, yield stress, and thixotropy, each contributing to the extrudability and post-print integrity of the printed constructs [28,29].

The bioink's apparent viscosity, which changes with the shear rate, requires a careful balance. It needs to be low enough for smooth extrusion, but high enough to keep the filament's shape and prevent it from spreading after printing. Shear-thinning behavior is especially valuable, it allows the viscosity to decrease during printing and recover quickly after deposition, ensuring structure retention and minimizing shear-induced cell damage [4,30].

Viscoelastic materials, such as hydrogels, exhibit both solid-like (elastic) and fluid-like (viscous) characteristics. Ideal bioinks transition through three rheological states during printing: a pre-extrusion gel state, a flow-dominated phase during extrusion, and a restructured state post-deposition. This cycle supports shape fidelity while protecting cell integrity [27,31].

The rheological profile is influenced by formulation parameters like polymer concentration, temperature, crosslinking chemistry, and cell density. Measurement of storage modulus (G') and loss modulus (G'') through rheometry helps characterize gelation behavior, with the sol–gel transition identified when G' exceeds G'' [30].

A bioink's rheological performance significantly impacts the printing process. Formulations that are either overly elastic or too viscous can hinder printability or compromise cell viability. Therefore, understanding and tuning rheological behavior is fundamental to developing functional, high-resolution bioinks for diverse tissue engineering (TE) applications [27,32].

2.2.5 Surface Tension and Wettability

The behavior of bioinks during extrusion-based 3DBP is highly dependent on their surface tension and wettability. Surface tension refers to the cohesive forces at the interface of the bioink that impact filament formation. High surface tension can lead to droplet formation at the nozzle tip, whereas upon deposition, it can aid in maintaining filament shape and structural fidelity [4].

A bioink's wettability, quantified by the contact angle with the printing substrate, presents a key trade-off for print quality. A large contact angle is beneficial for achieving vertical dimensional fidelity, while a smaller angle promotes substrate anchoring, which prevents unwanted displacement and deformation of the printed structure during the process [30].

Since most bioinks are hydrogel-based and contain living cells, their surface interaction is governed by the balance between hydrophilicity and hydrophobicity. Hydrophilic surfaces enhance initial spreading and cell–substrate interaction, while hydrophobic surfaces can facilitate easier detachment post-crosslinking. Mastering surface tension and wettability parameters is key to preserving fine structural features and long-term integrity in biofabricated constructs [4,30].

2.2.6 Mechanical Strength

To promote tissue-specific differentiation and maturation, bioprinted constructs must be exposed to appropriate environmental stimuli. For example, air–liquid interface culture is essential for the stratification and keratinization of 3D human skin models [33], whereas electromechanical stimulation is indispensable for the maturation and contractility of engineered muscle tissues [34,35]. In this context, 3DBP emerges as a strategic interface with mechanobiology, offering a robust and versatile platform to examine how exogenous mechanical cues affect cellular behaviors, fate decisions, and phenotypic modulation [36].

A fundamental requirement in bioink design is the ability to mimic the mechanical properties of native tissues [4,21]. These mechanical characteristics are largely dictated by the type and extent of crosslinking within the hydrogel network [37]. In extrusion-based and inkjet 3DBP platforms, bioinks must exhibit shear-thinning properties to facilitate flow during deposition while allowing for rapid post-printing gelation to preserve the construct's shape [38,39]. Crosslinking strategies range from ionic (e.g., Ca^{2+}-mediated gelation of alginate) to enzymatic, thermal, and photopolymerization methods (e.g., ultraviolet (UV)-initiated crosslinking of gelatin methacryloyl – GelMA) [40]. Polymers like collagen, hyaluronic acid (HA), and polyethylene glycol (PEG) can be chemically modified to enable photocrosslinking, thereby improving their printability and mechanical performance [36].

The mechanical microenvironment exerts a direct influence on cellular responses. A recent study demonstrated that dermal fibroblasts encapsulated in thiol-ene photo-clickable bioinks with varying stiffness responded distinctly: in soft matrices (814.0 ± 129.1 Pa), cells exhibited significant elongation after 24 hours; in intermediate matrices (1156.0 ± 49.13 Pa), cell morphology was heterogeneous; and in stiff bioinks (2169.0 ± 194.8 Pa), cells remained rounded with minimal spreading. After

14 days, cells in high-stiffness matrices demonstrated reduced cytoplasmic projection and limited cell–cell interactions, underscoring the centrality of mechanotransduction and the potential risk of triggering fibrotic or maladaptive responses when mechanical stimuli deviate from physiological norms [41].

Optimizing the physicochemical properties of bioinks is therefore necessary. A recent investigation revealed that the concentration of constituents and the degree of chemical functionalization strongly influenced the agarose bioink's rheological and mechanical performance. The optimized formulation presented a storage modulus (G′) of 11.6 Pa at 37°C and a Young's modulus of 1.4 ± 0.10 MPa following crosslinking. This bioink supported high cell viability (111% at 72 hours) and induced osteogenic differentiation in human mesenchymal stem cells, as evidenced by the upregulation of lineage-specific markers [42]. Another example of enhanced functionality was a hybrid bioink composed of poly(lactic-co-glycolic acid), hydroxyapatite, and PEG-based microparticles coprinted with an extracellular matrix (ECM)-derived hydrogel. Upon thermal sintering at 37°C, the composite generated rigid, porous scaffolds that supported neovascularization and osteoinduction, significantly improving bone regeneration in a rat femoral defect model [43] (Figure 2.3).

In comprehensive TE applications, scaffold mechanical properties must emulate the biomechanical profile of the native tissue. For skeletal muscle, optimal matrix stiffness approximates 10 kPa to sustain contractile performance and preserve satellite cell functionality [44]. Cartilage and osteotendinous interfaces, in contrast, exhibit complex mechanical gradients, demanding scaffolds with spatially resolved stiffness patterns to replicate native transitions [45]. Hydrogel-based bioinks can be tailored to reproduce the mechanical microenvironment, including stiffness, compressive resistance, and shear stress, parameters that significantly influence not only cell behavior and matrix remodeling but also pathological phenomena such as tumor progression [46]. Ultimately, the integrated effects of mechanical (e.g., elasticity and modulus), structural (e.g., topology and anisotropy), chemical (e.g., adhesion ligands), and crosslinking variables guide the cellular response in 3D systems, affirming the necessity for precision bioink engineering [47]. For instance, the combination of κ-carrageenan, a thermosensitive, sulfated polysaccharide with poly(vinyl alcohol) (PVA) has resulted in bioinks with adjustable porosity, mechanical resilience, and temperature-responsive gelation. This approach has proven effective in enabling cellular infiltration and nutrient diffusion, fundamental for the fabrication of anatomically and functionally relevant auricular cartilage constructs [48,49].

2.2.7 Oxygen Permeability

Oxygen permeability is a critical property of bioinks that directly influences cell viability, metabolic activity, and construct functionality in 3DBP. As bioprinted constructs increase in complexity and thickness, oxygen diffusion becomes a limiting factor, particularly in the absence of vascularization [50].

Bioinks with high oxygen permeability allow for adequate oxygen transport to encapsulated cells, supporting aerobic metabolism and reducing hypoxic zones within the printed structure. This property is largely governed by the porosity and molecular diffusivity of the bioink material. Hydrogels, due to their hydrated and porous nature, are often favored for their relatively good oxygen diffusion capabilities [51–53].

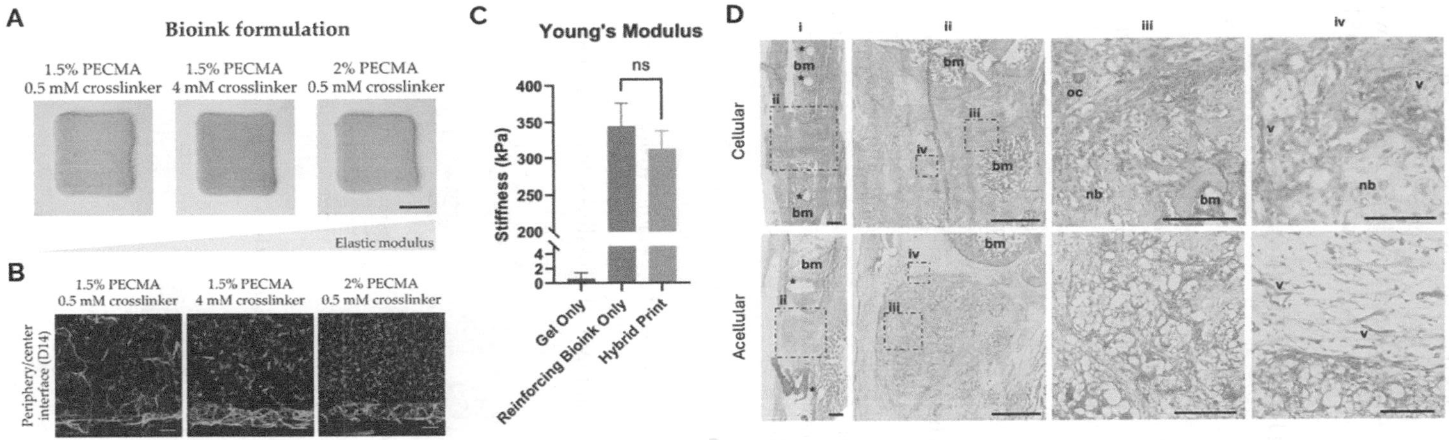

FIGURE 2.3 (a) Macroscopic images of bioprinted 3D dermal equivalents using bioinks with varying composition after 14 days of culture (scale bar: 2 mm). (Reproduced from Ref. [41].) (b) Cross-section confocal images of cells within bioprinted hydrogels stained for F-actin and nuclei at day 14 (scale bar: 100 µm), showing the morphology of cells located at the hydrogel center and periphery. (Reproduced from Ref. [41].) (c) *Compressive modulus* of constructs fabricated using gel-only, reinforcing bioink only, and hybrid printing approaches (n = 3). (Reproduced from Ref. [43].) (d) Bioprinted hybrid bone tissue supports new bone formation and *blood vessel formation*. Representative H&E-stained cryosection of explanted tissues three weeks after surgery. (i) Low-magnification image of explanted femurs showing the defect area (dashed box) and plate fixation screws (asterisk) and bone marrow (bm). Scale bar: 1 mm. (ii–iv) Higher-magnification images showing new bone (nb) formation with *osteoclasts* (oc) and blood vessels (v). Scale bar: ii: 1 mm, iii: 200 µm, iv: 100 µm, (Reproduced from Ref. [43].)

The architecture of the printed construct also plays a role: pore size, distribution, and interconnectivity impact fluid and gas exchange. Materials with tunable microstructure, such as dual-crosslinked or nanocellulose-reinforced hydrogels, have shown promise in enhancing oxygen permeability while maintaining mechanical integrity [54].

2.3 CROSSLINKING METHODS FOR BIOINKS

Crosslinking is a core process in 3DBP that governs the transition of bioinks from a flowable state to a stable three-dimensional structure post-printing. This transformation is important for maintaining the geometry, mechanical strength, and biological functionality of printed constructs. Depending on the application and bioink composition, crosslinking can be achieved through ionic interactions, thermal transitions, photo-initiated polymerization, or enzymatic reactions [21,22]. Each method has its own advantages, such as faster gel formation, better cell compatibility, greater control over where the gel forms, and the ability to adjust its properties. It is important to highlight that the way the material is crosslinked directly affects key factors such as cell survival, nutrient transport, and the rate at which the material degrades. Therefore, choosing the crosslinking strategy is a crucial step in the development of bioinks for TE applications [23,25].

In this section, we highlight the primary crosslinking mechanisms used in 3DBP: ionic, thermal, photo, and enzymatic. For each, we'll cover its core principles, specific applications, and inherent limitations (Figure 2.4).

2.3.1 Ionic Crosslinking

Ionic crosslinking is a widely favored method for creating hydrogels used in 3DBP due to its rapid gelation kinetics, cytocompatibility, and the absence of toxic by-products [55]. This process involves forming physical crosslinks between anionic polymers

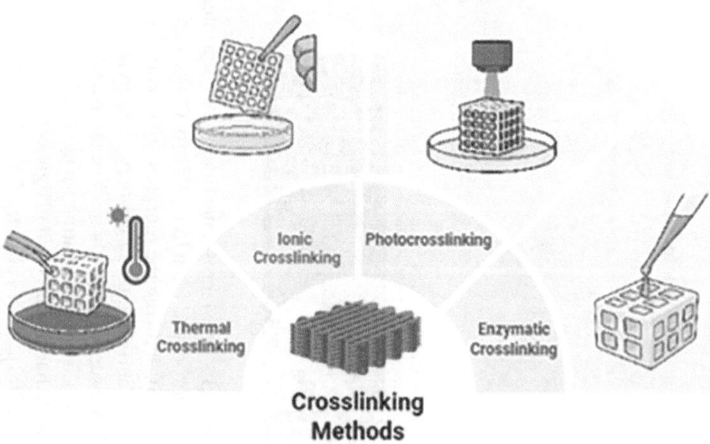

FIGURE 2.4 Crosslinking methods.

and various cations, including monovalent (e.g., K^+), divalent (e.g., Ca^{2+}, Ba^{2+}, and Sr^{2+}), or trivalent (e.g., Al^{3+}) [56,57].

Among these polymers, sodium alginate stands out as the most commonly used. Its linear structure, composed of β-D-mannuronic (M) and α-L-guluronic (G) acid blocks, allows the G blocks to preferentially bind with divalent cations. This interaction forms a 3D hydrogel network via the well-known egg-box model [58,59]. In this model, calcium ions effectively bridge guluronic acid residues on adjacent alginate chains, leading to efficient gelation and structural integrity [60,61]. In 3DBP, Ca^{2+} ions are typically supplied by aqueous solutions of calcium chloride ($CaCl_2$), calcium sulfate ($CaSO_4$), or calcium carbonate ($CaCO^3$), with the choice depending on the desired gelation rate and mechanical properties [59]. The resulting calcium-crosslinked alginate hydrogels typically exhibit an elastic modulus ranging from 1 to 100 kPa, influenced by both ionic concentration and the M/G ratio of the alginate backbone [62–64].

However, ionic crosslinking demands precise control. Excessive or uneven crosslinking can result in overly compact networks, decreased biodegradability in biological systems, and increased stiffness, all of which hinder cell migration and spreading [62,65]. Furthermore, while alternatives like barium chloride can create more stable and exchange-resistant hydrogels, their use is limited due to toxicity concerns [66,67]. Another significant limitation of simple ionic crosslinking is its instability in biological environments. This instability is particularly evident in the presence of calcium chelators (e.g., phosphates), monovalent ions (e.g., Na^+ and K^+), or non-crosslinking divalent ions (e.g., Mg^{2+}), which can displace the crosslinking ions and lead to hydrogel destabilization [62,68].

Recent studies have also highlighted cytotoxicity concerns linked to prolonged or high-concentration exposure to Ca^{2+}. For instance, extended treatment (30 minutes) of alginate-based bioprinted constructs with $CaCl_2$ solutions has been shown to compromise cell viability due to osmotic stress [62,69]. Elevated calcium levels can disrupt cellular electrolyte balance, induce morphological changes, damage cell membranes, rearrange the cytoskeleton (e.g., bleb formation), cause mitochondrial dysfunction, and activate apoptotic and inflammatory signaling pathways [70–72]. While ionic crosslinking enables rapid hydrogel solidification, these findings underscore the critical need to finely modulate salt exposure to preserve cell viability and ensure optimal construct performance.

Beyond alginate, other anionic biopolymers are gaining traction in biofabrication for their ionic crosslinking capabilities. Pectin, a polysaccharide from plant cell walls, forms stable, biocompatible hydrogels by coordinating efficiently with divalent cations like Ca^{2+} via its galacturonic acid residues, also forming "egg-box" structures [73,74]. Carrageenans, sulfated polysaccharides from seaweeds, can be crosslinked by K^+ or Ca^{2+} depending on the type (kappa, iota, lambda), with kappa-carrageenan notably forming rigid gels with potassium ions [75–77]. These diverse materials offer promising avenues for tailoring hydrogel characteristics, such as stiffness, degradation rate, and release profiles for drugs or growth factors, to suit specific biomedical applications.

2.3.2 Thermal Crosslinking

Thermal crosslinking involves the induction of gelation in polymeric systems through heating or cooling, making it one of the simplest crosslinking methods employed in 3DBP. This approach is suitable for thermoresponsive polymers that undergo conformational transitions at specific temperatures, enabling network formation without the need for external chemical agents [78].

Polymers such as collagen, gelatin, agarose, alginate, and κ-carrageenan are frequently utilized in this context. Agarose, for instance, transitions from a random coil to a helical conformation upon cooling below 32°C, forming a stable 3D gel network. As the polymer concentration increases, the transition tends to occur more quickly, which may result in improvements in gel fidelity and shape retention, although the relationship between concentration and performance depends on other factors, such as the specific formulation and processing conditions [79].

Despite its biocompatibility and simplicity, thermal crosslinking presents challenges, including prolonged gelation times and limited control over the crosslinking degree. Without proper control, the elevated temperatures needed for gelation may compromise cell viability and function [80]. Therefore, thermally responsive bioinks must be carefully tailored to balance mechanical integrity with biological safety.

Innovative techniques, such as using heated printheads or laser-based localized heating, allow for real-time gelation during extrusion. These strategies enhance print fidelity while reducing post-processing steps, making thermal crosslinking a valuable method for scaffold fabrication, particularly for applications requiring gentle processing conditions.

2.3.3 Photocrosslinking

Photocrosslinking refers to the light-induced formation of covalent bonds between macromolecules, facilitating the formation of crosslinked hydrogel networks. This method is particularly useful in 3D BP due to its spatial and temporal control over gelation. Photocurable polymers, when combined with suitable photoinitiators, can be solidified by exposure to light sources such as UV, visible, or near-infrared radiation [81].

Biopolymers like gelatin, fibrin, and collagen can be made photocrosslinkable through chemical modification (e.g., methacrylation), enabling them to be crosslinked using photoinitiators such as riboflavin or eosin Y under light exposure [82,83]. Acrylate-based derivatives are particularly responsive to UV light in the range of 320–365 nm [84].

However, the use of UV light poses potential risks to cellular viability due to DNA damage. As an alternative, visible light (400–700 nm) offers greater tissue penetration and reduced cytotoxicity. Recent research supports the use of visible-light photoinitiators like eosin Y and riboflavin activated by blue light (450–495 nm), which have shown high efficiency and minimal cellular impact [85,86].

Optimizing wavelength and photoinitiator choice is crucial for minimizing cytotoxic effects while ensuring adequate crosslinking efficiency, especially when working with cell-laden bioinks. Visible-light systems are increasingly preferred for applications requiring high cell viability and functional tissue outcomes [87].

2.3.4 Enzymatic Crosslinking

Enzymatic crosslinking offers a biologically inspired approach for hydrogel formation in 3DBP, providing mild reaction conditions, high specificity, and excellent biocompatibility. Enzymes such as horseradish peroxidase, transglutaminase, and tyrosinase catalyze crosslinking reactions that result in stable networks suitable for cell encapsulation and TE applications [88].

Horseradish peroxidase catalyzes the oxidative coupling of phenol- or tyramine-functionalized polymers in the presence of hydrogen peroxide (H_2O_2), enabling rapid *in situ* gelation. This reaction has been widely employed with polymers such as gelatin, HA, and PEG to create hydrogels with tunable mechanical and degradation properties [89].

Transglutaminase promotes the formation of covalent ε-(γ-glutamyl) lysine isopeptide bonds between proteins, particularly in gelatin- and fibrin-based systems. Its use in bioinks enhances elasticity and stability without the need for exogenous chemical initiators [90].

Tyrosinase catalyzes the oxidation of phenolic groups, facilitating crosslinking in polymers like silk fibroin (SF) and gelatin. It has demonstrated potential for controlled gelation rates and improved biocompatibility, supporting applications in neural and soft TE [91].

Enzymatic crosslinking provides distinct advantages over physical or photocrosslinking, particularly for bioinks requiring gentle conditions to maintain cellular viability. Its specificity allows precise modulation of network architecture, and ongoing research continues to expand the enzymatic toolkit for designing functional bioinks.

2.4 NATURAL BIOMATERIALS FOR 3D BIOPRINTING

2.4.1 Polysaccharide-Based Biomaterials

2.4.1.1 Alginate

Alginate is a natural anionic polysaccharide primarily derived from brown seaweed species such as *Laminaria hyperborea*, *Macrocystis pyrifera*, and *Ascophyllum nodosum*, although it can also be bacterially synthesized [92,93]. Its linear copolymer structure consists of M and G units, arranged in homopolymeric and heteropolymeric blocks, which confer diverse mechanical and gelation properties [94] (Figure 2.5).

Valued for its biocompatibility, biodegradability, and cost-effectiveness, alginate is extensively used in biomedical and bioprinting applications. It offers high water retention, oxygen permeability, and shear-thinning behavior, traits favorable for extrusion-based 3DBP [95,96].

Gelation typically occurs via ionic crosslinking with divalent cations such as Ca^{2+}, forming the well-known "egg-box" structure that provides mechanical stability [97]. However, crosslinking with Zn^{2+} or Mg^2+ or via covalent strategies like glutaraldehyde further tunes its performance [98,99]. Alginate's mechanical properties depend heavily on the crosslinking method and polymer composition [100].

Due to its mild gelation conditions and cytocompatibility, alginate is frequently used in combination with collagen or fibrin for engineering bone [101], cartilage [102], hepatic [103], and ocular [104] tissues [105]. Despite not being ideal for stereolithography, it remains a staple for extrusion and inkjet printing.

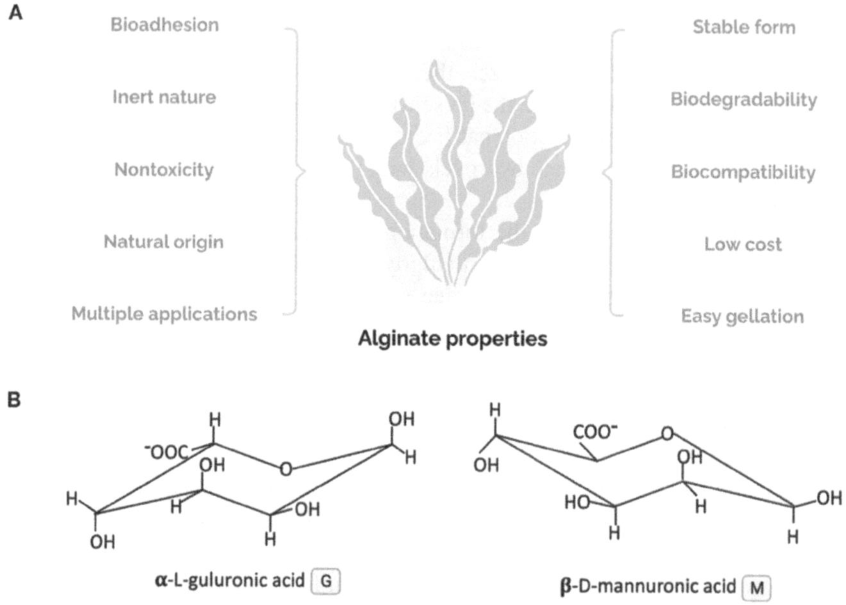

FIGURE 2.5 (a) Schematic presentation of alginate properties. (b) The structure of α-L-guluronic acid and ß-D-mannuronic acid. (Reproduced from Ref. [92].)

2.4.1.2 Agarose

Agarose is a natural polysaccharide derived mainly from red algae and composed of repetitive units of D-galactose and 3,6-anhydro-L-galactose. Its hydroxyl-rich structure promotes extensive hydrogen bonding, enabling reversible gelation and high thermal stability; key properties for biomedical and biofabrication applications [106,107].

Upon heating to 90°C–100°C, agarose dissolves in water, forming random coils; upon cooling to 30°C –40°C, it transitions into a double-helix network, producing stable hydrogels [108]. These hydrogels are widely applied in 3DBP due to their biocompatibility, structural integrity, and simple preparation [109].

Despite these advantages, native agarose has limitations, including low mechanical strength and poor cell adhesion [110]. To overcome such drawbacks, modification strategies are employed. Biological approaches, such as enzymatic desulfation, improve biointeraction but may lack scalability [105]. Physical methods, including ultrasonication and high-pressure homogenization, modulate gel architecture without altering the covalent structure [111,112]. Chemical modifications, particularly the addition of functional groups like sulfate or carboxymethyl, enhance solubility and cellular responses [113,114].

This is supported by biocompatibility studies showing that agarose-based hydrogels maintain near-100% cell viability, especially in endothelial cultures [115]. Furthermore, hybrid formulations combining agarose with HA have improved extracellular matrix (ECM) deposition and chondrocyte proliferation in cartilage TE [116].

2.4.1.3 Chitosan

Chitosan is a linear aminopolysaccharide composed of glucosamine and N-acetylglucosamine units linked via β-1,4-glycosidic bonds. It is derived through the deacetylation of chitin, which is abundantly found in the exoskeletons of crustaceans and insects [117,118]. This biopolymer is soluble in dilute acidic solutions due to its degree of deacetylation exceeding 50%, which distinguishes it from chitin and confers important functional properties [119,120].

Chitosan exhibits high viscosity and molecular rigidity, which stem from its partially deacetylated structure. Its unique physicochemical profile makes it attractive for biomedical applications. Classified as Generally Recognized as Safe (GRAS) by the U.S. Food and Drug Administration (FDA), chitosan has been widely used in pharmaceuticals and biomedicine [121].

Biologically, chitosan displays antimicrobial, antifungal, antioxidant, wound healing, mucoadhesive, and antitumoral properties [122,123]. It is also biodegradable, biocompatible, nontoxic, and nonimmunogenic [124,125].

In biofabrication, chitosan-based hydrogels are employed for extrusion-based 3DBP. Their ability to mimic ECM components facilitates cellular adhesion and proliferation, which makes them suitable for scaffold fabrication [126]. Moreover, chitosan's cationic nature allows interactions with negatively charged cell membranes and biomolecules, enhancing its biofunctionality [127].

Its *in vivo* degradation occurs via enzymes such as lysozyme, and its structure allows for chemical modifications to tailor its mechanical and biological behavior [128]. When combined with other polysaccharides such as alginate or agarose, chitosan contributes to structural support for layer-by-layer deposition in bone and soft TE [117].

2.4.1.4 Hyaluronic Acid (HA)

HA is a non-sulfated glycosaminoglycan naturally present in the ECM of connective tissues, synovial fluid, skin, and other soft tissues [129,130]. Structurally, it consists of repeating disaccharide units of N-acetyl-D-glucosamine and D-glucuronic acid linked via alternating β-1,4 and β-1,3 glycosidic bonds [131]. It exhibits a strong hydrophilic capacity and forms viscoelastic solutions due to extensive hydrogen bonding and a coiled tertiary structure stabilized by electrostatic and hydrophobic interactions.

HA-based hydrogels demonstrate shear-thinning behavior, which is desirable for extrusion-based 3DBP, and their rheological properties can be tuned by molecular weight and environmental factors like pH and ionic strength [132,133]. Enzymatic degradation *in vivo* primarily occurs via hyaluronidase, β-D-glucuronidase, and β-N-acetyl-hexosaminidase [134].

For bioprinting applications, HA can be crosslinked using physical, chemical, or enzymatic methods. Common techniques include Diels–Alder click chemistry, UV-photo crosslinking, and enzyme-mediated crosslinking using tyramine-functionalized HA and horseradish peroxidase [135,136]. These properties make HA an attractive candidate for bioinks aimed at soft TE and regenerative medicine.

2.4.1.5 Dextran

Dextran is a branched polysaccharide composed predominantly of α-(1→6)-linked D-glucopyranose units, with occasional branches arising from α-(1→2), α-(1→3), or α-(1→4) linkages [137]. It is naturally synthesized by lactic acid (LA) bacteria such as *Leuconostoc mesenteroides*, and commercially produced from sucrose through microbial fermentation [138].

Its chemical versatility and hydroxyl-rich backbone allow extensive functionalization, enabling the development of dextran-based hydrogels and composites for 3DBP. Chemical modification, e.g., methacrylation, permits photocrosslinking to form stable hydrogels, while aldehyde-functionalized dextran can be used for Schiff base reactions [139,140].

Dextran hydrogels show biocompatibility, with applications in soft TE, drug delivery, and wound healing. However, its mechanical weakness and low cell-adhesion capacity often require blending with other biopolymers such as gelatin or HA to improve printability and biofunctionality [141]. Recent strategies include hybrid bioinks using dextran-alginate or dextran-PEG systems to enhance mechanical strength and biological activity.

2.4.1.6 Cellulose and Nanocellulose

Cellulose, a natural linear polysaccharide composed of β(1→4)-linked D-glucose units, is one of the most abundant biopolymers in nature. Its derivative, nanocellulose (either nanofibrillated cellulose or cellulose nanocrystals (CNC)), offers unique physicochemical properties such as high aspect ratio, large surface area, and excellent mechanical strength [142].

Nanocellulose materials are biocompatible and biodegradable, and their highly tunable surface chemistry allows for a range of modifications to improve gelation, printability, and biological interactions [143]. The rheological properties of nanocellulose-based bioinks can be adjusted by concentration, degree of polymerization, and ionic content, resulting in formulations suitable for extrusion-based 3DBP [144].

Due to the intrinsic shear-thinning behavior and thixotropy of nanocellulose suspensions, they can form self-supporting filaments after extrusion, ensuring high shape fidelity. Although nanocellulose lacks inherent bioactivity, it is often combined with other biomaterials such as alginate, gelatin, or fibrin to enhance cellular adhesion and viability [145]. These composite inks have shown potential in cartilage, bone, and skin TE applications.

2.4.1.7 Starch

Starch is a natural polysaccharide composed of two types of glucose polymers: amylose (linear chains) and amylopectin (branched chains). It is abundantly found in plants such as corn, potato, wheat, and cassava. Due to its renewability, biocompatibility, and cost-effectiveness, starch has been explored as a bioink component in 3DBP [146].

However, native starch lacks ideal mechanical properties and printability, which often requires chemical or physical modifications. These modifications aim to improve solubility, rheological behavior, and gelation ability. Common strategies include hydroxypropylation, oxidation, or blending with other biopolymers such as gelatin or alginate [146,147].

Modified starch-based bioinks show enhanced extrusion behavior, shear-thinning properties, and better post-printing shape fidelity. Additionally, they can support cell viability and proliferation when appropriately crosslinked and hydrated [148]. Their biodegradability and tunable mechanical performance make them candidates for TE applications, particularly in soft tissues [146,148].

Despite these benefits, starch-based bioinks still face challenges such as low native cell-adhesion capacity and limited structural integrity under physiological conditions, prompting their frequent use in hybrid formulations [147].

2.4.2 Protein-Based Biomaterials

2.4.2.1 Collagen

Collagen is a protein abundantly found in mammals and other species such as amphibians, birds, fish, and marine animals [149]. It is the most prevalent protein in the human body, with 28 different types identified, localized primarily in tendons, ligaments, skin, bones, corneas, and other ECM-rich tissues [150,151].

Structurally, collagen is composed of three alpha-chains in a triple-helix conformation, typically repeating the sequence Gly–X–Y, where X and Y are often proline and hydroxyproline. This structure confers mechanical strength and is stabilized by 4-hydroxyproline. Type I collagen can be homotrimeric or heterotrimeric, though the heterotrimeric form is more prevalent in human tissues [150].

For bioink formulation, collagen offers high biocompatibility, water retention, and fibrous architecture favorable for cellular adhesion, proliferation, and migration [152,153]. Collagen hydrogels derived primarily from animal sources, such as bovine and porcine tissues, require careful processing to minimize the risk of zoonotic contamination and immune rejection [152].

Despite being mechanically weak when used in isolation, collagen's structural integrity during extrusion and its responsiveness to modifications in concentration and porosity make it a valuable component for tailoring rheology and biological function in bioprinting applications [154]. Crosslinking strategies, such as chemical or enzymatic methods, are employed to modulate its degradation rate and stiffness [155].

Nutrient and oxygen diffusion through collagen-based hydrogels is critical, and optimal filament thickness (~200 μm) and collagen concentration are essential for maintaining cell viability in printed constructs [154].

2.4.2.2 Gelatin

Gelatin is a denatured form of collagen obtained through partial hydrolysis, resulting in the breakdown of its triple-helix structure into smaller peptides and proteins [156]. As a natural biopolymer, gelatin is widely used in bioinks due to its inherent biocompatibility, biodegradability, and ability to support cell adhesion and proliferation [157].

The source of collagen influences the properties of the resulting gelatin. While porcine and bovine sources dominate global production, accounting for approximately 46% and 29.4% respectively, marine sources such as fish, sponges, and jellyfish are gaining attention for biomedical applications due to their lower immunogenicity [158–160].

Gelatin-based bioinks typically exhibit thermoresponsive behavior, allowing them to gel at physiological temperatures, which is a required property for extrusion-based 3DBP systems. However, gelatin's mechanical properties and stability under physiological conditions are limited, prompting its combination with other polymers or the use of chemical crosslinkers to enhance print fidelity and structural integrity [158].

Overall, gelatin remains a cornerstone in the development of bioinks for applications in TE and regenerative medicine, especially for soft tissues, owing to its versatility and compatibility with various cell types [160].

2.4.2.3 GelMA

GelMA is a photoreactive hydrogel derived from gelatin, widely employed in cell culture and TE [161]. Its inherent biological advantages stem from natural Arg-Gly-Asp (RGD) tripeptides, which promote cell attachment, spreading, and differentiation, and matrix metalloproteinase sequences, enabling enzymatic degradation. These features collectively contribute to GelMA's excellent biocompatibility and degradability [162–164].

GelMA is synthesized by reacting gelatin with methacrylic anhydride, which substitutes amine and hydroxyl groups with methacryloyl moieties [162]. These methacryloyl groups enable crosslinking of the hydrogel in the presence of photoinitiators (e.g., Irgacure 2959 and lithium phenyl-2,4,6-trimethylbenzoylphosphinate (LAP)) and light (UV/visible), ensuring structural integrity and stability under physiological conditions [162,165]. The degree of methacryloyl substitution (DS) offers flexibility in processing, allowing for precise control over GelMA's physicochemical characteristics [166], while processing temperature also significantly impacts its mechanical properties due to its thermoresponsive nature [167].

As a prominent bioink for 3DBP [165], GelMA's tunable mechanical and biological properties make it suitable for diverse applications. These range from simple cell culture scaffolds to intricate TE platforms and advanced delivery systems for drugs, genes, or growth factors [164,168]. For instance, it has been successfully used to create 3D-bioprinted human sensory models, supporting high cell viability and significant neurite outgrowth for functional neuron differentiation [169]. GelMA is also extensively utilized to mimic the ECM in 3D cell models for various diseases, including arthritis [170], ovarian cancer [171], and liver cancer [107].

However, the successful implementation of GelMA in 3DBP necessitates careful modulation of its physicochemical properties. Critical factors influencing the viscosity and printability of GelMA-based bioinks include polymer concentration, temperature, and the degree of methacrylation [172]. While higher GelMA concentrations can improve structural fidelity, they may compromise cell viability due to denser crosslinked networks. Furthermore, GelMA's thermoresponsive behavior demands tight temperature control for optimal printability; for example, a 10% w/v GelMA solution performs best between 18°C and 19°C for extrusion-based 3DBP, exhibiting self-healing and shear-thinning properties [173,174].

Photocrosslinking during extrusion is a common strategy to enhance viscosity and stabilize printed structures. The choice of photoinitiator is crucial, based on cytocompatibility, cost, availability, efficiency, solubility, and compatibility with the bioprinter's light system [175,176]. The DS profoundly impacts crosslinking potential and rheological behavior; insufficient DS leads to inadequate viscosity, while higher DS values improve both viscosity and shear-thinning properties. DS is influenced by factors like gelatin source, reaction conditions (temperature, duration, pH, and solvent), and gelatin-to-methacrylic anhydride ratio [175]. Moreover, incorporating secondary components like methylcellulose can further enhance GelMA's printability and structural stability [177]. Effectively addressing these challenges through sustained research and precise parameter refinement is fundamental to advancing GelMA's widespread application in TE.

2.4.2.4 Fibrin/Fibrinogen

Fibrin and its precursor fibrinogen are key natural biopolymers involved in the final stages of the coagulation cascade. Fibrinogen is a soluble glycoprotein that is converted into insoluble fibrin through thrombin-mediated enzymatic cleavage, forming a fibrous network that plays a critical role in hemostasis [178].

These biopolymers have gained prominence in 3DBP due to their excellent biocompatibility, intrinsic cell-binding motifs, and capacity to mimic the ECM, thereby promoting cell proliferation, migration, and differentiation [179]. Fibrin-based hydrogels exhibit fast polymerization under physiological conditions and are especially useful for applications involving vascularized and soft tissues [180].

However, their rapid degradation by proteolytic enzymes such as plasmin poses a limitation for long-term applications, often requiring blending with more stable biomaterials or the use of inhibitors to control degradation rates [181]. Despite this, their use in combination with other natural or synthetic polymers enhances mechanical strength and structural stability while retaining biological functionality [179].

In 3DBP, fibrin and fibrinogen are primarily used in extrusion-based and inkjet-based modalities due to their fast gelation kinetics and mild crosslinking requirements. They are often used to fabricate tissues such as skin, liver, and vascular networks, and have been incorporated into bioinks for both *in vitro* tissue models and regenerative medicine applications [182].

2.4.2.5 Silk Fibroin

SF is a natural, water-insoluble protein that has gained increasing attention as a promising biomaterial for TE applications. Its biocompatibility, biodegradability, and lack of immunogenicity make it ideal for biomedical use [183]. Derived primarily from the silkworm *Bombyx mori*, SF is composed of heavy (H-chain) and light chains (L-chain), connected via disulfide bridges, forming a stable H–L complex that contributes to its exceptional mechanical properties [184,185].

Initially approved by the FDA in 1993 for use in sutures and wound dressings, SF has since expanded into various biomedical applications [186,187]. The sericin coating that naturally envelops silk filaments must be removed through a degumming process, as sericin can provoke inflammatory responses and reduce mechanical strength [188].

SF exhibits remarkable tensile strength (300–740 MPa), strain at break (4%–26%), and toughness (70–78 MJ/m^3), making it suitable for load-bearing applications such as musculoskeletal TE [183]. These properties have led to widespread interest in incorporating SF into bioinks for 3DBP.

In the context of 3DBP, SF can be processed using multiple strategies, including shear-induced β-sheet crystallization, enzymatic crosslinking, chemical modification, and the addition of copolymers or plasticizers to enhance rheological performance [189–191]. Due to its low inherent viscosity, SF is often combined with materials such as gelatin or gellan gum to enable efficient extrusion-based printing.

Recent advances have also enabled the photopolymerization of SF through methacrylation, making it compatible with light-assisted bioprinting technologies [91,133,192,193]. In preclinical models, SF has been demonstrated to support osteogenesis in cranial defect repair and shows promising results as an ECM substitute scaffold [194,195].

Additionally, SF has recently emerged as a candidate for food engineering applications. For instance, [196] used SF-based hydrogels in cultured meat bioprinting, demonstrating favorable outcomes for myogenic differentiation and tissue formation when combined with GelMA.

Collectively, the mechanical strength, versatility, and biocompatibility of SF make it a highly attractive biomaterial for developing functional bioinks tailored to both regenerative medicine and novel biomanufacturing applications.

2.4.2.6 Decellularized Extracellular Matrix (dECM)

Decellularized extracellular matrix (dECM) bioinks represent a promising strategy to replicate the biochemical and structural complexity of native tissues for 3DBP applications. Derived from animal or human sources, dECM retains essential extracellular components, such as collagen, elastin, and glycosaminoglycans, that provide biological cues necessary for cell adhesion, proliferation, and differentiation [197,198].

The decellularization process aims to eliminate immunogenic cellular material while preserving the ultrastructure and functionality of the ECM. Methods include chemical (e.g., detergents like SDS and Triton X-100), enzymatic, and physical treatments (e.g., freeze–thaw cycles) [199]. Achieving effective decellularization without excessive damage to ECM integrity remains a key challenge.

Once processed into printable hydrogels, dECM-based bioinks can simulate tissue-specific microenvironments, supporting applications in liver, cartilage, cardiac, and adipose TE [197]. However, these hydrogels typically lack mechanical robustness and require blending with materials such as gelatin or alginate or crosslinking with agents like genipin or transglutaminase to enhance their printability [198].

An advancement in the field has been reported by the Brazilian company Quantis Biotecnologia, which applies 3DBP as a bioreactor system to generate dermis-like constructs from human fibroblasts [200]. These tissues are processed via homogenization, centrifugation, and filtration to extract high-purity ECM proteins, including fibrillar collagens (types I and II), elastin, fibronectin, and glycosaminoglycans (Figure 2.6). The products achieve protein purities of 97%–99%, eliminating the need for animal-derived components or enzymatic steps, and are suitable for use in biomedical, pharmaceutical, and cosmetic applications (WO2022073090) [201] (Figure 2.6).

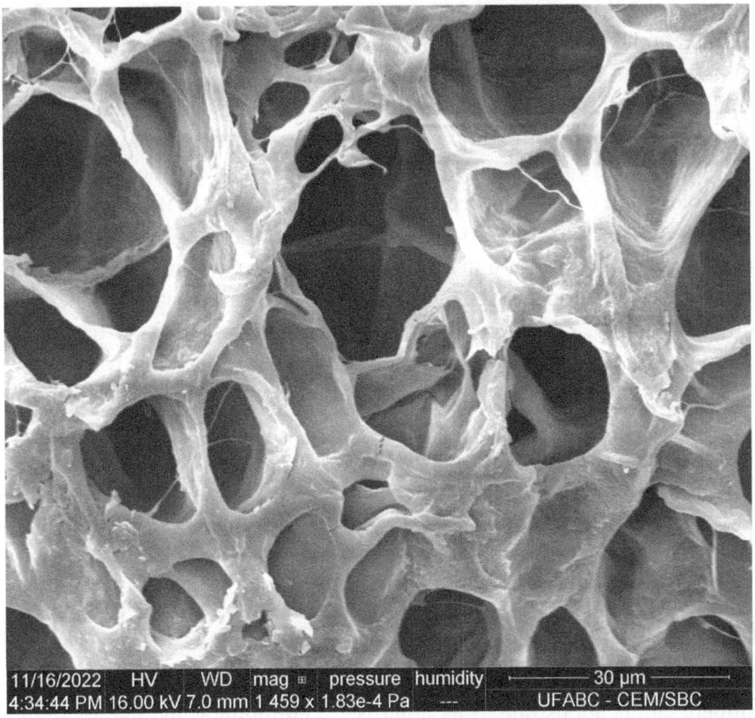

FIGURE 2.6 ECM proteins – including fibrillar collagens (types I and II), elastin, fibronectin, and glycosaminoglycans – produced. (Kindly provided by Quantis Biotechnology.)

2.5 SYNTHETIC BIOMATERIALS FOR 3D BIOPRINTING

2.5.1 Poly(ε-Caprolactone) (PCL)

Synthetic biodegradable polymers are essential in TE due to their accessibility, tunable physicochemical properties, and reproducible quality, which reduce immune response risks. Their controlled manufacturing enables tailored morphologies for diverse applications [202–204]. Among these, PCL stands out as a semicrystalline polyester containing polar ester and nonpolar methylene units [205,206]. With crystallinity reaching 69% and molecular weights ranging from 3,000 to 90,000 g/mol, PCL's structural features directly influence its thermal, mechanical, and degradation behavior [207–210]. Synthesized via ring-opening polymerization of ε-caprolactone using various catalysts [210,211], PCL exhibits specific solvent affinities, being soluble in aromatic solvents but insoluble or poorly soluble in most polar and aliphatic media [210,212,213].

In TE, PCL is widely applied for scaffold fabrication owing to its proven *in vitro* and *in vivo* biocompatibility, leading to FDA approval for multiple medical devices and drug delivery platforms [214–218]. However, its hydrophobic nature, slow degradation rate, and limited cell adhesion often necessitate modification through copolymerization or blending with other biomaterials [219]. Complete degradation under physiological conditions may take two to three years, controlled by molecular weight, crystallinity, and hydrophilicity, with hydrolysis proceeding through water diffusion, fragmentation, and metabolic clearance [211,217].

Recent advances integrate PCL with natural polymers (e.g., collagen, gelatin, and chitosan) [105,220,221], inorganic components (e.g., hydroxyapatite and strontium) [222–224], and metallic phases (e.g., magnesium and zinc oxides) [225,226] to generate scaffolds with enhanced mechanical, structural, and biochemical performance [227]. These multimaterial approaches, often realized through advanced 3DBP platforms [228], enable fabrication of complex, mechanically adaptive tissue constructs.

In multimaterial bioprinting, thermoplastic PCL is typically shaped via fused deposition modeling, complemented by hydrogel microextrusion to create hybrid scaffolds [229–231]. This design combines a rigid load-bearing framework with a soft, ECM-mimicking phase, achieving a balance of mechanical stability and bioactivity [231,232]. Applications include cartilage models supporting chondrogenesis and vascularization [233], GelMA/PCL growth plates enhancing mechanical strength for cartilage repair [234], and patterned tubular scaffolds for spinal cord regeneration [229], highlighting PCL's versatility in regenerative medicine and its potential for next-generation biofabrication strategies (Figure 2.7).

2.5.2 Polyethylene Glycol (PEG)

PEG is a synthetic, hydrophilic polymer widely utilized in biomedical, pharmaceutical, and cosmetic applications due to its nontoxic, nonimmunogenic nature and excellent biocompatibility, leading to FDA approval for human use [235]. Structurally, PEG possesses a flexible backbone terminated with hydroxyl groups, enabling conjugation with

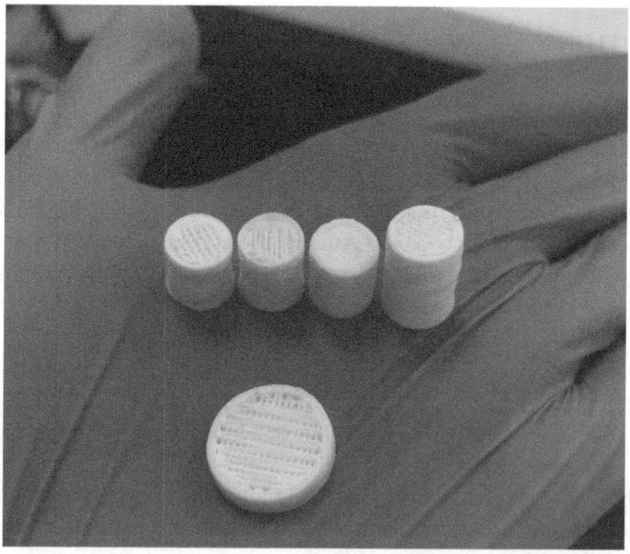

FIGURE 2.7 3D-printed bone graft composed of poly(ε-caprolactone) (PCL), β-tricalcium phosphate (β-TCP), and QMatrix® (Quantis). (Image courtesy of Quantis Biotechnology.)

diverse functional moieties [236,237]. This modification capacity enhances the solubility of hydrophobic compounds [235]. PEG is resistant to degradation by hydrolysis, with limited *in vivo* metabolism, and its elimination depends on molecular weight [238]. For TE applications, molecular weights below 50 kDa are preferred, with renal clearance predominating under 30 kDa and hepatic clearance above this threshold [239,240].

PEG hydrogels can be chemically tailored to suit specific applications. Acrylate or methacrylate functionalization allows photopolymerization, a light-driven process conducted under physiological conditions that produces mechanically stable, spatially, and temporally controlled 3D structures [241–243]. This approach is particularly suitable for encapsulating cells and labile biomolecules [236,244,245]. Biofunctionalization with RGD peptides or growth factors further enhances cell adhesion and ECM production, overcoming PEG's intrinsic bioinertness [237,246].

Additional crosslinking chemistries, such as Michael addition and click reactions, enable the fabrication of PEG hydrogels with tunable degradability, stiffness, and permeability [236,247]. Click-based hydrogels have gained prominence in 3DBP [248,249]. PEG can also be copolymerized with natural macromolecules such as gelatin [250], chitosan [251], heparin [252], and collagen [253], yielding biosynthetic matrices with enhanced biological performance [254].

In TE, PEG hydrogels facilitate ECM deposition and support the chondrogenic differentiation of stem cells for cartilage repair [255,256]. In wound healing, PEG serves as a biocompatible barrier to reduce inflammation, prevent postoperative adhesions, and limit organ-to-organ contact [257–259]. It is also fundamental in 3DBP and in culturing patient-derived cancer samples, including breast [260] and prostate tumors [261]. Incorporation of ECM proteins and degradable ligands allows PEG scaffolds to mimic native tissue architecture, reduce material heterogeneity, and improve reproducibility, making them a versatile alternative to Matrigel® [261,262].

2.5.3 Pluronic

Pluronic, also referred to as poloxamer, is a synthetic nonionic triblock copolymer consisting of alternating segments of poly(ethylene oxide) (PEO) and poly(propylene oxide) (PPO) in a PEO–PPO–PEO configuration [263]. This amphiphilic arrangement, with hydrophilic PEO ends and a hydrophobic PPO core, underlies its unique temperature- and concentration-dependent self-assembly behaviors, including micellization and hydrogel formation [264]. The physicochemical profile of each pluronic variant depends on its molecular weight and PEO/PPO ratio; for instance, Pluronic F127 (Poloxamer 407) contains approximately 70% PEO, granting high aqueous solubility and thermosensitive gelation [265]. Other types, such as F68, L61, and P85, vary in block length, influencing gelation temperature, viscosity, and hydrophobicity [266].

A defining feature of pluronics is their reversible, temperature-triggered gelation. At low temperatures and dilute concentrations, polymer chains remain dispersed in solution; upon heating past a threshold, PPO block interactions promote micelle formation with hydrophobic cores and hydrophilic coronas, leading to a sol–gel transition [267]. This property, coupled with biocompatibility, biodegradability, and encapsulation capacity for drugs or cells, supports their extensive use in controlled drug delivery, TE, gene therapy, and wound repair [265]. Pluronic F127 is particularly valuable in *in situ* gelling systems, remaining fluid at room temperature for easy drug loading and forming a depot gel at physiological temperature for sustained release [268].

Chemical functionalization, such as incorporating carboxyl, amine, or acrylate groups, has enabled covalent crosslinking to produce hydrogels with enhanced mechanical performance and responsiveness to stimuli including light, pH, and enzymes [269]. Such modifications are especially relevant for engineered cartilage and nerve scaffolds, where degradation rate, cell adhesion, and targeted bioactive factor release are critical. In oncology, pluronics have been explored as adjuvants due to their capacity to inhibit P-glycoprotein activity, improving intracellular retention of chemotherapeutics and overcoming multidrug resistance. When integrated into nanoparticles, they facilitate tumor-targeted delivery with reduced systemic toxicity [270].

In advanced biofabrication, particularly 3DBP, pluronics serve as bioinks due to their rapid, tunable sol–gel transitions, enabling high-resolution, multilayer constructs while maintaining cell viability [271]. Pluronic F127 has been employed as a sacrificial bioink for creating vascular channels [272] and, alongside F68, as a surfactant or stabilizer in pharmaceutical formulations [270,273]. Combining Pluronic F127 with natural biopolymers such as gelatin has shown promise in wound healing, providing adjustable rheology, transparency, and a regenerative microenvironment [274]. The adaptability of these copolymers, guided by precise selection and functionalization strategies, underpins their role as key materials in next-generation drug delivery, TE, and regenerative medicine [269].

2.5.4 Polylactic Acid (PLA)

PLA is an organic polymer obtained from LA (2-hydroxypropionic acid, $CH_3CHOHCOOH$), which contains carboxylic and hydroxyl functional groups. It is produced from renewable sources such as corn and sugarcane through either chemical synthesis or microbial fermentation, the latter offering advantages in production efficiency [275,276]. PLA synthesis requires the use of catalysts and prolonged polymerization periods, which increase the overall energy demand of the production process.

LA must undergo a high degree of purification before the polymerization of its monomer into PLA, as impurities can interfere with the polymerization process and alter the resulting polymer properties [276].

Despite its relatively high production cost, the use of PLA in medical applications continues to advance due to its biocompatibility, biodegradability, and mechanical strength. Variations in LA composition allow the development of PLA derivatives with tunable performance characteristics. These derivatives possess mechanical properties suitable for biofabrication, enabling the creation of scaffolds for supporting biomaterials [277]. Additionally, PLA exhibits satisfactory physical and barrier properties compared to petroleum-based polymers [276] and shows degradation rates that vary according to its degree of crystallinity [278].

PLA is approved by regulatory agencies such as the FDA and European Union authorities for specific healthcare applications, which enhances its competitiveness in the market [276].

2.6 COMPOSITE BIOINKS

Composite bioinks, combining polymeric matrices with inorganic or nanoscale additives, offer a strategic means to simultaneously enhance mechanical integrity, bioactivity, and long-term stability; surpassing the limitations of single-component systems [279]. For instance, the incorporation of nano-hydroxyapatite within gellan gum and PVA matrices has been demonstrated to enhance printing fidelity markedly, while reducing biodegradation rates from approximately 27% to 16% over a three-week period. Moreover, these composites exhibit viscoelastic behavior conducive to load-bearing applications and facilitate osteogenic differentiation, as evidenced by elevated alkaline phosphatase activity and ECM mineralization [280]. Similarly, alginate methacrylate hydrogels enriched with micron- and nano-scaled particles derived from decellularized human bone allograft exhibit substantial improvements in compressive modulus, rising from 21 ± 6.2 kPa in pure gels to 51 ± 7.1 kPa in composites, without compromising cellular viability, which remains above 90% for mesenchymal stem cells cultured up to 28 days. This mechanical reinforcement concurrently promotes significant osteogenic lineage commitment, as indicated by increased calcium deposition and osteocalcin expression [281]. Such strategies reinforce the importance of particulate inclusion for improving both scaffold architecture and cell-instructive cues (Figure 2.8).

Composite bioinks also offer enhanced rheological properties essential for extrusion-based bioprinting. Colloidal fillers, such as nanoclays, graphene oxide (GO), and CNC, can increase shear-thinning behavior and storage modulus, facilitating filament stability and fidelity postextrusion. The synergistic coupling of these fillers with biopolymers such as GelMA, alginate, chitosan, and methacrylated HA confers shear-thinning rheology and rapid viscosity recovery, properties fundamental to extrusion-based bioprinting techniques demanding high shape fidelity and structural integrity [282].

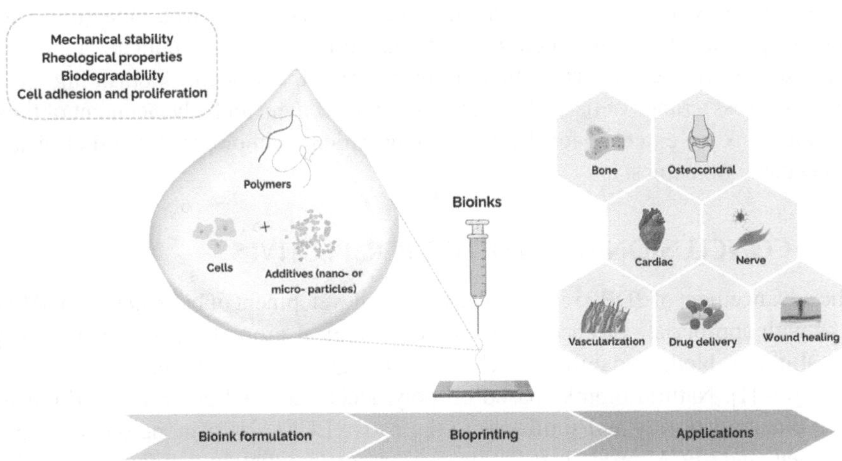

FIGURE 2.8 Bioink functionality in 3DBP: formulations combine polymers, cells, and additives to ensure mechanical stability, rheological control, biodegradability, and cell adhesion/proliferation. These bioinks enable applications in bone, osteochondral, cardiac, and nerve regeneration, as well as vascularization, drug delivery, and wound healing.

In the context of soft TE, particularly in cardiac regenerative medicine, composite bioinks incorporating electroconductive polymers have emerged as a promising strategy to enhance electrical signal propagation and synchronous contractility in engineered heart tissues [283,284]. Effective electrophysiological coupling is essential to prevent arrhythmogenic events postimplantation [285,286]. Among recent developments, biohybrid hydrogels composed of collagen, alginate, and poly(3,4-ethylenedioxythiophene)polystyrene sulfonate (PEDOT:PSS) have demonstrated improved electrical conductivity and ECM-mimetic architecture. The incorporation of PEDOT:PSS facilitates enhanced electrical integration among cardiomyocytes, reduces arrhythmic activity, and promotes cellular alignment, sarcomeric organization, and gap junction maturation. Notably, human-induced pluripotent stem cell-derived cardiomyocytes cultured within these constructs exhibit sarcomere lengths approaching 1.9 μm and spontaneous beating rates exceeding 200 bpm [287], highlighting the potential of electroconductive composite bioinks for the fabrication of physiologically relevant cardiac tissues.

Recent progress in neural TE has leveraged the electroactive properties of GO nanoparticles incorporated into GelMA-based hydrogels to address the poor electrical conductivity of gelatin-derived scaffolds. The integration of GO substantially enhances both the mechanical stiffness and electrical conductivity of the composite bioinks, critical parameters for engineered neural constructs that depend on efficient electrical signal transduction. These GO/GelMA formulations preserve favorable rheological characteristics, including pronounced shear-thinning behavior and reliable viscosity recovery, which collectively support high-resolution, and shape-fidelity bioprinting. In addition, GO nanoparticles confer UV shielding during *in situ* photocrosslinking, reducing phototoxic effects and maintaining cellular viability [288].

In conclusion, composite bioinks constitute a versatile platform for engineering scaffolds with reinforced mechanical performance, improved bioactivity, and tunable physicochemical functionalities, including electrical, optical, and other stimulus-responsive properties, thereby broadening the scope of bioprinting applications across a range of tissue types. Ongoing refinement and advancement of these formulations are essential for driving biofabrication technologies toward clinically translatable outcomes.

2.7 CONCLUSION AND FUTURE PERSPECTIVES

The advancement of 3DBP relies directly on the development of biomaterials and bioinks with appropriate physicochemical and biological properties, such as viscosity, crosslinking, biodegradability, mechanical strength, bioactivity, and cellular compatibility [1]. Natural bioinks based on polysaccharides and proteins stand out for their biocompatibility and similarity to the native ECM [21]. Among them, gelatin, collagen, and dECM promote cell adhesion and differentiation, but face mechanical limitations that have been mitigated through chemical modification, crosslinking, and hybrid formulations [289].

Current trends include multifunctional bioinks with tunable properties, multi-component printing, and the incorporation of bioactive agents and nanoparticles to produce more complex tissues [290]. An example is Quantis Biotecnologia, which employs bioprinting as a bioreactor to produce high-purity ECM proteins from human cells, creating customized and sustainable bioinks [201].

In the future, tailoring bioinks for specific target tissues, combined with precise printing control and integration with computational modeling, artificial intelligence, and microfluidic microenvironments, is expected to enhance the sophistication of biofabricated constructs [1]. However, challenges remain in standardization, reproducibility, scaling, and regulatory compliance [289], requiring ongoing collaboration between researchers, industry, and regulatory bodies.

The future trajectory points toward intelligent, biomimetic, and safe bioinks capable of transforming the manufacturing and regeneration of living tissues.

ACKNOWLEDGMENTS

The authors gratefully acknowledge the financial support provided by Quantis Biotechnology, the São Paulo Research Foundation (FAPESP) (project no. 2021/12156-1, 2021/14955-9, 2023/02636-1, and 2025/01402-2), and the Minas Gerais Research Foundation (FAPEMIG) (project no. APQ-04441-22), which made possible the collection and analysis of the data presented in this chapter.

REFERENCES

1. Ashammakhi, N., Ahadian, S., Xu, C., Montazerian, H., Ko, H., Nasiri, R., … & Khademhosseini, A. (2019). Bioinks and bioprinting technologies to make heterogeneous and biomimetic tissue constructs. *Materials Today Bio*, 1, 100008. https://doi.org/10.1016/j.mtbio.2019.100008.
2. Groll, J., Burdick, J. A., Cho, D. W., Derby, B., Gelinsky, M., Heilshorn, S. C., … & Woodfield, T. B. F. (2018). A definition of bioinks and their distinction from biomaterial inks. *Biofabrication*, 11(1), 013001. https://doi.org/10.1088/1758-5090/aaec52.
3. Williams, D. F. (2009). On the nature of biomaterials. *Biomaterials*, 30(30), 5897–5909. https://doi.org/10.1016/j.biomaterials.2009.07.027.
4. Chen, X. B., Fazel Anvari-Yazdi, A., Duan, X., Zimmerling, A., Gharraei, R., Sharma, N. K., … & Ning, L. (2023). Biomaterials/bioinks and extrusion bioprinting. *Bioactive Materials*, 28, 511–536. https://doi.org/10.1016/j.bioactmat.2023.06.006.
5. Li, J., Wu, C., Chu, P. K., & Gelinsky, M. (2020). 3D printing of hydrogels: Rational design strategies and emerging biomedical applications. *Materials Science and Engineering: R: Reports*, 140, 100543. https://doi.org/10.1016/j.mser.2020.100543.
6. Mateu-Sanz, M., Fuenteslópez, C. V., Uribe-Gomez, J., Haugen, H. J., Pandit, A., Ginebra, M.-P., … & Samara, A. (2024). Redefining biomaterial biocompatibility: Challenges for artificial intelligence and text mining. *Trends in Biotechnology*, 42(4), 402–417. https://doi.org/10.1016/j.tibtech.2023.09.015.
7. Huzum, B., Puha, B., Necoara, R. M., Gheorghevici, S., Puha, G., Filip, A., … & Alexa, O. (2021). Biocompatibility assessment of biomaterials used in orthopedic devices: An overview (review). *Experimental and Therapeutic Medicine*, 22(5), 1315. https://doi.org/10.3892/etm.2021.10750.

8. Rahmati, M., Silva, E. A., Reseland, J. E., Heyward, C. A., & Haugen, H. J. (2020). Biological responses to physicochemical properties of biomaterial surface. *Chemical Society Reviews*, 49(15), 5178–5224. https://doi.org/10.1039/D0CS00103A.
9. Ratner, B. D. (2011). The biocompatibility manifesto: Biocompatibility for the twenty-first century. *Journal of Cardiovascular Translational Research*, 4(5), 523–527. https://doi.org/10.1007/s12265-011-9287-x.
10. Ferreira, M. R., Santos, G. A., Biagi, C. A., Silva Junior, W. A., & Zambuzzi, W. F. (2021). GSVA score reveals molecular signatures from transcriptomes for biomaterials comparison. *Journal of Biomedical Materials Research. Part A*, 109(6), 1004–1014. https://doi.org/10.1002/jbm.a.37090.
11. Wang, Z., Dahaja, R., Chen, L., & Banu, M. (2023). Machine learning unifies flexibility and efficiency of spinodal structure generation for stochastic biomaterial design. *Scientific Reports*, 13(1), 5414. https://doi.org/10.1038/s41598-023-31677-7.
12. Middleton, J. C., & Tipton, A. J. (2000). Synthetic biodegradable polymers as orthopedic devices. *Biomaterials*, 21(23), 2335–2346. https://doi.org/10.1016/s0142-9612(00)00101-0.
13. Anderson, J. M., Rodriguez, A., & Chang, D. T. (2008). Foreign body reaction to biomaterials. *Seminars in Immunology*, 20(2), 86–100. https://doi.org/10.1016/j.smim.2007.11.004.
14. Lei, M., & Wang, X. (2016). Biodegradable polymers and stem cells for bioprinting. *Molecules*, 21(5), 539. https://doi.org/10.3390/molecules21050539.
15. Makadia, H. K., & Siegel, S. J. (2011). Poly lactic-co-glycolic acid (PLGA) as biodegradable controlled drug delivery carrier. *Polymers*, 3(3), 1377–1397. https://doi.org/10.3390/polym3031377.
16. Woodruff, M. A., & Hutmacher, D. W. (2010). The return of a forgotten polymer – Polycaprolactone in the 21st century. *Progress in Polymer Science*, 35(10), 1217–1256. https://doi.org/10.1016/j.progpolymsci.2010.04.002.
17. Hospodiuk, M., Dey, M., Sosnoski, D., & Ozbolat, I.T., 2017. The bioink: A comprehensive review on bioprintable materials. *Biotechnology Advances*, 35(2), 217–239. https://doi.org/10.1016/j.biotechadv.2016.12.006.
18. Kretlow, J. D., Klouda, L., & Mikos, A. G. (2007). Injectable matrices and scaffolds for drug delivery in tissue engineering. *Advanced Drug Delivery Reviews*, 59(4–5), 263–273. https://doi.org/10.1016/j.addr.2007.03.013.
19. Lu, L., Peter, S. J., Lyman, M. D., Lai, H. L., Leite, S. M., Tamada, J. A., … & Mikos, A. G. (2000). In vitro and in vivo degradation of porous poly(dl-lactic-co-glycolic acid) foams. *Biomaterials*, 21(18), 1837–1845. https://doi.org/10.1016/s0142-9612(00)00047-8.
20. Seal, B. L., Otero, T. C., & Panitch, A. (2001). Polymeric biomaterials for tissue and organ regeneration. *Materials Science and Engineering: R: Reports*, 34(4–5), 147–230. https://doi.org/10.1016/S0927-796X(01)00035-3.
21. Gungor-Ozkerim, P. S., Inci, I., Zhang, Y. S., Khademhosseini, A., & Dokmeci, M. R., (2018). Bioinks for 3D bioprinting: An overview. *Biomaterials Science*, 6(5), 915–946. https://doi.org/10.1039/c7bm00765e.
22. Chimene, D., Lennox, K. K., Kaunas, R. R., & Gaharwar, A. K. (2016). Advanced bioinks for 3D printing: A materials science perspective. *Annals of Biomedical Engineering*, 44(6), 2090–2102. https://doi.org/10.1007/s10439-016-1638-y.
23. Ozbolat, I. T., & Hospodiuk, M. (2016). Current advances and future perspectives in extrusion-based bioprinting. *Biomaterials*, 76, 321–343. https://doi.org/10.1016/j.biomaterials.2015.10.076.
24. Ribeiro, A., Blokzijl, M. M., Levato, R., Visser, C. W., Castilho, M., Hennink, W. E., … & Malda, J. (2017). Assessing bioink shape fidelity to aid material development in 3D bioprinting. *Biofabrication*, 10(1), 014102. https://doi.org/10.1088/1758-5090/aa90e2.

25. Gudapati, H., Dey, M., & Ozbolat, I. (2016). A comprehensive review on droplet-based bioprinting: Past, present and future. *Biomaterials*, 102, 20–42. https://doi.org/10.1016/j.biomaterials.2016.06.012.
26. Ouyang, L., Yao, R., Zhao, Y., & Sun, W. (2016). Effect of bioink properties on printability and cell viability for 3D bioplotting of embryonic stem cells. *Biofabrication*, 8(3), 035020. https://doi.org/10.1088/1758-5090/8/3/035020.
27. Gillispie, G. J., Copus, J., Uzun-Per, M., Yoo, J. J., Atala, A., Niazi, M. K. K., & Lee, S. J. (2023). The correlation between rheological properties and extrusion-based printability in bioink artifact quantification. *Materials & Design*, 233, 112237. https://doi.org/10.1016/j.matdes.2023.112237.
28. Sánchez-Sánchez, R., Rodríguez-Rego, J. M., Macías-García, A., Mendoza-Cerezo, L., & Díaz-Parralejo, A. (2023). Relationship between shear-thinning rheological properties of bioinks and bioprinting parameters. *International Journal of Bioprinting*, 9(2), 687. https://doi.org/10.18063/ijb.687.
29. Budai, L., Budai, M., Fülöpné Pápay, Z. E., Vilimi, Z., & Antal, I. (2023). Rheological considerations of pharmaceutical formulations: Focus on viscoelasticity. *Gels*, 9(6), 469. https://doi.org/10.3390/gels9060469.
30. Chopin-Doroteo, M., Mandujano-Tinoco, E. A., & Krötzsch, E. (2021). Tailoring of the rheological properties of bioinks to improve bioprinting and bioassembly for tissue replacement. *Biochimica et Biophysica Acta. General Subjects*, 1865(2), 129782. https://doi.org/10.1016/j.bbagen.2020.129782.
31. Amorim, P. A., d'Ávila, M. A., Anand, R., Moldenaers, P., Van Puyvelde, P., & Bloemen, V. (2021). Insights on shear rheology of inks for extrusion-based 3D bioprinting. *Bioprinting*, 22, e00129. https://doi.org/10.1016/j.bprint.2021.e00129.
32. Habib, M. A., & Khoda, B. (2022). Rheological analysis of bio-ink for 3D bio-printing processes. *Journal of Manufacturing Processes*, 76, 708–718. https://doi.org/10.1016/j.jmapro.2022.02.048.
33. Yan, W.-C., Davoodi, P., Vijayavenkataraman, S., Tian, Y., Ng, W. C., Fuh, J. Y. H., ... & Wang, C.-H. (2018). 3D bioprinting of skin tissue: From pre-processing to final product evaluation. *Advanced Drug Delivery Reviews*, 132, 270–295. https://doi.org/10.1016/j.addr.2018.07.016.
34. Bliley, J. M., Stang, M. A., Behre, A., & Feinberg, A. W. (2024). Advances in 3D bioprinted cardiac tissue using stem cell-derived cardiomyocytes. *Stem Cells Translational Medicine*, 13(5), 425–435. https://doi.org/10.1093/stcltm/szae014.
35. Kupfer, M. E., Lin, W.-H., Ravikumar, V., Qiu, K., Wang, L., Gao, L., ... & Ogle, B. M. (2020). In situ expansion, differentiation, and electromechanical coupling of human cardiac muscle in a 3D bioprinted, chambered organoid. *Circulation Research*, 127(2), 207–224. https://doi.org/10.1161/CIRCRESAHA.119.316155.
36. Hagenbuchner, J., Nothdurfter, D., & Ausserlechner, M. J. (2021). 3D bioprinting: novel approaches for engineering complex human tissue equivalents and drug testing. *Essays in Biochemistry*, 65(3), 417–427. https://doi.org/10.1042/EBC20200153.
37. Martinez, A. W., Caves, J. M., Ravi, S., Li, W., & Chaikof, E. L. (2014). Effects of crosslinking on the mechanical properties, drug release and cytocompatibility of protein polymers. *Acta Biomaterialia*, 10(1), 26–33. https://doi.org/10.1016/j.actbio.2013.08.029.
38. Karvinen, J., & Kellomäki, M. (2023). Design aspects and characterization of hydrogel-based bioinks for extrusion-based bioprinting. *Bioprinting*, 32, e00274. https://doi.org/10.1016/j.bprint.2023.e00274.
39. Seymour, A. J., Kilian, D., Navarro, R. S., Hull, S. M., & Heilshorn, S. C. (2023). 3D printing microporous scaffolds from modular bioinks containing sacrificial, cell-encapsulating microgels. *Biomaterials Science*, 11(21), 4495–4507. https://doi.org/10.1039/D3BM00721A.

40. Augustine, R., Alhussain, H., Zahid, A.A., Raza Ur Rehman, S., Ahmed, R., & Hasan, A. (2021). Crosslinking strategies to develop hydrogels for biomedical applications. In: Jose, J., Thomas, S., & Thakur, V. K. (eds) *Nano Hydrogels. Gels Horizons: From Science to Smart Materials.* Springer, Singapore. https://doi.org/10.1007/978-981-15-7138-1_2.
41. Bebiano, L. B., Presa, R., Vieira, F., Lourenço, B. N., & Pereira, R. F. (2024). Bioinspired and photo-clickable thiol-ene bioinks for the extrusion bioprinting of mechanically tunable 3D skin models. *Biomimetics*, 9(4), 228. https://doi.org/10.3390/biomimetics9040228.
42. Mukundan, L. M., Rajasekaran, R., Das, S., Seesala, V. S., Ganguly, D., Kumar, N., … & Chattopadhyay, S. (2025). Tailoring of agarose hydrogel to modulate its 3D bioprintability and mechanical properties for stem cell mediated bone tissue engineering. *International Journal of Biological Macromolecules*, 309(Pt 1), 142795. https://doi.org/1 0.1016/j.ijbiomac.2025.142795.
43. Machour, M., Meretzki, R., Haizler, Y. M., Shuhmaher, M., Safina, D., Levy, M. M., & Levenberg, S. (2025). A stiff bioink for hybrid bioprinting of vascularized bone tissue with enhanced mechanical properties. *Biomaterials*, 322, 123406. https://doi.org/10.1016/j.biomaterials.2025.123406.
44. Wang, Z., Wang, L., Li, T., Liu, S., Guo, B., Huang, W., & Wu, Y. (2021). 3D bioprinting in cardiac tissue engineering. *Theranostics*, 11(16), 7948–7969. https://doi.org/10.7150/thno.61621.
45. Chen, K., Liu, Z., Zhou, X., Zheng, W., Cao, H., Yang, Z., … & Zhao, H. (2025). Hierarchy reproduction: Multiphasic strategies for tendon/ligament-bone junction repair. *Biomaterials Research*, 29, 0132. https://doi.org/10.34133/bmr.0132.
46. Sahan, A. Z., Baday, M., & Patel, C. B. (2022). Biomimetic hydrogels in the study of cancer mechanobiology: Overview, biomedical applications, and future perspectives. *Gels*, 8(8), 496. https://doi.org/10.3390/gels8080496.
47. Morales, X., Cortés-Domínguez, I., & Ortiz-de-Solorzano, C. (2021). Modeling the mechanobiology of cancer cell migration using 3D biomimetic hydrogels. *Gels*, 7(1), 17. https://doi.org/10.3390/gels7010017.
48. Muscolino, E., Di Stefano, A.B., Toia, F., Sabatino, M.A., Moschella, F., Cordova, A., … & Dispenza, C. (2021). k-Carrageenan and PVA blends as 3D printing bioinks for cartilage reconstruction scaffolding. *International Journal of Biological Macromolecules*, 222(B), 1861. https://doi.org/10.1016/j.ijbiomac.2022.09.275.
49. Di Stefano, A. B., Urrata, V., Schilders, K., Franza, M., Di Leo, S., Moschella, F., … & Toia, F. (2025). Three-dimensional bioprinting techniques in skin regeneration: Current insights and future perspectives. *Life*, 15(5), 787. https://doi.org/10.3390/life15050787.
50. Monfared, M., Mawad, D., Rnjak-Kovacina, J., & Stenzel, M. (2021). 3D bioprinting of dual-crosslinked nanocellulose hydrogels for tissue engineering applications. *Journal of Materials Chemistry B*, 9, 6163–6175. https://doi.org/10.1039/D1TB00624J.
51. Dell, A. C., Wagner, G., Own, J., & Geibel, J. P. (2022). 3D bioprinting using hydrogels: Cell inks and tissue engineering applications. *Pharmaceutics*, 14(12), 2596. https://doi.org/10.3390/pharmaceutics14122596.
52. Ghosh, S., & Yi, H. G. (2022). A review on bioinks and their application in plant bioprinting. *International Journal of Bioprinting*, 8(4), 612. https://doi.org/10.18063/ijb.v8i4.612.
53. Donderwinkel, Ilze & Hest, Jan & Cameron, Neil. (2017). Bio-inks for 3D bioprinting: Recent advances and future prospects. *Polymer Chemistry*, 8, 4451–4471. https://doi.org/10.1039/C7PY00826K.
54. Bandyopadhyay, A., Mandal, B. B., & Bhardwaj, N. (2022). 3D bioprinting of photo-crosslinkable silk methacrylate (SilMA)-polyethylene glycol diacrylate (PEGDA) bioink for cartilage tissue engineering. *Journal of Biomedical Materials Research. Part A*, 110(4), 884–898. https://doi.org/10.1002/jbm.a.37336.

55. Anaya-Sampayo, L. M., Roa, N. S., Martínez-Cardozo, C., García-Robayo, D. A., & Rodríguez-Lorenzo, L. M. (2024). Influence of hydroxyapatite and gelatin content on crosslinking dynamics and HDFn cell viability in alginate bioinks for 3D bioprinting. *Polymers*, 16(22), 3224. https://doi.org/10.3390/polym16223224.
56. Mørch, Y. A., Donati, I., Strand, B. L., & Skjåk-Braek, G. (2006). Effect of Ca^{2+}, Ba^{2+}, and Sr^{2+} on alginate microbeads. *Biomacromolecules*, 7(5), 1471–1480. https://doi.org/10.1021/bm060010d.
57. Ručigaj, A., Golobič, J., & Kopač, T. (2024). The role of multivalent cations in determining the cross-linking affinity of alginate hydrogels: A combined experimental and modeling study. *Chemical Engineering Journal Advances*, 20, 100678. https://doi.org/10.1016/j.ceja.2024.100678.
58. Skopinska-Wisniewska, J., Tuszynska, M., Kaźmierski, Ł., Bartniak, M., & Bajek, A. (2024). Gelatin–sodium alginate hydrogels cross-linked by squaric acid and dialdehyde starch as a potential bio-ink. *Polymers*, 16(18), 2560. https://doi.org/10.3390/polym16182560.
59. Lee, J. E., Heo, S. W., Kim, C. H., Park, S. J., Park, S. H., & Kim, T. H. (2023). In-situ ionic crosslinking of 3D bioprinted cell-hydrogel constructs for mechanical reinforcement and improved cell growth. *Biomaterials Advances*, 147, 213322. https://doi.org/10.1016/j.bioadv.2023.213322.
60. Borgogna, M., Skjåk-Bræk, G., Paoletti, S., & Donati, I. (2013). On the initial binding of alginate by calcium ions. The tilted egg-box hypothesis. *The Journal of Physical Chemistry B*, 117(24), 7277–7282. https://doi.org/10.1021/jp4030766.
61. Hecht, H., & Srebnik, S. (2016). Structural characterization of sodium alginate and calcium alginate. *Biomacromolecules*, 17(6), 2160–2167. https://doi.org/10.1021/acs.biomac.6b00378.
62. Jahani Kadousaraei, M., Yamada, S., Aydin, M. S., Rashad, A., Cabeza, N. M., Mohamed-Ahmed, S., … & Mustafa, K. (2025). Bioprinting of mesenchymal stem cells in low concentration gelatin methacryloyl/alginate blends without ionic crosslinking of alginate. *Scientific Reports*, 15(1), 6609. https://doi.org/10.1038/s41598-025-90389-2.
63. Nützl, M., Schrottenbaum, M., Müller, T., & Müller, R. (2022). Mechanical properties and chemical stability of alginate-based anisotropic capillary hydrogels. *Journal of the Mechanical Behavior of Biomedical Materials*, 134, 105397. https://doi.org/10.1016/j.jmbbm.2022.105397.
64. Schütz, K., Placht, A. M., Paul, B., Brüggemeier, S., Gelinsky, M., & Lode, A. (2017). Three-dimensional plotting of a cell-laden alginate/methylcellulose blend: towards biofabrication of tissue engineering constructs with clinically relevant dimensions. *Journal of Tissue Engineering and Regenerative Medicine*, 11(5), 1574–1587. https://doi.org/10.1002/term.2058.
65. Boretti, G., Baldursson, H. E., Buonarrivo, L., Simonsson, S., Brynjólfsson, S., Gargiulo, P., & Sigurjónsson, Ó. E. (2024). Mechanical and biological characterization of ionic and photo-crosslinking effects on gelatin-based hydrogel for cartilage tissue engineering applications. *Polymers*, 16(19), 2741. https://doi.org/10.3390/polym16192741.
66. Mørch, Y.A., Qi, M., Gundersen, P.O.M., Formo, K., Lacik, I., Skjåk-Bræk, G., … & Strand, B.L. (2012), Binding and leakage of barium in alginate microbeads†. *Journal of Biomedical Materials Research*, 100A, 2939–2947. https://doi.org/10.1002/jbm.a.34237.
67. Antunes, M., Bonani, W., Reis, R. L., Migliaresi, C., Ferreira, H., Motta, A., & Neves, N. M. (2022). Development of alginate-based hydrogels for blood vessel engineering. *Biomaterials Advances*, 134, 112588. https://doi.org/10.1016/j.msec.2021.112588.
68. Nie, L., Sun, Y., Okoro, O., Deng, Y., Jiang, G., & Shavandi, A. (2023). Click chemistry for 3D bioprinting. *Materials Horizons*, 10, 2727–2763. https://doi.org/10.1039/D3MH00516J.

69. Cao, N., Chen, X., & Schreyer, D. (2012). Influence of calcium ions on cell survival and proliferation in the context of an alginate hydrogel. *ISRN Chemical Engineering*, 2012, 6. https://doi.org/10.5402/2012/516461.
70. Orrenius, S., McConkey, D. J., Bellomo, G., & Nicotera, P. (1989). Role of Ca^{2+} in toxic cell killing. *Trends in Pharmacological Sciences*, 10(7), 281–285. https://doi.org/10.1016/0165-6147(89)90029-1.
71. Nicotera, P., Hartzell, P., Davis, G., & Orrenius, S. (1986). The formation of plasma membrane blebs in hepatocytes exposed to agents that increase cytosolic Ca^{2+} is mediated by the activation of a non-lysosomal proteolytic system. *FEBS Letters*, 209(1), 139–144. https://doi.org/10.1016/0014-5793(86)81099-7.
72. Dong, Z., Saikumar, P., Weinberg, J. M., & Venkatachalam, M. A. (2006). Calcium in cell injury and death. *Annual Review of Pathology*, 1, 405–434. https://doi.org/10.1146/annurev.pathol.1.110304.100218.
73. Lee, H. W., Chen, K. T., Li, Y. E., Yeh, Y. C., Chiang, C. Y., & Lee, I. C. (2024). Dual crosslinking silk fibroin/pectin-based bioink development and the application on neural stem/progenitor cells spheroid laden 3D bioprinting. *International Journal of Biological Macromolecules*, 269(Pt 2), 131720. https://doi.org/10.1016/j.ijbiomac.2024.131720.
74. Said, N. S., Olawuyi, I. F., & Lee, W. Y. (2023). Pectin hydrogels: gel-forming behaviors, mechanisms, and food applications. *Gels*, 9(9), 732. https://doi.org/10.3390/gels9090732.
75. Lim, W., Kim, G. J., Kim, H. W., Lee, J., Zhang, X., Kang, M. G., … & Bae, H. (2020). Kappa-carrageenan-based dual crosslinkable bioink for extrusion type bioprinting. *Polymers*, 12(10), 2377. https://doi.org/10.3390/polym12102377.
76. Campo, V., Kawano, D., Júnior, D., & Ivone, C. (2009). Carrageenans: Biological properties, chemical modifications and structural analysis – A review. *Carbohydrate Polymers*, 77, 167–180. https://doi.org/10.1016/j.carbpol.2009.01.020.
77. Lai, V. M. F., Wong, P. A.-L., & Lii, C.-Y. (2006). Effects of cation properties on sol-gel transition and gel properties of κ-carrageenan. *Journal of Food Science*, 65, 1332–1337. https://doi.org/10.1111/j.1365-2621.2000.tb10607.x.
78. Ghavaminejad, A., Ashammakhi, N., Wu, X. Y., & Khademhosseini, A. (2020). Crosslinking strategies for 3D bioprinting of polymeric hydrogels. *Small*, 16(35), e2002931. https://doi.org/10.1002/smll.202002931.
79. Yang, X., Li, S., Ren, Y., Qiang, L., Liu, Y., Wang, J., & Dai, K. (2022). 3D printed hydrogel for articular cartilage regeneration. *Composites Part B: Engineering*, 237, 109863. https://doi.org/10.1016/j.compositesb.2022.109863.
80. Daly, A. C., Critchley, S. E., Rencsok, E. M., & Kelly, D. J. (2016). A comparison of different bioinks for 3D bioprinting of fibrocartilage and hyaline cartilage. *Biofabrication*, 8(4), 045002. https://doi.org/10.1088/1758-5090/8/4/045002.
81. Ma, H., Peng, Y., Zhang, S., Zhang, Y., & Min, P. (2022). Effects and progress of photo-crosslinking hydrogels in wound healing improvement. Gels, 8(10), 609. https://doi.org/10.3390/gels8100609.
82. Tan, G., Xu, J., Yu, Q., Zhang, J., Hu, X., Sun, C., & Zhang, H. (2022). Photo-crosslinkable hydrogels for 3D bioprinting in the repair of osteochondral defects: A review of present applications and future perspectives. *Micromachines*, 13(7), 1038. https://doi.org/10.3390/mi13071038.
83. Diamantides, N., Wang, L., Pruiksma, T., Siemiatkoski, J., Dugopolski, C., Shortkroff, S., … & Bonassar, L. J. (2017). Correlating rheological properties and printability of collagen bioinks: The effects of riboflavin photocrosslinking and pH. *Biofabrication*, 9(3), 034102. https://doi.org/10.1088/1758-5090/aa780f.

84. Pepelanova, I., Kruppa, K., Scheper, T., & Lavrentieva, A. (2018). Gelatin-methacryloyl (GelMA) hydrogels with defined degree of functionalization as a versatile toolkit for 3D cell culture and extrusion bioprinting. *Bioengineering*, 5(3), 55. https://doi.org/10.3390/bioengineering5030055.
85. Xue, X., Hu, Y., Wang, S., Chen, X., Jiang, Y., & Su, J. (2022). Fabrication of physical and chemical crosslinked hydrogels for bone tissue engineering. *Bioactive Materials*, 12, 327–339. https://doi.org/10.1016/j.bioactmat.2021.10.029.
86. Li, Y., Zhang, X., Zhang, X., Zhang, Y., & Hou, D. (2023). Recent progress of the vat photopolymerization technique in tissue engineering: A brief review of mechanisms, methods, materials, and applications. *Polymers*, 15, 3940. https://doi.org/10.3390/polym15193940.
87. Pitton, M., Urzì, C., Farè, S., & Negrini, N. C. (2024). Visible light photo-crosslinking of biomimetic gelatin-hyaluronic acid hydrogels for adipose tissue engineering. *Journal of the Mechanical Behavior of Biomedical Materials*, 158, 106675. https://doi.org/10.1016/j.jmbbm.2024.106675.
88. Rusu, A. G., Niță, L. E., Simionescu, N., Ghilan, A., Chiriac, A. P., & Mititelu-Tărâu, L. (2023). Enzymatically-crosslinked gelatin hydrogels with nanostructured architecture and self-healing performance for potential use as wound dressings. *Polymers*, 15(4), 780. https://doi.org/10.3390/polym15040780.
89. Naranjo-Alcázar, R., Bendix, S., Groth, T., & Gallego Ferrer, G. (2023). Research progress in enzymatically cross-linked hydrogels as injectable systems for bioprinting and tissue engineering. *Gels*, 9(3), 230. https://doi.org/10.3390/gels9030230.
90. Moreira Teixeira, L. S., Bijl, S., Pully, V. V., Otto, C., Jin, R., Feijen, J., … & Karperien, M. (2012). Self-attaching and cell-attracting in situ forming dextran-tyramine conjugate hydrogels for arthroscopic cartilage repair. *Biomaterials*, 33(11), 3164–3174. https://doi.org/10.1016/j.biomaterials.2012.01.001.
91. Choi, H., Young Ryu, I., Choi, I., Ullah, S., Jin Jung, H., Park, Y., … & Ryong Moon, H. (2022). Identification of (Z)-2-benzylidene-dihydroimidazothiazolone derivatives as tyrosinase inhibitors: Anti-melanogenic effects and in silico studies. *Computational and Structural Biotechnology Journal*, 20, 899–912. https://doi.org/10.1016/j.csbj.2022.02.007.
92. Adamiak, K., & Sionkowska, A. (2023). State of innovation in alginate-based materials. *Marine Drugs*, 21(6), 353. https://doi.org/10.3390/md21060353.
93. Fernando, I. P. S., Lee, W., Han, E. J., & Ahn, G. (2020). Alginate-based nanomaterials: Fabrication techniques, properties, and applications. *Chemical Engineering Journal*, 391, 123823. https://doi.org/10.1016/j.cej.2019.123823.
94. Abka-khajouei, R., Tounsi, L., Shahabi, N., Patel, A. K., Abdelkafi, S., & Michaud, P. (2022). Structures, properties and applications of alginates. *Marine Drugs*, 20(6), 364. https://doi.org/10.3390/md20060364.
95. Axpe, E., & Oyen, M. L. (2016). Applications of alginate-based bioinks in 3D bioprinting. *International Journal of Molecular Sciences*, 17(12), 1976. https://doi.org/10.3390/ijms17121976.
96. Panwar, A., & Tan, L. P. (2016). Current status of bioinks for micro-extrusion-based 3D bioprinting. *Molecules*, 21(6), 685. https://doi.org/10.3390/molecules21060685.
97. Hurtado, A., Aljabali, A. A. A., Mishra, V., Tambuwala, M. M., & Serrano-Aroca, Á. (2022). Alginate: Enhancement strategies for advanced applications. *International Journal of Molecular Sciences*, 23(9), 4486. https://doi.org/10.3390/ijms23094486.
98. Frígols, B., Martí, M., Salesa, B., Hernández-Oliver, C., Aarstad, O., Ulset, A.-S.T., … & Serrano-Aroca, A. (2019). Graphene oxide in zinc alginate films: Antibacterial activity, cytotoxicity, zinc release, water sorption/diffusion, wettability and opacity. *PLoS One*, 14, e0212819. https://doi.org/10.1371/journal.pone.0212819.

99. Hennink, W. E., & van Nostrum, C. F. (2012). Novel crosslinking methods to design hydrogels. *Advanced Drug Delivery Reviews*, 64, 223–236. https://doi.org/10.1016/j.addr.2012.09.009.
100. Rosiak, P., Latanska, I., Paul, P., Sujka, W., & Kolesinska, B. (2021). Modification of alginates to modulate their physic-chemical properties and obtain biomaterials with different functional properties. *Molecules*, 26(23), 7264. https://doi.org/10.3390/molecules26237264.
101. Amini-Mosleh-Abadi, S., Yazdanpanah, Z., Ketabat, F., Saadatifar, M., Mohammadi, M., Salimi, N., … & Sadeghianmaryan, A. (2025). In vitro characterization of 3D printed polycaprolactone/graphene oxide scaffolds impregnated with alginate and gelatin hydrogels for bone tissue engineering. *Journal of Biomaterials Applications*, 40(3), 374–388. https://doi.org/10.1177/08853282251336552.
102. Sundaram, M., Karthikeyan, B., Saravanakumar, I., Jayaraman, G., & Muthuvijayan, V. (2025). Recombinant hyaluronic acid-incorporated self-healing injectable hydrogel for cartilage tissue engineering: A case study on effects of molecular weight. *Journal of Materials Chemistry B*, 13, 9589–9606. https://doi.org/10.1039/D5TB00248F.
103. Jin, Y., Zhang, J., Chen, X., Li, F., Xue, T., Yi, K., … & Tao, Y. (2025). 3D printing incorporating gold nanozymes with mesenchymal stem cell-derived hepatic spheroids for acute liver failure treatment. *Biomaterials*, 315, 122895. https://doi.org/10.1016/j.biomaterials.2024.122895.
104. Wong, F. S. Y., Tsang, K. K., Chan, B. P., & Lo, A. C. Y. (2023). Both non-coated and polyelectrolytically-coated intraocular collagen-alginate composite gels enhanced photoreceptor survival in retinal degeneration. *Biomaterials*, 293, 121948. https://doi.org/10.1016/j.biomaterials.2022.121948.
105. Zhang, Y., Zhou, D., Chen, J., Zhang, X., Li, X., Zhao, W., & Xu, T. (2019). Biomaterials based on marine resources for 3D bioprinting applications. *Marine Drugs*, 17(10), 555. https://doi.org/10.3390/md17100555.
106. Jiang, W., Wang, J., Yuan, D., Gao, Z., Hu, B., Li, Y., & Wu, Y. (2023). Fabrication, characterization and emulsifying properties of agarose microgel. *International Journal of Biological Macromolecules*, 241, 124565. https://doi.org/10.1016/j.ijbiomac.2023.124565.
107. Wang, X., Yang, X., Liu, Z., Shen, Z., Li, M., Cheng, R., … & Sang, S. (2024). 3D bioprinting of an in vitro hepatoma microenvironment model: Establishment, evaluation, and anticancer drug testing. *Acta Biomaterialia*, 185, 173–189. https://doi.org/10.1016/j.actbio.2024.07.019.
108. Pokusaev, B., Vyazmin, A., Zakharov, N., Karlov, S., Nekrasov, D., Reznik, V., & Khramtsov, D. (2020). Thermokinetics and rheology of agarose gel applied to bioprinting technology. *Thermal Science*, 24(1 Part A), 347–353. https://doi.org/10.2298/TSCI191101453P.
109. Su, T., Zhang, M., Zeng, Q., Pan, W., Huang, Y., Qian, Y., … & Shen, J. (2021). Mussel-inspired agarose hydrogel scaffolds for skin tissue engineering. *Bioactive Materials*, 6(3), 579–588. https://doi.org/10.1016/j.bioactmat.2020.09.004.
110. Mandal, S., Nagi, G. K., Corcoran, A. A., Agrawal, R., Dubey, M., & Hunt, R. W. (2023). Algal polysaccharides for 3D printing: A review. *Carbohydrate Polymers*, 300, 120267. https://doi.org/10.1016/j.carbpol.2022.120267.
111. Punia, S. (2020). Barley starch modifications: Physical, chemical and enzymatic – A review. *International Journal of Biological Macromolecules*, 144, 578–585. https://doi.org/10.1016/j.ijbiomac.2019.12.088.

112. Krömmelbein, C., Mütze, M., Konieczny, R., Schönherr, N., Griebel, J., Gerdes, W., ... & Riedel, S. (2021). Impact of high-energy electron irradiation on mechanical, structural and chemical properties of agarose hydrogels. *Carbohydrate Polymers*, 263, 117970. https://doi.org/10.1016/j.carbpol.2021.117970.
113. Zhang, B., Lan, W., & Xie, J. (2022). Chemical modifications in the structure of marine polysaccharide as serviceable food processing and preservation assistant: A review. *International Journal of Biological Macromolecules*, 223(Pt A), 1539–1555. https://doi.org/10.1016/j.ijbiomac.2022.11.034.
114. Forget, A., & Shastri, V. P. (2024). Sulfated and phosphorylated agarose as biomaterials for a biomimetic paradigm for FGF-2 release. *Biomimetics*, 10(1), 12. https://doi.org/10.3390/biomimetics10010012.
115. Zhang, H., Shi, L. W. E., & Zhou, J. (2023). Recent developments of polysaccharide-based double-network hydrogels. *Journal of Polymer Science*, 61(1), 7–43. https://doi.org/10.1002/pol.20220510.
116. Choi, J. H., Kim, J. S., Kim, W. K., Lee, W., Kim, N., Song, C. U., ... & Khang, G. (2020). Evaluation of hyaluronic acid/agarose hydrogel for cartilage tissue engineering biomaterial. *Macromolecular Research*, 28(11), 979–985. https://doi.org/10.1007/s13233-020-8137-6.
117. Zhang, Y.H., Song, X.-N, Lin, Y., Xiao, Q., Du, X.-D., ... & Xiao, A.-F. (2019). Antioxidant capacity and prebiotic effects of Gracilaria neoagaro oligosaccharides prepared by agarase hydrolysis. *International Journal of Biological Macromolecules*, 137, 177–186. https://doi.org/10.1016/j.ijbiomac.2019.06.207.
118. Xu, H., Zhang, L., Zhang, H., Luo, J., & Gao, X. (2021). Green fabrication of chitin/chitosan composite hydrogels and their potential applications. *Macromolecular Bioscience*, 21(3), e2000389. https://doi.org/10.1002/mabi.202000389.
119. Shariatinia, Z. (2019). Pharmaceutical applications of chitosan. *Advances in Colloid and Interface Science*, 263, 131–194. https://doi.org/10.1016/j.cis.2018.11.008.
120. Novikov, V. Y., Derkach, S. R., Konovalova, I. N., Dolgopyatova, N. V., & Kuchina, Y. A. (2023). Mechanism of heterogeneous alkaline deacetylation of chitin: A review. *Polymers*, 15(7), 1729. https://doi.org/10.3390/polym15071729.
121. FDA. (2022). Substances generally recognized as safe. U.S. Food & Drug Administration. https://www.fda.gov/food/food-ingredients-packaging/generally-recognized-safe-gras.
122. Baharlouei, P., & Rahman, A. (2022). Chitin and chitosan: Prospective biomedical applications in drug delivery, cancer treatment, and wound healing. *Marine Drugs*, 20(7), 460. https://doi.org/10.3390/md20070460.
123. Dash, M., Chiellini, F., Ottenbrite, R. M., & Chiellini, E., 2011. Chitosan – A versatile semi-synthetic polymer in biomedical applications. *Progress in Polymer Science*, 36(8), 981–1014. https://doi.org/10.1016/j.progpolymsci.2010.11.001.
124. Chouhan, D., Dey, N., Bhardwaj, N., & Mandal, B. B. (2019). Emerging and innovative approaches for wound healing and skin regeneration: Current status and advances. *Biomaterials*, 216, 119267. https://doi.org/10.1016/j.biomaterials.2019.119267.
125. Muthu, M., Gopal, J., Chun, S., Devadoss, A. J. P., Hasan, N., & Sivanesan, I. (2021). Crustacean waste-derived chitosan: Antioxidant properties and future perspective. *Antioxidants*, 10(2), 228. https://doi.org/10.3390/antiox10020228
126. Islam, M. M., Shahruzzaman, M., Biswas, S., Sakib, M. N., & Rashid, T. U. (2020). Chitosan based bioactive materials in tissue engineering applications – A review. *Bioactive Materials*, 5(1), 164–183. https://doi.org/10.1016/j.bioactmat.2020.01.012.
127. Troy, E., Tilbury, M. A., Power, A. M., & Wall, J. G. (2021). Nature-based biomaterials and their application in biomedicine. *Polymers*, 13(19), 3321. https://doi.org/10.3390/polym13193321.

128. Zhao, L., Zhou, Y., Zhang, J., Liang, H., Chen, X., & Tan, H. (2023). Natural polymer-based hydrogels: From polymer to biomedical applications. *Pharmaceutics*, 15(10), 2514. https://doi.org/10.3390/pharmaceutics15102514.
129. Necas, J., Bartosikova, L., Brauner, P., & Kolar, J. (2008). Hyaluronic acid (hyaluronan): A review. *Veterinary Medicine*, 53, 397–411.
130. Shimojo, A. A. M. (2011). Modificações químicas do ácido hialurônico para a produção de géis reticulados e de fosfolipídios derivatizados. Tese de Doutorado. [sn].
131. Xu, X., Jha, A. K., Harrington, D. A., Farach-Carson, M. C., & Jia, X. (2012). Hyaluronic acid-based hydrogels: from a natural polysaccharide to complex networks. *Soft Matter*, 8(12), 3280–3294.
132. Fallacara, A., Baldini, E., Manfredini, S., & Vertuani, S. (2018). Hyaluronic acid in the third millennium. *Polymers*, 10(7), 701.
133. Kim, J., Chang, J.-Y., Kim, Y.-Y., Kim, M.-J., & Kho, H.-S. (2018). Effects of molecular weight of hyaluronic acid on its viscosity and enzymatic activities of lysozyme and peroxidase. *Archives of Oral Biology*, 89, 55–64.
134. Baier Leach, J., Bivens, K. A., Patrick Jr, C. W., & Schmidt, C. E. (2003). Photocrosslinked hyaluronic acid hydrogels: natural, biodegradable tissue engineering scaffolds. *Biotechnology and Bioengineering*, 82(5), 578–589.
135. Jin, R., Moreira Teixeira, L. S., Dijkstra, P. J., van Blitterswijk, C. A., Karperien, M., & Feijen, J. (2010). Enzymatically-crosslinked injectable hydrogels based on biomimetic dextran–hyaluronic acid conjugates for cartilage tissue engineering. *Biomaterials*, 31(11), 3103–3113.
136. Gholamali, I., Vu, T. T., Jo, S.-H., Park, S.-H., & Lim, K. T. (2024). Exploring the progress of hyaluronic acid hydrogels: synthesis, characteristics, and wide-ranging applications. *Materials*, 17(10), 2439.
137. Cumpstey, I. (2013). Chemical modification of polysaccharides. *ISRN Organic Chemistry*, 2013, Article ID 417672. https://doi.org/10.1155/2013/417672.
138. Naessens, M., Cerdobbel, A., Soetaert, W., & Vandamme, E. J. (2005). Leuconostoc dextransucrase and dextran: Production, properties and applications. *Journal of Chemical Technology & Biotechnology*, 80(8), 845–860. https://doi.org/10.1002/jctb.1278.
139. Liu, Z., Wei, Z., Zhu, X., Huang, G., Xu, F., Hai, J., ... & Chen, Y. (2015). Dextran-based hydrogel formed by thiol-Michael addition reaction for 3D cell encapsulation. *Colloids and Surfaces B: Biointerfaces*, 128C, 140–148. https://doi.org/10.1016/j.colsurfb.2015.02.005.
140. Sun, G., & Mao, J. J. (2012). Engineering dextran-based scaffolds for drug delivery and tissue repair. *Nanomedicine (London, England)*, 7(11), 1771–1784. https://doi.org/10.2217/nnm.12.149.
141. Masri, S., Maarof, M., Aziz, I. A., Idrus, R., & Fauzi, M. B. (2023). Performance of hybrid gelatin-PVA bioinks integrated with genipin through extrusion-based 3D bioprinting: An in vitro evaluation using human dermal fibroblasts. *International Journal of Bioprinting*, 9(3), 677. https://doi.org/10.18063/ijb.677.
142. Moon, R.J., Martini, A., Nairn, J., Simonsen, J., & Youngblood, J. (2011). Cellulose nanomaterials review: Structure, properties and nanocomposites. *Chemical Society Reviews*, 40(7), 3941–3994. https://doi.org/10.1039/C0CS00108B.
143. Lin, N., & Dufresne, A. (2014). Nanocellulose in biomedicine: Current status and future prospect. *European Polymer Journal*, 59, 302–325. https://doi.org/10.1016/j.eurpolymj.2014.07.025.
144. Bhattacharya, M., Malinen, M., Laurén, P., Lou, Y.-R., Kuisma, S., Kanninen, L., ... & Yliperttula, M. (2012). Nanofibrillar cellulose hydrogel promotes three-dimensional liver cell culture. *Journal of Controlled Release: Official Journal of the Controlled Release Society*, 164, 291–298. https://doi.org/10.1016/j.jconrel.2012.06.039.

145. Bhattacharya, M., Malinen, M.M., Lauren, P., Lou, Y.-R., Kuisma, S. W., Kanninen, L., …& Yliperttula, M. (2019). Nanofibrillar cellulose hydrogel promotes three-dimensional liver cell culture. *Journal of Controlled Release*, 295, 75–88. https://doi.org/10.1016/j.jconrel.2012.06.039..
146. Silva, L., Scheibel, J., & Soares, R. (2023). Starch-based nanocomposite hydrogels for biomedical applications. *Functional Nanocomposite Hydrogels*, 2023, 311–338. https://doi.org/10.1016/B978-0-323-99638-9.00013-7.
147. Pereira, R. F., Barrias, C. C., Bártolo, P. J., & Granja, P. L., 2018. Cell-instructive pectin hydrogels crosslinked via thiol-norbornene photo-click chemistry for skin tissue engineering. *Acta Biomaterialia*, 66, 282–293. https://doi.org/10.1016/j.actbio.2017.11.030.
148. Li, X., Wang, H., Li, D., Long, S., Zhang, G., Wu, Z. L. (2018). Dual ionically cross-linked double-network hydrogels with high strength, toughness, swelling resistance, and improved 3D printing processability. *ACS Applied Materials & Interfaces*, 10, 31198–31207. https://doi.org/10.1021/acsami.8b13038.
149. León-López, A., Morales-Peñaloza, A., Martínez-Juárez, V. M, Vargas-Torres, A., Zeugolis, D. I., & Aguirre-Álvarez, G. (2019). Hydrolyzed collagen – Sources and applications. *Molecules*, 24(22), 4031.
150. Ricard-Blum, S., 2011. The collagen family. *Cold Spring Harbor Perspectives in Biology*, 3(1), a004978. https://doi.org/10.1101/cshperspect.a004978.
151. Frantz, C., Stewart, K. M., & Weaver, V. M. (2010). The extracellular matrix at a glance. *Journal of Cell Science*, 123(24), 4195–4200. https://doi.org/10.1242/jcs.023820.
152. Mao, A. S., Shin, J. W., & Mooney, D. J. (2020). Effects of substrate stiffness and cell-cell contact on mesenchymal stem cell differentiation. *Biomaterials*, 232, 119734. https://doi.org/10.1016/j.biomaterials.2019.119734.
153. Osidak, E. O., Karalkin, P. A., Osidak, M. S., Parfenov, V. A., Sivogrivov, D. E., Pereira, F. D. A. S., & Domogatsky, S. P. (2019). Viscoll collagen solution as a novel bioink for direct 3D bioprinting. *Journal of Materials Science: Materials in Medicine*, 30, 1–12.
154. Beketov, E. E., Isaeva, E. V., Yakovleva, N. D., Demyashkin, G. A., Arguchinskaya, N. V., Kisel, A. A., … & Kaprdin, A. D. (2021). Bioprinting of cartilage with bioink based on high-concentration collagen and chondrocytes. *International Journal of Molecular Sciences*, 22(21), 11351.
155. Parenteau-Bareil, R., Gauvin, R., & Berthod, F. (2010). Collagen-based biomaterials for tissue engineering applications. *Materials*, 3(3), 1863–1887. https://doi.org/10.3390/ma3031863.
156. Lueyot, A., Rungsardthong, V., Vatanyoopaisarn, S., Hutangura, P., Wonganu, B., Wongsa-Ngasri, P., … & Thumthanaruk, B. (2021). Influence of collagen and some proteins on gel properties of jellyfish gelatin. *PLoS One*, 16(6), e0253254. https://doi.org/10.1371/journal.pone.0253254.
157. Al-Nimry, S., Dayah, A.A., Hasan, I., & Daghmash, R. (2021). Cosmetic, biomedical and pharmaceutical applications of fish gelatin/hydrolysates. *Marine Drugs*, 19(3), 145. https://doi.org/10.3390/md19030145.
158. AnilKumar, S., Allen, S.C., Tasnim, N., Akter, T., Park, S., Kumar, A., … & Joddar, B. (2019). The applicability of furfuryl-gelatin as a novel bioink for tissue engineering applications. *Journal of Biomedical Materials Research Part B: Applied Biomaterials*, 107(2), 314–323. https://doi.org/10.1002/jbm.b.34123.
159. Khrunyk, Y., Lach, S., Petrenko, I., & Ehrlich, H. (2020). Progress in modern marine biomaterials research. *Marine Drugs*, 18(12), 589. https://doi.org/10.3390/md18120589.
160. Derkach, S. R., Voron'ko, N. G., Yuliya, A., Kuchina, Y. A., & Kolotova, D. S. (2020). Modified fish gelatin as an alternative to mammalian gelatin in modern food technologies. *Polymers*, 12(12), 3051. https://doi.org/10.3390/polym12123051.

161. Chalard, A. E., Porritt, H., Lam Po Tang, E. J., Taberner, A. J., Winbo, A., Ahmad, A. M., … & Malmström, J. (2024). Dynamic composite hydrogels of gelatin methacryloyl (GelMA) with supramolecular fibers for tissue engineering applications. *Biomaterials Advances*, 163, 213957. https://doi.org/10.1016/j.bioadv.2024.213957.
162. Zhang, Y., Chen, H., & Li, J. (2022). Recent advances on gelatin methacrylate hydrogels with controlled microstructures for tissue engineering. *International Journal of Biological Macromolecules*, 221, 91–107. https://doi.org/10.1016/j.ijbiomac.2022.08.171.
163. Zhu, B., Wang, D., Pan, H., Gong, T., Ren, Q., Wang, Z., & Guo, Y. (2023). Three-in-one customized bioink for islet organoid: GelMA/ECM/PRP orchestrate pro-angiogenic and immunoregulatory function. *Colloids and Surfaces. B, Biointerfaces*, 221, 113017. https://doi.org/10.1016/j.colsurfb.2022.113017.
164. Kurian, A. G., Singh, R. K., Patel, K. D., Lee, J. H., & Kim, H. W. (2021). Multifunctional GelMA platforms with nanomaterials for advanced tissue therapeutics. *Bioactive Materials*, 8, 267–295. https://doi.org/10.1016/j.bioactmat.2021.06.027.
165. de Barros, N. R., Gomez, A., Ermis, M., Falcone, N., Haghniaz, R., Young, P., … & Li, B. (2023). Gelatin methacryloyl and laponite bioink for 3D bioprinted organotypic tumor modeling. *Biofabrication*, 15(4), 045005. https://doi.org/10.1088/1758-5090/ace0db.
166. Pramanik, S., Alhomrani, M., Alamri, A. S., Alsanie, W. F., Nainwal, P., Kimothi, V., … & Sargsyan, A. S. (2024). Unveiling the versatility of gelatin methacryloyl hydrogels: A comprehensive journey into biomedical applications. *Biomedical Materials*, 19(4), 042008. https://doi.org/10.1088/1748-605X/ad4df7.
167. Mendoza-Cerezo, L., Rodríguez-Rego, J. M., Macías-García, A., Callejas-Marín, A., Sánchez-Guardado, L., & Marcos-Romero, A. C. (2024). Three-dimensional bioprinting of GelMA hydrogels with culture medium: Balancing printability, rheology and cell viability for tissue regeneration. *Polymers*, 16(10), 1437. https://doi.org/10.3390/polym16101437.
168. Salisbury, E., Rawlings, T. M., Efstathiou, S., Tryfonos, M., Makwana, K., Fitzgerald, H. C., … & Eissa, A. M. (2024). Photo-cross-linked gelatin methacryloyl hydrogels enable the growth of primary human endometrial stromal cells and epithelial gland organoids. *ACS Applied Materials & Interfaces*, 16(30), 39140–39152. https://doi.org/10.1021/acsami.4c08763.
169. St Clair-Glover, M., Finol-Urdaneta, R. K., Maddock, M., Wallace, E., Miellet, S., Wallace, G., … & Dottori, M. (2024). Efficient fabrication of 3D bioprinted functional sensory neurons using an inducible Neurogenin-2 human pluripotent stem cell line. *Biofabrication*, 16(4), 045022. https://doi.org/10.1088/1758-5090/ad69c4.
170. Liang, Z., Han, Y., Chen, T., Wang, J., Lin, K., Yuan, L., … & Liang, Q. (2024). Application of 3D bioprinting technology apply to assessing Dangguiniantongtang (DGNT) decoctions in arthritis. *Chinese Medicine*, 19(1), 96. https://doi.org/10.1186/s13020-024-00948-4.
171. Xiang, Y., Zhao, Z., Yao, E. J., Balayan, A., Fiering, S. N., Steinmetz, N. F., & Chen, S. (2024). Multifaceted cancer alleviation by cowpea mosaic virus in a bioprinted ovarian cancer peritoneal spheroid model. *Biomaterials*, 311, 122663. https://doi.org/10.1016/j.biomaterials.2024.122663.
172. Rajabi, N., Rezaei, A., Kharaziha, M., Bakhsheshi-Rad, H. R., Luo, H., RamaKrishna, S., & Berto, F. (2021). Recent advances on bioprinted gelatin methacrylate-based hydrogels for tissue repair. *Tissue Engineering. Part A*, 27(11–12), 679–702. https://doi.org/10.1089/ten.TEA.2020.0350.
173. Zhu, Y., Yu, X., Liu, H., Li, J., Gholipourmalekabadi, M., Lin, K., … & Wang, P. (2024). Strategies of functionalized GelMA-based bioinks for bone regeneration: Recent advances and future perspectives. *Bioactive Materials*, 38, 346–373. https://doi.org/10.1016/j.bioactmat.2024.04.032.

174. Gu, Y., Zhang, L., Du, X., Fan, Z., Wang, L., Sun, W., … & Chen, C. (2018). Reversible physical crosslinking strategy with optimal temperature for 3D bioprinting of human chondrocyte-laden gelatin methacryloyl bioink. *Journal of Biomaterials Applications*, 33(5), 609–618. https://doi.org/10.1177/0885328218805864.
175. Das, S., Jegadeesan, J. T., & Basu, B. (2024). Gelatin methacryloyl (GelMA)-based biomaterial inks: Process science for 3D/4D printing and current status. *Biomacromolecules*, 25(4), 2156–2221. https://doi.org/10.1021/acs.biomac.3c01271.
176. Yue, K., Trujillo-de Santiago, G., Alvarez, M. M., Tamayol, A., Annabi, N., & Khademhosseini, A. (2015). Synthesis, properties, and biomedical applications of gelatin methacryloyl (GelMA) hydrogels. *Biomaterials*, 73, 254–271. https://doi.org/10.1016/j.biomaterials.2015.08.045.
177. Rastin, H., Ormsby, R. T., Atkins, G. J., & Losic, D. (2020). 3D bioprinting of methylcellulose/gelatin-methacryloyl (MC/GelMA) bioink with high shape integrity. *ACS Applied Bio Materials*, 3(3), 1815–1826. https://doi.org/10.1021/acsabm.0c00169.
178. Weisel, J. W., & Litvinov, R. I. (2017). Fibrin formation, structure and properties. *Subcellular Biochemistry*, 82, 405–456. https://doi.org/10.1007/978-3-319-49674-0_13.
179. Ahmed, T. A. E., Dare, E. V., & Hincke, M. (2020). Fibrin: A versatile scaffold for tissue engineering applications. *Tissue Engineering Part B: Reviews*, 24(4), 373–391. https://doi.org/10.1089/ten.teb.2017.0463.
180. Gsib, O., Egles, C., & Bencherif, S. (2017). Fibrin: An underrated biopolymer for skin tissue engineering. *Journal of Molecular Biology and Biotechnology*, 1, 1.
181. Jockenhoevel, S., Zund, G., Hoerstrup, S. P., Chalabi, K., Sachweh, J. S., Demircan, L., … & Turina, M. (2001). Fibrin gel – Advantages of a new scaffold in cardiovascular tissue engineering. *European Journal of Cardio-Thoracic Surgery*, 19(4), 424–430. https://doi.org/10.1016/s1010-7940(01)00624-8.
182. Poldervaart, M.T., Wang, H., van der Stok, J., Weinans, H. H., Leeuwenburgh, S. C. G., Öner, F. C., … & Alblas, J. (2013). Sustained release of BMP-2 in bioprinted alginate for osteogenicity in mice and rats. *PLoS One*, 8(8), e72610. https://doi.org/10.1371/journal.pone.0072610.
183. Xu, L., Wu, C., Yap, P. L., Losic, D., Zhu, J., Yang, Y., … & Wang, H. (2023). Recent advances of silk fibroin materials: From molecular modification and matrix enhancement to possible encapsulation-related functional food applications. *Food Chemistry*, 438, 137964. https://doi.org/10.1016/j.foodchem.2023.137964.
184. Wang, K., Ma, Q., Zhou, H., Zhao, J.-M., Cao, M., & Wang, S.-D. (2023). Review on fabrication and application of regenerated Bombyx mori silk fibroin materials. *AUTEX Research Journal*, 23(2), 164–183. https://doi.org/10.2478/aut-2021-0059.
185. De Giorgio, G., Matera, B., Vurro, D., Manfredi, E., Galstyan, V., Tx, G., … & D'Angelo, P. (2024). Silk fibroin materials: Biomedical applications and perspectives. *Bioengineering*, 11, 167. https://doi.org/10.3390/bioengineering11020167.
186. Minoura, N., Tsukada, M., & Nagura, M., 1995. Physico-chemical properties of silk fibroin and its application to biomaterials. *Journal of Biomaterials Science, Polymer Edition*, 6(3), 173–183. https://pubmed.ncbi.nlm.nih.gov/7695601/.
187. Lin, Y., Zhao, L., Jin, H., Gu, Q., Lei, L., Fang, C., & Pan, X. (2025). Multifunctional applications of silk fibroin in biomedical engineering: A comprehensive review on innovations and impact. *International Journal of Biological Macromolecules*, 309(Pt 4), 143067. https://doi.org/10.1016/j.ijbiomac.2025.143067.
188. Ma, L., Dong, W., Lai, E., & Wang, J. (2024). Silk fibroin-based scaffolds for tissue engineering. *Frontiers in Bioengineering and Biotechnology*, 12, 1381838. https://doi.org/10.3389/fbioe.2024.1381838.
189. Sakai, S., Yoshii, A., Sakurai, S., Horii, K., & Nagasuna, O. (2020). Silk fibroin nanofibers: A promising ink additive for extrusion three-dimensional bioprinting. *Materials Today Bio*, 8, 100078. https://doi.org/10.1016/j.mtbio.2020.100078.

190. Du, X., Wei, D., Huang, L., Zhu, M., Zhang, Y., & Zhu, Y. (2019). 3D printing of mesoporous bioactive glass/silk fibroin composite scaffolds for bone tissue engineering. *Materials Science & Engineering. C, Materials for Biological Applications*, 103, 109731. https://doi.org/10.1016/j.msec.2019.05.016.
191. Trucco, D., Sharma, A., Manferdini, C., Gabusi, E., Petretta, M., Desando, G., … & Lisignoli, G. (2021). Modeling and fabrication of silk fibroin-gelatin-based constructs using extrusion-based three-dimensional bioprinting. *ACS Biomaterials Science & Engineering*, 7(7), 3306–3320. https://doi.org/10.1021/acsbiomaterials.1c00410.
192. Dan, X., Chen, H., Li, S., Xue, P., Liu, B., Zhang, Z., … & Fan, X. (2025). Silk fibroin as a 3D printing bioink for tissue engineering applications. *Applied Materials Today*, 44, 102775. https://doi.org/10.1016/j.apmt.2025.102775.
193. Amirian, J., Wychowaniec, J. K., Amel Zendehdel, E., Sharma, G., Brangule, A., & Bandere, D. (2023). Versatile potential of photo-cross-linkable silk fibroin: Roadmap from chemical processing toward regenerative medicine and biofabrication applications. *Biomacromolecules*, 24(7), 2957–2981. https://doi.org/10.1021/acs.biomac.3c00098.
194. Mulas, C., Hodgson, A. C., Kohler, T. N., Agley, C. C., Humphreys, P., Kleine-Brüggeney, H., … & Chalut, K. J. (2020). Microfluidic platform for 3D cell culture with live imaging and clone retrieval. *Lab on a Chip*, 20(14), 2580–2591. https://doi.org/10.1039/d0lc00165a.
195. Zhang, T., Zhang, R., Zhang, Y., Kannan, P. R., Li, Y., Lv, Y., … & Kong, X. (2025). Silk-based biomaterials for tissue engineering. *Advances in Colloid and Interface Science*, 338, 103413. https://doi.org/10.1016/j.cis.2025.103413.
196. Patel, K., Lamarra, K., Sawadkar, P., Ludwig, A., & Perriman, A. (2025). Silk fibroin/GelMA-based hydrogels as a platform for tissue adhesives and tissue engineering. *ACS Biomaterials Science & Engineering*, 11, 3893–3931. https://doi.org/10.1021/acsbiomaterials.5c00286.
197. Pati, F., Jang, J., Ha, D.-H., Kim, S. W., Rhie, J.-W., Shim, J.-H., … & Cho, D.-W. (2014). Printing three-dimensional tissue analogues with decellularized extracellular matrix bioink. *Nature Communications*, 5, 3935. https://doi.org/10.1038/ncomms4935.
198. Kim, S., Min, S., Choi, Y. S., Jo, S.-H., Jung, J. H., Han, K., … & Cho, S.-W. (2020). Tissue extracellular matrix hydrogels as alternatives to Matrigel for culturing gastrointestinal organoids. *Nature Communications*, 13, 1692. https://doi.org/10.1038/s41467-022-29279-4.
199. Crapo, P. M., Gilbert, T. W., & Badylak, S. F. (2011). An overview of tissue and whole organ decellularization processes. *Biomaterials*, 32(12), 3233–3243. https://doi.org/10.1016/j.biomaterials.2011.01.057.
200. Dernowsek, J. (2024). Bioimpressão 3D. In N. Volpato (Org.), *Tecnologias e aplicações da manufatura aditiva* (pp. 507–529). São Paulo: Blucher.
201. Quantis Biotecnologia. (2022). Method for producing high-purity extracellular matrix proteins from human cells via 3D bioprinting (Patent WO2022073090A1). World Intellectual Property Organization. https://patentscope.wipo.int/search/en/detail.jsf?docId=WO2022073090&_cid=P12-L.
202. Asadi, N., Del Bakhshayesh, A. R., Davaran, S., & Akbarzadeh, A. (2020). Common biocompatible polymeric materials for tissue engineering and regenerative medicine. *Materials Chemistry and Physics*, 242, 122528.
203. Panchal, S. S., & Vasava, D. V. (2020). Biodegradable polymeric materials: Synthetic approach. *ACS Omega*, 5(9), 4370–4379. https://doi.org/10.1021/acsomega.9b04422.
204. Terzopoulou, Z., Zamboulis, A., Koumentakou, I., Michailidou, G., Noordam, M. J., & Bikiaris, D. N. (2022). Biocompatible synthetic polymers for tissue engineering purposes. *Biomacromolecules*, 23(5), 1841–1863.

205. Wei, X., Gong, C., Gou, M., Fu, S., Guo, Q., Shi, S., … & Qian, Z. (2009). Biodegradable poly (ε-caprolactone)–poly (ethylene glycol) copolymers as drug delivery system. *International Journal of Pharmaceutics*, 381(1), 1–18.
206. Christodoulou, E., Notopoulou, M., Nakiou, E., Kostoglou, M., Barmpalexis, P., & Bikiaris, D. N. (2022). Branched poly (ε-caprolactone)-based copolyesters of different architectures and their use in the preparation of anticancer drug-loaded nanoparticles. *International Journal of Molecular Sciences*, 23(23), 15393.
207. Labet, M., & Thielemans, W. (2009). Synthesis of polycaprolactone: A review. *Chemical Society Reviews*, 38(12), 3484–3504.
208. Wang, W., Caetano, G. F., Wei-Hung, C., Braz, A. L., Blaker, J. J., Frade, M. A. C., & Bartolo, P. J. D. S. (2016). Morphological, mechanical and biological assessment of PCL/pristine graphene scaffolds for bone regeneration. *International Journal of Bioprinting*, 2(2), 95–105.
209. Mirbagheri, M., Mohebbi-Kalhori, D., & Jirofti, N. (2017). Evaluation of mechanical properties and medical applications of polycaprolactone small diameter artificial blood vessels. *International Journal of Basic Science in Medicine*, 2(1), 58–70.
210. Rahimkhoei, V., Padervand, M., Hedayat, M., Seidi, F., Dawi, E. A., & Akbari, A. (2023). Biomedical applications of electrospun polycaprolactone-based carbohydrate polymers: A review. *International Journal of Biological Macromolecules*, 253, 126642.
211. Obisesan, O. S., Ajiboye, T. O., Mhlanga, S. D., & Mufhandu, H. T. (2023). Biomedical applications of biodegradable polycaprolactone-enhanced magnetic iron oxides nanoparticles and their polymer nanocomposites. *Colloids and Surfaces B: Biointerfaces*, 227, 113342.
212. Archer, E., Torretti, M., & Madbouly, S. (2023). Biodegradable polycaprolactone (PCL) based polymer and composites. *Physical Sciences Reviews*, 8(11), 4391–4414.
213. Azari, A., Golchin, A., Maymand, M. M., Mansouri, F., & Ardeshirylajimi, A. (2022). Electrospun polycaprolactone nanofibers: Current research and applications in biomedical application. *Advanced Pharmaceutical Bulletin*, 12(4), 658.
214. Backes, E. H., Harb, S. V., Beatrice, C. A. G., Shimomura, K. M. B., Passador, F. R., Costa, L. C., & Pessan, L. A. (2022). Polycaprolactone usage in additive manufacturing strategies for tissue engineering applications: A review. *Journal of Biomedical Materials Research Part B: Applied Biomaterials*, 110(6), 1479–1503.
215. Murugan, S., & Parcha, S. R. (2021). Fabrication techniques involved in developing the composite scaffolds PCL/HA nanoparticles for bone tissue engineering applications. *Journal of Materials Science: Materials in Medicine*, 32(8), 93.
216. Shahverdi, M., Seifi, S., Akbari, A., Mohammadi, K., Shamloo, A., & Movahhedy, M. R. (2022). Melt electrowriting of PLA, PCL, and composite PLA/PCL scaffolds for tissue engineering application. *Scientific Reports*, 12(1), 19935.
217. Homaeigohar, S., & Boccaccini, A. R. (2022). Nature-derived and synthetic additives to poly (ε-caprolactone) nanofibrous systems for biomedicine; an updated overview. *Frontiers in Chemistry*, 9, 809676.
218. Mokhena, T. C., Chabalala, M. B., Mapukata, S., Mtibe, A., Hlekelele, L., Cele, Z., … & Shingange, K. (2024). Electrospun PCL-based materials for health-care applications: An overview. *Macromolecular Materials and Engineering*, 309, 2300388.
219. Sadeghianmaryan, A., Ahmadian, N., Wheatley, S., Sardroud, H. A., Nasrollah, S. A. S., Naseri, E., & Ahmadi, A. (2024). Advancements in 3D-printable polysaccharides, proteins, and synthetic polymers for wound dressing and skin scaffolding – A review. *International Journal of Biological Macromolecules*, 266, 131207.
220. Chen, D., Zhu, T., Fu, W., & Zhang, H. (2019). Electrospun polycaprolactone/collagen nanofibers cross-linked with 1-ethyl-3-(3-dimethylaminopropyl) carbodiimide/N-hydroxysuccinimide and genipin facilitate endothelial cell regeneration and may be a promising candidate for vascular scaffolds. *International Journal of Nanomedicine*, 14, 2127–2144.

221. Sawadkar, P., Mohanakrishnan, J., Rajasekar, P., Rahmani, B., Kohli, N., Bozec, L., & Garcia-Gareta, E. (2020). A synergistic relationship between polycaprolactone and natural polymers enhances the physical properties and biological activity of scaffolds. *ACS Applied Materials & Interfaces*, 12(12), 13587–13597.
222. Mohandesnezhad, S., Pilehvar-Soltanahmadi, Y., Alizadeh, E., Goodarzi, A., Davaran, S., Khatamian, M., ... & Akbarzadeh, A. (2020). In vitro evaluation of zeolite-nHA blended PCL/PLA nanofibers for dental tissue engineering. *Materials Chemistry and Physics*, 252, 123152.
223. Yedekçi, B., Tezcaner, A., Yılmaz, B., Demir, T., & Evis, Z. (2022). 3D porous PCL-PEG-PCL/strontium, magnesium and boron multi-doped hydroxyapatite composite scaffolds for bone tissue engineering. *Journal of the Mechanical Behavior of Biomedical Materials*, 125, 104941.
224. Gharibshahian, M., Salehi, M., Beheshtizadeh, N., Kamalabadi-Farahani, M., Atashi, A., Nourbakhsh, M. S., & Alizadeh, M. (2023). Recent advances on 3D-printed PCL-based composite scaffolds for bone tissue engineering. *Frontiers in Bioengineering and Biotechnology*, 11, 1168504.
225. Harikrishnan, P., & Sivasamy, A. (2020). Preparation, characterization of electrospun polycaprolactone-nano zinc oxide composite scaffolds for osteogenic applications. *Nano-Structures & Nano-Objects*, 23, 100518.
226. Niknam, Z., Azarbayjani, A. F., Rafaei, S. M., Rasmi, Y., & Tayebi, L. (2024). Polycaprolactone/graphene oxide/magnesium oxide as a novel composite scaffold for bone tissue engineering: Preparation and physical/biological assessment. *Journal of Drug Delivery Science and Technology*, 95, 105531.
227. Alharbi, N., Brigham, A., & Guthold, M. (2023). The mechanical properties of blended fibrinogen: Polycaprolactone (PCL) nanofibers. *Nanomaterials*, 13(8), 1359.
228. Park, H. S., Lee, J. S., Kim, C. B., Lee, K. H., Hong, I. S., Jung, H., ... & Park, C. H. (2023). Fluidic integrated 3D bioprinting system to sustain cell viability towards larynx fabrication. *Bioengineering & Translational Medicine*, 8(2), e10423.
229. Hamid, O. A., Eltaher, H. M., Sottile, V., & Yang, J. (2021). 3D bioprinting of a stem cell-laden, multi-material tubular composite: An approach for spinal cord repair. *Materials Science and Engineering: C*, 120, 111707.
230. Mukherjee, P., Chung, J., Cheng, K., Gupta, R., Haag, H., Williams, Z., & Wallace, G. (2021). Invitro and invivo study of PCL-hydrogel scaffold to advance bioprinting translation in microtia reconstruction. *Journal of Craniofacial Surgery*, 32(5), 1931–1936.
231. Koch, F., Thaden, O., Conrad, S., Tröndle, K., Finkenzeller, G., Zengerle, R., ... & Koltay, P. (2022). Mechanical properties of polycaprolactone (PCL) scaffolds for hybrid 3D-bioprinting with alginate-gelatin hydrogel. *Journal of the Mechanical Behavior of Biomedical Materials*, 130, 105219.
232. Jia, L., Hua, Y., Zeng, J., Liu, W., Wang, D., Zhou, G., ... & Jiang, H. (2022). Bioprinting and regeneration of auricular cartilage using a bioactive bioink based on microporous photocrosslinkable acellular cartilage matrix. *Bioactive Materials*, 16, 66–81.
233. Pitacco, P., Sadowska, J. M., O'Brien, F. J., & Kelly, D. J. (2023). 3D bioprinting of cartilaginous templates for large bone defect healing. *Acta Biomaterialia*, 156, 61–74.
234. Fan, M., Qiang, L., Wang, Y., Liu, Y., Zhuang, H., Guo, R., ... & Zheng, P. (2023). 3D bioprinted hydrogel/polymer scaffold with factor delivery and mechanical support for growth plate injury repair. *Frontiers in Bioengineering and Biotechnology*, 11, 1210786.
235. Li, Y., He, R., Huang, Y., Zhang, T., Xiao, L., Xiao, Y., ... & Gao, J. (2025). A 3R (remove-remodel-repair)-integrated self-assembled Chlorella-gelatin-PEG hydrogel for diabetic wound healing. *Materials Today Bio*, 33, 101935. https://dx.doi.org/10.1016/j.mtbio.2025.101935.

236. Zhu, J. (2010). Bioactive modification of poly(ethylene glycol) hydrogels for tissue engineering. *Biomaterials*, 31(17), 4639–4656. https://doi.org/10.1016/j.biomaterials.2010.02.044.
237. He, C., Wang, Y., Fang, X., Jiang, W., Liu, S., Yi, X., … & Zhang, X. (2025). Charge microenvironment and bioactivity of in situ-formed PEG-RGD dual hydrogel dressings promote wound healing. *Journal of Materials Chemistry B*, 13. https://doi.org/10.1039/D5TB00683J.
238. Makharadze, D., del Valle, L. J., Katsarava, R., & Puiggalí, J. (2025). The art of PEGylation: From simple polymer to sophisticated drug delivery system. *International Journal of Molecular Sciences*, 26(7), 3102. https://doi.org/10.3390/ijms26073102.
239. Tessmar, J. K., & Göpferich, A. M. (2007). Customized PEG-derived copolymers for tissue-engineering applications. *Macromolecular Bioscience*, 7(1), 23–39. https://doi.org/10.1002/mabi.200600096.
240. Veronese, F. M., & Pasut, G. (2005). PEGylation, successful approach to drug delivery. *Drug Discovery Today*, 10(21), 1451–1458. https://doi.org/10.1016/S1359-6446(05)03575-0.
241. Eddine, M. A., Carvalho, A., Schmutz, M., Salez, T., de Chateauneuf-Randon, S., Bresson, B., … & Monteux, C. (2023). Sieving and clogging in PEG-PEGDA hydrogel membranes. *Langmuir: The ACS Journal of Surfaces and Colloids*, 39(42), 15085–15094. https://doi.org/10.1021/acs.langmuir.3c02153.
242. Roquart, M., Kharlamova, A., Marcos Celada, L., Norvez, S., Nicolaÿ, R., & Corté, L. (2023). PEG-based photo-cross-linked networks with adjustable topologies and mechanical properties. *Biomacromolecules*, 24(10), 4454–4464. https://doi.org/10.1021/acs.biomac.2c01265.
243. Fourniols, T., Randolph, L. D., Staub, A., Vanvarenberg, K., Leprince, J. G., Préat, V., … & Danhier, F. (2015). Temozolomide-loaded photopolymerizable PEG-DMA-based hydrogel for the treatment of glioblastoma. *Journal of Controlled Release: Official Journal of the Controlled Release Society*, 210, 95–104. https://doi.org/10.1016/j.jconrel.2015.05.272.
244. Jang, L. K., Ahlquist, J. T., Ye, C., Trujillo, J., Triplett, M., Moya, M. L., … & Wasson, E. M. (2024). Rapid curing dynamics of PEG-thiol-ene resins allow facile 3D bioprinting and in-air cell-laden microgel fabrication. *Biomedical Materials*, 20(1), 015009. https://doi.org/10.1088/1748-605X/ad8540.
245. Piluso, S., Skvortsov, G. A., Altunbek, M., Afghah, F., Khani, N., Koç, B., & Patterson, J. (2021). 3D bioprinting of molecularly engineered PEG-based hydrogels utilizing gelatin fragments. *Biofabrication*, 13(4), 045008. https://doi.org/10.1088/1758-5090/ac0ff0.
246. Ziani, K., Saenz-Del-Burgo, L., Pedraz, J. L., & Ciriza, J. (2025). Advances in cryopreservation strategies for 3D biofabricated constructs: From hydrogels to bioprinted tissues. *International Journal of Molecular Sciences*, 26(14), 6908. https://doi.org/10.3390/ijms26146908.
247. Kim, M. H., & Lin, C. C. (2023). Poly(ethylene glycol)-norbornene as a photoclick bioink for digital light processing 3D bioprinting. *ACS Applied Materials & Interfaces*, 15(2), 2737–2746. https://doi.org/10.1021/acsami.2c20098.
248. Zhang, I. W., Choi, L. S., Friend, N. E., McCoy, A. J., Midekssa, F. S., Hu, M. M., … & Putnam, A. J. (2025). Clickable PEG-norbornene microgels support suspension bioprinting and microvascular assembly. *Acta Biomaterialia*, 201, 283–296. https://doi.org/10.1016/j.actbio.2025.06.006.
249. Hammer, T., Yang, K., Spirig, T., Meier-Schiesser, B., Rottmar, M., Maniura, K., … & Wei, K. (2025). Mechanically robust non-swelling cold water fish gelatin hydrogels for 3D bioprinting. *Materials Today Bio*, 32, 101701. https://doi.org/10.1016/j.mtbio.2025.101701.

250. Moon, Y.-W., Dobroski, T., Willson, K., Jeong, J.-O., Bishop, C., Atala, A., … & Lee, S. J. (2025). 3D bioprinted thick hepatic constructs with vascular network as a physiologically relevant in vitro organ model. *Materials Today Bio*, 32, 101786. https://doi.org/10.1016/j.mtbio.2025.101786.
251. Magli, S., Rossi, G. B., Risi, G., Bertini, S., Cosentino, C., Crippa, L., … & Russo, L. (2020). Design and synthesis of chitosan-gelatin hybrid hydrogels for 3D printable in vitro models. *Frontiers in Chemistry*, 8, 524. https://doi.org/10.3389/fchem.2020.00524.
252. Kast, V. J., Hauser, S., Nadernezhad, A., Pette, D., Maitz, M. F., Petzold, A., … & Loessner, D. (2026). A biomaterial-based platform of pancreatic cancer reveals kallikrein-related peptidase 6 (KLK6) as a mediator of neutrophil recruitment and immunosuppression. *Biomaterials*, 324, 123456. https://doi.org/10.1016/j.biomaterials.2025.123456.
253. Hou, C., Lei, Y., Li, N., Wei, M., Wang, S., Rahman, S. U., … & Wu, W. (2023). Collagen from Iris squid grafted with polyethylene glycol and collagen peptides promote the proliferation of fibroblast through PI3K/AKT and Ras/RAF/MAPK signaling pathways. *International Journal of Biological Macromolecules*, 247, 125772. https://doi.org/10.1016/j.ijbiomac.2023.125772.
254. Simaan-Yameen, H., Bar-Am, O., Saar, G., & Seliktar, D. (2023). Methacrylated fibrinogen hydrogels for 3D cell culture and delivery. *Acta Biomaterialia*, 164, 94–110. https://doi.org/10.1016/j.actbio.2023.03.046.
255. Ravi, S., Chokkakula, L. P. P., Giri, P. S., Korra, G., Dey, S. R., & Rath, S. N. (2023). 3D bioprintable hypoxia-mimicking PEG-based nano bioink for cartilage tissue engineering. *ACS Applied Materials & Interfaces*, 15(16), 19921–19936. https://doi.org/10.1021/acsami.3c00389.
256. Wang, J., Zhang, F., Tsang, W. P., Wan, C., & Wu, C. (2017). Fabrication of injectable high strength hydrogel based on 4-arm star PEG for cartilage tissue engineering. *Biomaterials*, 120, 11–21. https://doi.org/10.1016/j.biomaterials.2016.12.015.
257. Zhan, Y., Zhao, X., He, C., Bi, S., Liu, R., Gu, J., & Yan, B. (2025). Temperature-responsive and self-healing hydrogel: A novel approach to combat postoperative adhesions. *Polymers*, 17(14), 1925. https://doi.org/10.3390/polym17141925.
258. Hemati, H., Haghiralsadat, F., Hemati, M., Sargazi, G., & Razi, N. (2023). Design and evaluation of liposomal sulforaphane-loaded polyvinyl alcohol/polyethylene glycol (PVA/PEG) hydrogels as a novel drug delivery system for wound healing. *Gels*, 9, 748. https://doi.org/10.3390/gels9090748.
259. Li, J., Feng, X., Liu, B., Yu, Y., Sun, L., Liu, T., … & Chen, X. (2017). Polymer materials for prevention of postoperative adhesion. *Acta Biomaterials*, 61, 21–40. https://doi.org/10.1016/j.actbio.2017.08.002.
260. Bock, N., Forouz, F., Hipwood, L., Clegg, J., Jeffery, P., Gough, M., … & Meinert, C. (2023). GelMA, click-chemistry gelatin and bioprinted polyethylene glycol-based hydrogels as 3D ex vivo drug testing platforms for patient-derived breast cancer organoids. *Pharmaceutics*, 15(1), 261. https://doi.org/10.3390/pharmaceutics15010261.
261. Fong, E. L., Martinez, M., Yang, J., Mikos, A. G., Navone, N. M., Harrington, D. A., & Farach-Carson, M. C. (2014). Hydrogel-based 3D model of patient-derived prostate xenograft tumors suitable for drug screening. *Molecular Pharmaceutics*, 11(7), 2040–2050. https://doi.org/10.1021/mp500085p.
262. Lee, J. Y., & Chaudhuri, O. (2018). Regulation of breast cancer progression by extracellular matrix mechanics: Insights from 3D culture models. *ACS Biomaterials Science & Engineering*, 4(2), 302–313. https://doi.org/10.1021/acsbiomaterials.7b00071.
263. Li, S., Yang, C., Li, J., Zhang, C., Zhu, L., Song, Y., … & Su, H. (2023). Progress in Pluronic F127 derivatives for application in wound healing and repair. *International Journal of Nanomedicine*, 18, 4485–4505. https://doi.org/10.2147/IJN.S418534.

264. Naharros-Molinero, A., Caballo-González, M. Á., de la Mata, F. J., & García-Gallego, S. (2022). Direct and reverse Pluronic micelles: Design and characterization of promising drug delivery nanosystems. *Pharmaceutics*, 14(12), 2628. https://doi.org/10.3390/pharmaceutics14122628.
265. Jarak, I., Varela, C. L., Tavares da Silva, E., Roleira, F. F. M., Veiga, F., & Figueiras, A. (2020). Pluronic-based nanovehicles: Recent advances in anticancer therapeutic applications. *European Journal of Medicinal Chemistry*, 206, 112526. https://doi.org/10.1016/j.ejmech.2020.112526.
266. Sharun, K., Banu, S. A., Mamachan, M., Emmanuel, R. S., Kumar, R., Vinodhkumar, O. R., … & Pal, A. (2024). Thermoresponsive and injectable Pluronic F127 hydrogel for loading adipose-derived mesenchymal stem cells. *Discoveries in Medicine*, 36(181), 294–307. https://doi.org/10.24976/Discov.Med.202436181.28.
267. Shriky, B., Kelly, A., Isreb, M., Babenko, M., Mahmoudi, N., Rogers, S., … & Gough, T. (2020). Pluronic F127 thermosensitive injectable smart hydrogels for controlled drug delivery system development. *Journal of Colloid and Interface Science*, 565, 119–130. https://doi.org/10.1016/j.jcis.2019.12.096.
268. de Castro, K. C., Coco, J. C., dos Santos, E. M., Ataide, J. A., Martinez, R. M., Monteiro do Nascimento, M. H., … & Lopes, A. M. (2023). Pluronic® triblock copolymer-based nanoformulations for cancer therapy: A 10-year overview. *Journal of Controlled Release*, 353, 802–822. https://doi.org/10.1016/j.jconrel.2022.12.017.
269. Camana, G., Tavano, M., Li, M., Castiglione, F., Rossi, F., & Cellesi, F. (2023). Design of functional Pluronic-based precursors for tailoring hydrogel thermoresponsiveness and cell-adhesive properties. *Materials*, 16(7), 2749. https://doi.org/10.3390/ma16072749.
270. Khaliq, N. U., Lee, J., Kim, S., Sung, D., & Kim, H. (2023). Pluronic F-68 and F-127 based nanomedicines for advancing combination cancer therapy. *Pharmaceutics*, 15(8), 2102. https://doi.org/10.3390/pharmaceutics15082102.
271. Chen, S.-Y., Chao, Y.-C., Yang, T.-S., Ou, K.-L., Lan, W.-C., Huang, B.-H., … & Ruslin, M. (2021). A tailored biomimetic hydrogel as potential bioink to print a cell scaffold for tissue engineering applications: Printability and cell viability evaluation. *Applied Sciences*, 11(2), 829. https://doi.org/10.3390/app11020829.
272. Fang, Y., Guo, Y., Wu, B., Liu, Z., Ye, M., Xu, Y., … & Xiong, Z. (2023). Expanding embedded 3D bioprinting capability for engineering complex organs with freeform vascular networks. *Advanced Materials*, 35(22), e2205082. https://doi.org/10.1002/adma.202205082.
273. Bollenbach, L., Buske, J., Mäder, K., & Garidel, P. (2022). Poloxamer 188 as surfactant in biological formulations – An alternative for polysorbate 20/80? *International Journal of Pharmaceutics*, 620, 121706. https://doi.org/10.1016/j.ijpharm.2022.121706.
274. Zhang, T., Cheng, X., Xiu, J., Liu, M., Liu, S., Zhang, B., … & Zhao, X. (2023). pH-responsive injectable multifunctional Pluronic F127/gelatin-based hydrogels with hydrogen production for treating diabetic wounds. *ACS Applied Materials & Interfaces*, 15(48), 55392–55408. https://doi.org/10.1021/acsami.3c12672.
275. Lim, L.-T., Auras, R., & Rubino, M. (2008). Processing technologies for poly (lactic acid). *Progress in Polymer Science*, 33(8), 820–852. https://doi.org/10.1016/j.progpolymsci.2008.03.003.
276. Singhvi, M. S., Zinjarde, S. S., & Gokhale, D. V. (2019). Polylactic acid: Synthesis and biomedical applications. *Journal of Applied Microbiology*, 127(6), 1612–1626. https://doi.org/10.1111/jam.14398.
277. Galocha-León, C., Monzón, M. E., Ramírez-Tórrez, M. F., Moreno-Vega, L., Amezcua, M., Treviño-De la Rosa, B., & Ortega-Lara, W. (2024). Design and characterization of biomimetic hybrid construct based on hyaluronic acid and alginate bioink for regeneration of articular cartilage. *Pharmaceutics*, 16(11), 1422. https://doi.org/10.3390/pharmaceutics16111422.

278. Singhvi, M., & Gokhale, D. (2013). Biomass to biodegradable polymer (PLA). *RSC Advances*, 3(33), 13558–13568. https://doi.org/10.1039/C3RA44468A.
279. Lu, J., Gao, Y., Cao, C., Wang, H., Ruan, Y., Qin, K., ... & Chang, F. (2025). 3D bioprinted scaffolds for osteochondral regeneration: advancements and applications. *Materials Today Bio*, 32, 101834. https://doi.org/10.1016/j.mtbio.2025.101834.
280. Loukelis, K., Kontogianni, G. I., Vlassopoulos, D., & Chatzinikolaidou, M. (2025). Extrusion-based 3D bioprinted gellan gum/poly(vinyl alcohol)/nano-hydroxyapatite composite bioinks promote bone regeneration. *Advanced Healthcare Materials*, 14(19), e2500365. https://doi.org/10.1002/adhm.202500365.
281. Gharacheh, H., & Guvendiren, M. (2022). Cell-laden composite hydrogel bioinks with human bone allograft particles to enhance stem cell osteogenesis. *Polymers*, 14(18), 3788. https://doi.org/10.3390/polym14183788.
282. Kansız, S., Vurat, M. T., Parmaksiz, M., Elçin, A. E., & Elçin, Y. M. (2025). Methacrylated-κ-carrageenan/hydroxyapatite composite bioinks for extrusion-based bioprinting: Physicochemical, rheological, mechanical, and in vitro biological investigations. *International Journal of Biological Macromolecules*, 316(Pt 1), 144745. https://doi.org/10.1016/j.ijbiomac.2025.144745.
283. Tsui, J. H., Leonard, A., Camp, N. D., Long, J. T., Nawas, Z. Y., Chavanachat, R., ... & Kim, D. H. (2021). Tunable electroconductive decellularized extracellular matrix hydrogels for engineering human cardiac microphysiological systems. *Biomaterials*, 272, 120764. https://doi.org/10.1016/j.biomaterials.2021.120764.
284. Spencer, A. R., Shirzaei Sani, E., Soucy, J. R., Corbet, C. C., Primbetova, A., Koppes, R. A., & Annabi, N. (2019). Bioprinting of a cell-laden conductive hydrogel composite. *ACS Applied Materials & Interfaces*, 11(34), 30518–30533. https://doi.org/10.1021/acsami.9b07353.
285. Jackman, C. P., Ganapathi, A. M., Asfour, H., Qian, Y., Allen, B. W., Li, Y., & Bursac, N. (2018). Engineered cardiac tissue patch maintains structural and electrical properties after epicardial implantation. *Biomaterials*, 159, 48–58. https://doi.org/10.1016/j.biomaterials.2018.01.002.
286. Huethorst, E., Bishop, M. J., Burton, F. L., Denning, C., Gadegaard, N., Myles, R. C., & Smith, G. L. (2025). Evidence for intermittent coupling of intramyocardial small, engineered heart tissues acutely implanted into rabbit myocardium. *Cardiovascular Research*, cvaf034. https://doi.org/10.1093/cvr/cvaf034.
287. Roshanbinfar, K., Vogt, L., Greber, B., Diecke, S., Boccaccini, A., Scheibel, T., & Engel, F. (2018). Electroconductive biohybrid hydrogel for enhanced maturation and beating properties of engineered cardiac tissues. *Advanced Functional Materials*, 28. https://doi.org/10.1002/adfm.201803951.
288. Lai, J., Chen, X., Lu, H. H., & Wang, M. (2024). 3D bioprinting of graphene oxide-incorporated hydrogels for neural tissue regeneration. *3D Printing and Additive Manufacturing*, 11(6), e2022–e2032. https://doi.org/10.1089/3dp.2023.0150.
289. Malamatari, M., Wan, K.-W., & Baxevanis, F. (2024). Regulatory aspects of 3D-printed medicinal products. In D. A. Lamprou, D. Douroumis, & S. Qi (eds) *3D Printing of Pharmaceutical and Drug Delivery Devices: Progress from Bench to Bedside* (pp. 211–225). Hoboken, NJ: John Wiley & Sons, Inc. https://doi.org/10.1002/9781119836001.ch11.
290. Raei, F., Abdi, A., & Mashayekhan, S. (2025). 4D bioprinting: Materials, mechanisms, and mathematical modeling for next-generation tissue engineering. *Bioprinting*, 50, e00428. https://doi.org/10.1016/j.bprint.2025.e00428.

3 From Digital Models to Living Tissues
CAD Design in 3D Bioprinting

Gabriela Mendes da Rocha Vaz
and Luciano Paulino Silva

3.1 INTRODUCTION TO 3D BIOPRINTING AND CAD

3.1.1 Overview of 3D Bioprinting Technology

Three-dimensional (3D) bioprinting emerged as an extension of traditional 3D printing, adapting additive manufacturing principles for biological applications. Where traditional 3D printing constructs objects typically from inert materials like plastics or metals (Hull, 1984), bioprinting instead uses bioinks—complex blends of living cells, biomaterials, and growth factors (Murphy & Atala, 2014). This fundamental shift required a reimagining of digital design to incorporate biological constraints, such as cell viability, tissue microstructure, and dynamic maturation process that occurs after bioprinting. The result is a transformative synergy between engineering and biology, where digital blueprints must anticipate how living structures will grow and function beyond the print bed.

The foundations of this relatively new paradigm trace back to 2002, when Landers and colleagues pioneered a rapid prototyping technology specifically tailored for tissue engineering. Their work enabled the 3D dispensing of liquids and pastes while maintaining cell viability—a critical breakthrough that addressed both structural porosity and the translation of volumetric models into printing paths (Landers et al., 2002). This marked the inception of 3D bioprinting, demonstrating for the first time that hydrogels could serve as viable materials in additive manufacturing, with computer-aided design (CAD) models guiding free-form fabrication of biologically relevant structures.

The standard 3D bioprinting workflow begins with biomaterial selection. Here, bioinks—often hydrogel-based formulations—are chosen for their ability to mimic the native extracellular matrix while supporting embedded cells. The next and perhaps most critical stage is digital model creation, where computational designs are translated into biologically viable templates for fabrication. Medical imaging data, such as magnetic resonance imaging (MRI) or computed tomography (CT) scans, can be reconstructed into patient-specific 3D models, while *in silico* designs might

DOI: 10.1201/9781032638164-3

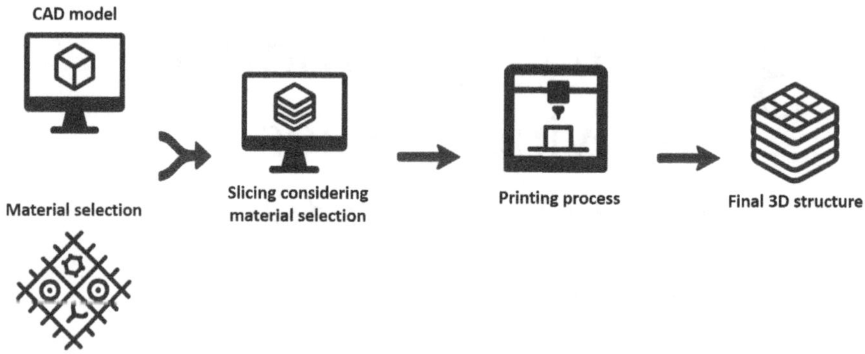

FIGURE 3.1 Workflow of the 3D bioprinting process. The procedure begins with (1) the digital design of a 3D model using CAD software. Concurrently, (2) bioink development is undertaken to ensure the material's biocompatibility and mechanical functionality. The digital model is then (3) processed and sliced into individual layers suitable to generate a printing path. The sliced model is subsequently (4) printed layer-by-layer using a bioprinter. The final step (5) yields a fabricated, functional bioprinted construct. This entire workflow illustrates the critical synergy between digital design and biological fabrication.

engineer intricate vascular networks or porous scaffolds optimized for cell migration; models can also be developed entirely *ab initio*. At this point, CAD software faces a unique challenge: balancing geometric precision with biological realism. Unlike traditional 3D printing, where a model's success is judged by its static form, a bioprinted design must also predict cellular behavior—how cells will proliferate, communicate, and remodel their environment over time. Once the digital blueprint and biocompatible material are prepared, the bioprinting process proceeds through layer-by-layer deposition, resulting in a preliminary construct (Figure 3.1). This bioprinted structure subsequently undergoes a maturation phase—often involving biochemical, mechanical, or cellular conditioning—to achieve the functional and structural properties required for its final biomedical application (Mironov et al., 2003; Murphy & Atala, 2014).

3.1.2 The Evolution and Expansion of CAD Technology

CAD originated within traditional manufacturing as a powerful tool for virtually modeling products prior to their physical fabrication (Figure 3.2). It is formally defined as the integrated use of computer systems to assist in the creation, modification, analysis, or optimization of a design (Groover & Zimmers, 1983; Elanchezhian & Sundar, 2007). This digital representation enabled not only the precise visualization of the intended object (Barr & Juricic, 1994) but also streamlined design optimization through iterative adjustments. Furthermore, CAD environments facilitated simulations that could predict structural behavior, mechanical performance, or material response under various virtual conditions, expressively reducing the reliance on physical prototyping (Schulz et al., 2017). When integrated with computer-aided manufacturing (CAM), CAD models transformed production workflows by directly

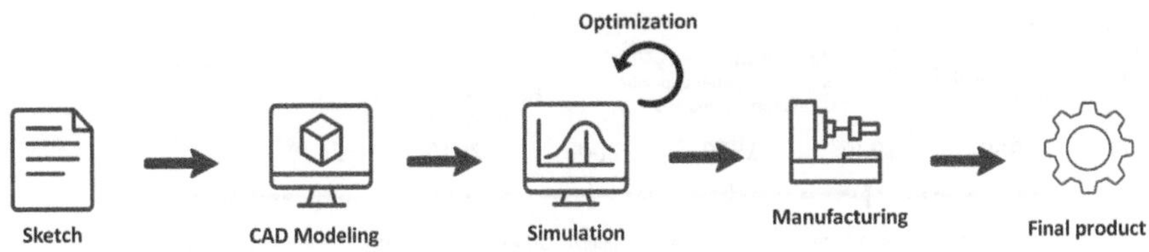

FIGURE 3.2 Schematic workflow of CAD-based design optimization, from initial sketch to final product, integrating 3D modeling and virtual simulation.

informing fabrication parameters, effectively bridging the gap between design intent and automated manufacturing execution (Groover & Zimmers, 1983; Elanchezhian & Sundar, 2007). This synergy between design and production laid the essential groundwork for advanced applications like bioprinting, where digital precision and adaptability are paramount.

CAD evolved from a niche drafting tool into a foundational technology driving innovation across a wide range of industries (Weisberg, 2008). Originally developed in the 1960s as a digital replacement for manual technical drawings, early CAD systems were limited to two-dimensional schematics and were primarily employed in aerospace and automotive engineering. The introduction of 3D modeling capabilities in the 1980s marked a transformative moment, enabling engineers to create and manipulate volumetric representations with unprecedented precision (Groover & Zimmers, 1983). This transition from flat blueprints to dynamic 3D environments revolutionized the product development cycle, allowing for virtual prototyping, interference detection, and finite element analysis long before the initiation of physical manufacturing. As computational power advanced and software became more sophisticated, CAD expanded beyond its mechanical engineering origins to become a universal platform for design, with domain-specific adaptations enhancing its utility across disciplines.

The expansion of CAD into diverse fields has been propelled by its ability to solve complex spatial and structural problems while integrating with complementary technologies. In architecture and construction, building information modeling represents the maturation of CAD into four-dimensional planning systems that incorporate temporal and financial parameters alongside geometric data (Teizer et al., 2018). In civil engineering, CAD is routinely used for infrastructure development—ranging from transportation networks to wastewater treatment facilities—and is often integrated with geographic information systems for large-scale environmental planning (Peachavanish et al., 2006). In electronics, specialized electronic CAD tools facilitate the design of circuit boards and microchips, combining nanometer-scale precision with electrical and thermal simulations (Son et al., 2014). Even the fashion industry has adopted CAD for digital pattern making and virtual garment prototyping, significantly reducing material waste and time to market (Papachrıstou & Bılalıs, 2015; Choi, 2022). This cross-disciplinary adoption has been further accelerated by cloud-based platforms that enable distributed

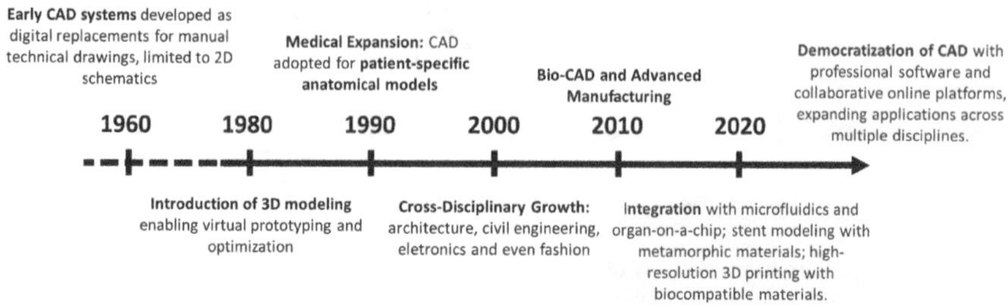

FIGURE 3.3 Evolution of computer-aided design (CAD): key technological milestones and cross-disciplinary applications (1960s to present).

collaboration, allowing teams to interact with shared models in real time, regardless of geographic or technical boundaries (Figure 3.3).

Notably, CAD has become indispensable in domains where digital design directly interfaces with biological systems. The medical field began adopting CAD in the 1990s, integrating data from CT and MRI to generate patient-specific anatomical models for surgical planning. One of the earliest applications was in craniofacial reconstruction (Vannier et al., 1985), where surgeons could virtually plan osteotomies and fabricate 3D-printed surgical guides based on individualized CT-derived CAD models (Parthasarathy, 2014). This advancement marked a paradigm shift from generic implants to personalized medical solutions—a trend exemplified by the U.S. Food and Drug Administration (FDA)'s clearance of the EXT 220 MED system by 3D Systems, a cleanroom-certified platform designed for the additive manufacturing of medical-grade polyether ether ketone (PEEK) cranial implants (3D Systems, 2023).

Soon thereafter, prosthetics and orthopedics embraced CAD's potential, combining anatomical fidelity with biomechanical optimization. Contemporary prosthetic sockets, for instance, are designed using parametric CAD models that adapt geometries based on residual limb pressure distribution (Ballit et al., 2022). Likewise, spinal implants increasingly feature lattice structures engineered to mimic patient-specific bone density gradients (Harrysson et al., 2007). This translation of CAD modeling into the virtual construction of human body components gave rise to the concept of Bio-CAD—a subfield dedicated to the design of biological and bioengineered systems.

The emergence of Bio-CAD for tissue engineering represents the most advanced frontier of CAD application. Here, geometric modeling must account for the dynamic behavior of living cells and biological tissues. In bioprinting, for example, CAD tools are used to design vascular networks with branching angles optimized for endothelial cell adhesion (Sun et al., 2020), and to create pore architectures that modulate stem cell differentiation through mechanobiological stimuli. These innovations underscore the shift from static, mechanical design to biologically informed modeling strategies.

This expansion into the life sciences highlights the extraordinary adaptability of CAD. The same parametric techniques used to engineer aircraft components are now employed to design coronary stents with auxetic metamaterials that expand in synchrony with arterial pulsation (Ren et al., 2016). Likewise, CAD plays a critical role in the design of microfluidic organ-on-chip platforms, enabling simulation of physiological shear stresses at capillary-scale resolutions (<100 μm), as well as the physical fabrication of these devices (Waldbaur et al., 2013). This is closely aligned with advances in 3D printing technologies, which now support the creation of complex microfluidic systems using biocompatible resins, transparent thermoplastics, and ultra-fine resolutions down to 50 μm layer thickness (Au et al., 2016).

The ongoing democratization of CAD—ranging from high-end professional software suites to browser-based, open-access platforms—ensures that this technology will continue to find novel applications across both established and emerging disciplines. What remains constant is CAD's core value: its capacity to transform abstract ideas into precise, executable models that push the boundaries of what we can design, build, and understand.

3.1.3 Role of Computer-Aided Design (CAD) in Bioprinting

Historically, computer-assisted modeling in tissue engineering has addressed multiple applications (Figure 3.4). These include surgical planning and simulation—where CAD facilitates preoperative visualization (Cutting et al., 1987); scaffold informatics—enabling the biomimetic design of hierarchical structures (Sun et al., 2004a); and 3D bioprinting blueprint generation—bridging digital models with physical constructs (Mironov et al., 2003). Despite its essential role in the bioprinting workflow, CAD modeling remains comparatively underexplored relative to the extensive research devoted to biocompatible materials, cell selection, and growth factor optimization. While these biological components are unquestionably critical, the computational frameworks that translate biological complexity into printable designs—collectively referred to as Bio-CAD—have received limited attention in the literature (Fay, 2020).

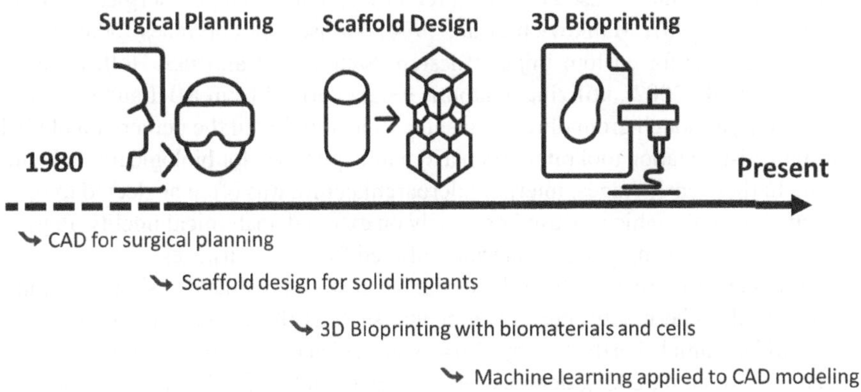

FIGURE 3.4 Historical progression of Bio-CAD applications, highlighting the shift from static anatomical modeling to the use of machine learning tools in the field.

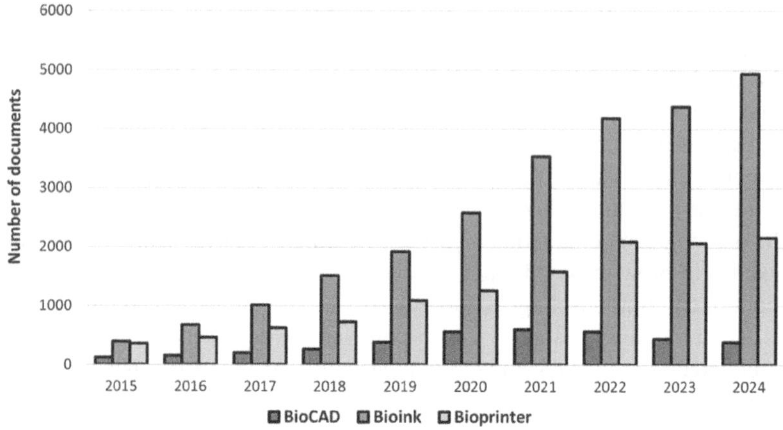

FIGURE 3.5 Bibliometric analysis of publication trends from 2015 to 2024, querying the terms "BioCAD," "Bioink," or "Bioprinter" in Google Scholar (search performed September 26, 2025; excluding patents and citations).

This disparity is clearly evident when examining scholarly publication trends. A bibliometric comparison among search terms such as "Bio-CAD," "Bioink," or "Bioprinter" reveals almost an order-of-magnitude difference in research output, despite the shared relevance of these domains to successful bioprinting (Figure 3.5). Although it can be argued that some relevant computational design studies may use the broader term "CAD" without the "Bio" prefix—a phenomenon that may also occur, although not necessarily to the same extent, with the other terms—this bibliometric snapshot nonetheless reflects a general perception among bioprinting practitioners. The underrepresentation of Bio-CAD is especially noticeable in the context of anatomically accurate, multiscale models that aim to replicate the intricate structural and functional features of native tissues.

The origins of this imbalance are partly historical. Early CAD applications in medicine were primarily used for visual reconstructions to support surgical planning (Cutting et al., 1987; Mankovich et al., 1994)—a use that continues today (Ghosh et al., 2022)—or for custom implant design (Saunders et al.,1985; Hollister et al., 2000; Lee et al., 2002), utilizing anatomical data derived from MRI and CT. These applications, although groundbreaking at the time, reinforced the perception of CAD as a static visualization tool rather than a dynamic platform for biologically informed design. In these early stages, internal microarchitecture was often neglected to surgical planning goals, which focused primarily on external anatomical fidelity. Physical models produced using plastic materials sufficed for these purposes.

Subsequent advances enabled the design of custom prosthetics using biocompatible materials. These solid custom implants, such as those used in spinal (Mobbs et al., 2017), cranial (Parthasarathy, 2014; Maricevich et al., 2019), and pelvic reconstructions (Xu et al., 2021), demonstrated the potential of CAD–CAM technologies in patient-specific medicine. However, these constructs lacked cellular integration in the manufacturing process, limiting their utility for regenerative applications.

A decisive turning point emerged with progress in both hardware and software for high-resolution modeling (Starly et al., 2005). These developments enabled CAD tools to meet the growing need for scaffold designs in tissue engineering, where functionality depends not only on macroscopic form but also on microscale and nanoscale features. Medical imaging continued to play a critical role, with micro-CT facilitating accurate mapping of scaffold microarchitecture (Ritman, 2004) and multimodal image registration enabling the integration of MRI and CT data for composite tissue modeling.

Nonetheless, the arrival of 3D bioprinting introduced a new set of challenges. CAD models now needed to accommodate not only anatomical fidelity but also a range of biological viability constraints. Parameters such as shear stress during bioink extrusion, oxygen diffusion limits in volumetric constructs, and the degradation kinetics of scaffolds became fundamental design considerations. Mironov's pioneering work in blueprint generation for bioprinting represented a major conceptual leap, yet even these initial approaches fell short in representing the dynamic, heterogeneous, and self-organizing nature of living tissues.

Traditional engineering design relies on deterministic assumptions—where materials behave in predictable ways under specific loads and conditions. In contrast, biological systems are adaptive, heterogeneous, and responsive to microenvironmental cues. These differences demand a fundamental rethinking of design principles. The central challenge for Bio-CAD is therefore not merely geometric modeling, but the integration of biologically relevant features such as spatial cell distribution, mechanical anisotropy, matrix composition, and dynamic remodeling potential.

Recent advances illustrate the growing maturity of Bio-CAD as a distinct field. For instance, vascularized tissue constructs now incorporate computationally generated angiogenic networks that are precisely aligned with parenchymal architectures. Machine learning algorithms are increasingly deployed to optimize scaffold parameters based on omics datasets and predictive models of cellular behavior (Jeznach et al., 2024). This pivotal transition—from static anatomical reconstruction to dynamic, biologically active design—highlights the emerging potential of Bio-CAD to finally close the gap between digital modeling and functional biological performance.

3.2 DESIGNING DIGITAL MODELS FOR BIOPRINTING

The initial CAD modeling of living tissues for 3D bioprinting typically follows two major distinct yet complementary strategies: CAD-based design and image-based design. The first involves creating models entirely from scratch using computational tools (Giannitelli et al., 2014; Ozbolat & Gudapati, 2016). This approach often employs basic geometric shapes or algorithmic patterns as building blocks (CAD-based unit cells), making it particularly useful for proof-of-concept studies or standardized tissue models (Giannitelli et al., 2014). While these designs can range from simple uniform structures to complex hierarchical architectures, they typically lack the anatomical specificity required for clinical applications. For personalized medicine, the second approach—image-based design—unlocks the true potential of bioprinting by combining engineered designs with patient-specific anatomical data.

Medical imaging techniques such as MRI and CT scans provide the foundation for creating biologically accurate, patient-specific models. These noninvasive methods capture detailed anatomical information in the form of 2D Digital Imaging and Communications in Medicine (DICOM) image slices, which then undergo a sophisticated transformation process (Sun et al., 2005). The workflow from medical images to printable CAD models begins with segmentation, where specific tissues or structures are identified and isolated using specialized software. This is followed by 3D reconstruction, which converts the segmented 2D data into volumetric models through computational algorithms. The resulting digital representation often requires additional refinement to optimize it for bioprinting—smoothing surfaces, adjusting wall thicknesses, or incorporating microarchitectural features that were not visible in the original scans. This image-to-model pipeline presents unique challenges, particularly in balancing the resolution limitations of clinical imaging with the need for biologically relevant detail.

Beyond these two primary strategies, other computational design paradigms offer additional tools for tailoring construct geometry and functionality. Free-form systems, for example, enable the creation of complex, nonuniform geometries using nonuniform rational B-splines and lofting techniques. These approaches allow for spatial control over architectural features and material composition, as well as spatiotemporal modulation of bioactive component release—beneficial for designing constructs with functional gradients and targeted biological responses (Giannitelli et al., 2014; Ozbolat & Gudapati, 2016).

Another promising direction is the use of implicit surface modeling, which relies on mathematical equations to define highly intricate internal structures, such as triply periodic minimal surfaces. These architectures, often used to mimic bone and cartilage microenvironments, provide both mechanical strength and interconnected porosity. Similarly, space-filling curve-based designs—such as Hilbert or Peano curves—use continuous extrusion paths to maximize surface area and structural integrity, particularly in extrusion-based bioprinting (Giannitelli et al., 2014; Ozbolat & Gudapati, 2016).

The most advanced applications often combine multiple approaches, using medical images as the anatomical foundation while employing computational design to enhance the model's functionality (Soellner et al., 2024). This hybrid approach leverages the strengths of both methods—the biological accuracy of medical imaging and the design flexibility of computational modeling. As the field progresses, the integration of artificial intelligence (AI) and advanced imaging techniques promises to further blur the lines between these approaches, potentially enabling automated generation of optimized designs that satisfy both anatomical and functional requirements. The ultimate goal remains the creation of digital models that not only resemble natural tissues but can also function as living biological systems once materialized through bioprinting.

3.2.1 Data Acquisition

3.2.1.1 Computed Tomography (CT)

CT provides high-resolution volumetric data of mineralized tissues through X-ray attenuation measurements. Its ability to differentiate variations in electron density makes it indispensable for modeling bone structures (Hounsfield, 1973). However, CT's limited soft tissue contrast (~5–20 Hounsfield units between similar tissues) often necessitates the use of contrast agents for effective visualization of vascular or parenchymal structures (Keklikoglou et al., 2019). A notable advantage of CT is that it is nondestructive and requires minimal sample preparation compared to conventional histological analysis, which is particularly beneficial when sample availability is limited. Furthermore, scaffold porosity—often estimated theoretically from CAD models or indirectly via deposition geometry or pycnometry—can be assessed with greater accuracy using micro-CT (μCT) (Bertoldi et al., 2011). This technique enables direct, spatially resolved evaluation of internal scaffold morphology (Tuan & Hutmacher, 2005), offering sufficient resolution for microarchitectural analysis of bone, including trabecular and cortical regions (Tellis et al., 2008; Bouxsein et al., 2010).

The integration of μCT with biomedical imaging and CAD software enhances scaffold characterization by enabling 3D visualization, digital manipulation, and quantification of architectural features such as porosity, density estimation, structure thickness, surface area-to-volume ratio, and interconnectivity (Keklikoglou et al., 2019). This noninvasive approach facilitates detailed evaluation of scaffold performance and the progression of bone regeneration in complex biological environments. In vascular imaging, contrast-enhancing techniques are being studied to generate stereolithography file format (STL)-compatible 3D mesh models suitable for direct import into CAD software, thereby improving the fidelity of vascular scaffold design (Mondy et al., 2009). Nonetheless, certain limitations persist; for example, in osteochondral models, not all scaffold or tissue components within the region of interest (ROI) may be fully captured during scanning (Tuan & Hutmacher, 2005). Even so, the combined application of μCT, CAD/CAM, and advanced contrast protocols has proven to be a powerful strategy for assessing mineralization patterns and fine-tuning scaffold architecture for regenerative applications.

3.2.1.2 Magnetic Resonance Imaging (MRI)

MRI excels in soft tissue characterization through proton density and relaxation time (T1/T2) mapping. It uses nuclear magnetic resonance to generate high-resolution two-dimensional images of the body, similar in structure to CT scans but based on fundamentally different physical principles. A key advantage of MRI over CT lies in its use of nonionizing radiofrequency energy within a strong magnetic field, which causes certain atomic nuclei to absorb and emit energy—eliminating the radiation risks associated with X-ray-based methods. This makes MRI especially suitable for longitudinal studies and *in vivo* imaging. Functional MRI, a specialized extension of this technology, monitors hemodynamic responses by repeatedly imaging the same area to capture changes in blood flow. This is particularly useful for assessing neurological activity in the brain and spinal cord (Kim & Bandettini, 2010). Although this process generates large and complex datasets, it provides valuable insights into dynamic organ-level behaviors that are highly relevant for reproducing biological functionality in bioprinting (Fay, 2020). However, despite its superior ability to delineate soft tissue boundaries, MRI may fail to resolve fine microvascular networks, which often must be artificially reconstructed or supplemented within the biofabrication design (Mangrulkar et al., 2020).

3.2.1.3 Ultrasound

Despite its advantages as a portable, cost-effective, and real-time medical imaging modality, ultrasound is not routinely employed for generating CAD models in bioprinting. Although it has been previously tested with some success—particularly for reconstructing external bone geometries—its broader adoption remains limited (Mehta et al., 1997). Compared to high-resolution imaging techniques such as CT and MRI, ultrasound lacks the spatial resolution and geometric fidelity required for detailed scaffold design and is more susceptible to signal noise and artifacts. Nevertheless, ultrasound presents unique advantages beyond anatomical imaging, particularly in modulating cellular behavior during biofabrication (Zhou, 2016). For example, ultrasound standing wave fields (USWF) can exert acoustic radiation forces that drive cells toward pressure nodes, enabling the rapid (within minutes) and reproducible formation of uniformly sized spheroids with homogeneous cell distribution—an essential feature for microtissue assembly. Furthermore, USWF-induced endothelial spheroids have been shown to enhance neovascularization, and low-intensity ultrasound stimulation can promote stem cell proliferation and differentiation. These biophysical effects, combined with ultrasound's affordability and compatibility with bioreactor systems, highlight its potential to address critical challenges in tissue engineering, such as vascularization and spatial cell patterning. While ultrasound may not yet serve as a primary imaging source for CAD modeling, its integration into bioprinting workflows can complement traditional imaging modalities by enhancing biological functionality and cellular organization in bioengineered constructs.

3.2.2 Image Processing

The conversion of medical imaging data into usable CAD models is a critical step in the bioprinting workflow, serving as a bridge between anatomical data acquisition and physical bioconstruct fabrication. This process begins with DICOM files obtained from imaging modalities such as CT, MRI, or ultrasound. These files consist of 2D image slices that undergo preprocessing and segmentation to isolate anatomical regions of interest from surrounding structures. Segmentation techniques include automated methods—such as thresholding, edge detection, and region-growing algorithms—often supplemented by manual refinement to enhance precision, particularly in cases of low contrast or irregular morphology (Sun et al., 2004b), a task commonly performed by anatomy specialists.

When these 2D slices are reconstructed, they form a volumetric representation from which 3D data can be extracted, generating a voxel-based model. While medical imaging software commonly used in clinical settings can visualize the general segmented area, detailed partitioning of the ROI often requires more advanced computational methods. 3D anatomical reconstruction can be achieved through either segmentation-based or volumetric representation approaches. In 2D segmentation, geometry is extracted slice by slice by identifying contours (e.g., via conjugate gradient algorithms) which are later stacked and converted into a solid model through skinning operations. Alternatively, 3D segmentation directly processes the volumetric dataset, identifying voxel boundaries and generating a polygonal mesh—often using triangulated surfaces (Sun et al., 2005). More recently, deep learning strategies have significantly enhanced segmentation performance. Supervised and unsupervised machine learning models have been successfully applied to delineate various anatomical structures in medical images (Lundervold & Lundervold, 2019), including the pancreas (Zhang et al., 2025), lungs and heart (Cao et al., 2021), and kidneys (Zhao et al., 2020), with some models capable of multi-organ segmentation (Ilesanmi et al., 2022).

The resulting 3D segmented anatomical model preserves voxel intensity data, enabling volume rendering, volumetric representation, and 3D visualization. These reconstructions facilitate anatomic modeling, supporting contour-based generation and shaded surface representations for CAD-based medical models. However, computational demands increase with mesh complexity, often requiring optimization for downstream applications (Sun et al., 2005).

Subsequently, the volumetric data is reconstructed into a 3D model using surface rendering algorithms and typically exported in STL format—a mesh composed of interconnected triangular facets. Although CAD software was originally designed for engineering applications, its adaptability has led to widespread use in medical imaging, supporting various file formats (e.g., STL, DXF, DWG, IGES, and STEP). CAD tools enable 3D solid modeling, rendering, and database-linked object manipulation, allowing medical images to be converted, modified, and visualized in three dimensions (Shapi'i et al., 2011). Finally, the STL file can be post-processed to repair errors and discontinuities, smooth surfaces, and append additional structures (Bücking et al., 2017; Ripley et al., 2017).

Some software frameworks have been proposed for this goal. For example, Im2CAD converted JPEG images (derived from DICOM via Medweb) into DXF files for CAD compatibility (Shapi'i et al., 2011). Tools such as 3D Slicer (Fedorov et al., 2012; Kikinis et al., 2013), Seg3D (Tate et al., 2016), the Medical Imaging Interaction Toolkit, and Materialise Mimics have been used to create models for surgical planning, enabling DICOM-to-STL conversion for further processing in software like Blender, Meshmixer, and FreeCAD (Nizamuddin & Kirthana, 2018; Bücking et al., 2017; Witowski et al., 2019; Abdullah et al., 2016).

A key challenge lies in balancing geometric fidelity with computational efficiency. High-resolution meshes improve anatomical accuracy but may hinder processing and 3D printing, whereas oversimplified meshes risk losing critical morphological details. To optimize this trade-off, mesh simplification, smoothing, and decimation algorithms are applied post-conversion to ensure printability without compromising essential features. Following image reconstruction, the CAD environment enables the design and optimization of biofunctional scaffolds tailored to the biological, mechanical, and architectural demands of the target tissue. Scaffold models must satisfy competing requirements, including mechanical stability, nutrient diffusion, and cell migration. To meet these needs, scaffold geometries are often customized using parametric design tools and topology optimization algorithms.

3.2.3 Modeling

Despite the ongoing advancement of medical imaging, the CAD models derived from these datasets often lack the resolution needed to accurately represent the microarchitecture of biological tissues. This limitation stems partly from the historical development of CAD tools, which were originally designed for surgical planning with an emphasis on macrostructural visualization rather than microstructural detail. Within this evolutionary trajectory, osseous surgical implants were among the first structures where porosity and microarchitecture became critical design considerations.

The early discourse on porosity marked a foundational step in regenerative medicine, particularly as synthetic implants and tissue grafts evolved into bioengineered constructs. These bioconstructs began to utilize porous scaffolds to integrate cells, signaling molecules, and extracellular matrix components to promote tissue regeneration (Hollister, 2005). At that time, CAD models were predominantly used to customize bone implants made from biocompatible materials without involving the printing of living cells. As classified by Groll et al. (2018), these early approaches relied on biomaterial inks rather than true bioinks—formulations that combine biomaterials with living cells.

Even when focusing solely on bone tissue, structural heterogeneity in porosity is evident, and it plays a fundamental role in scaffold design by directly influencing cell proliferation, migration, and tissue ingrowth. As early as 2005, researchers acknowledged the pressing need for enhanced 3D representation techniques due to the inherent complexity of fabricating such microarchitectural features in tissue engineering applications (Schroeder et al., 2005).

CAD modeling allows for precise control over porosity by manipulating unit cell geometry, pore size, and interconnectivity. Since 2009, automated approaches for pore generation in CAD models have been explored to streamline and optimize the design process (Ramin & Harris, 2009). More recently, mathematical modeling techniques have been used to create stochastic scaffolds that successfully support *in vitro* cell attachment and proliferation (Schroeder et al., 2005; Kanwar et al., 2022).

Pore sizes can vary widely depending on the target tissue and must be optimized to ensure proper nutrient diffusion, cellular interactions, and mechanical integrity (Trifonov et al., 2024). In the specific context of 3D bioprinting—where bioinks, typically hydrogel-based biomaterials containing cells, are used—the concept of porosity becomes multifaceted. Here, porosity arises from two main sources: (1) the intrinsic porosity of the hydrogel, governed by crosslinking mechanisms and primarily influenced by rheological properties, yielding pores ranging from 1 to 250 μm; and (2) the extrinsic porosity introduced by the deposition pattern defined within the CAD model (Figure 3.6). The latter enables modulation of voids and channels on the centimeter scale, depending on the printing process and the interplay between ink viscoelasticity and CAD configuration (Trifonov et al., 2024).

As highlighted by Trifonov et al., the terminology used to describe pore features is often inconsistent. Terms like "voids" and "channels" may better reflect porosity in the CAD-based context. This lack of standardized nomenclature complicates comparisons across studies and poses challenges in understanding and quantifying

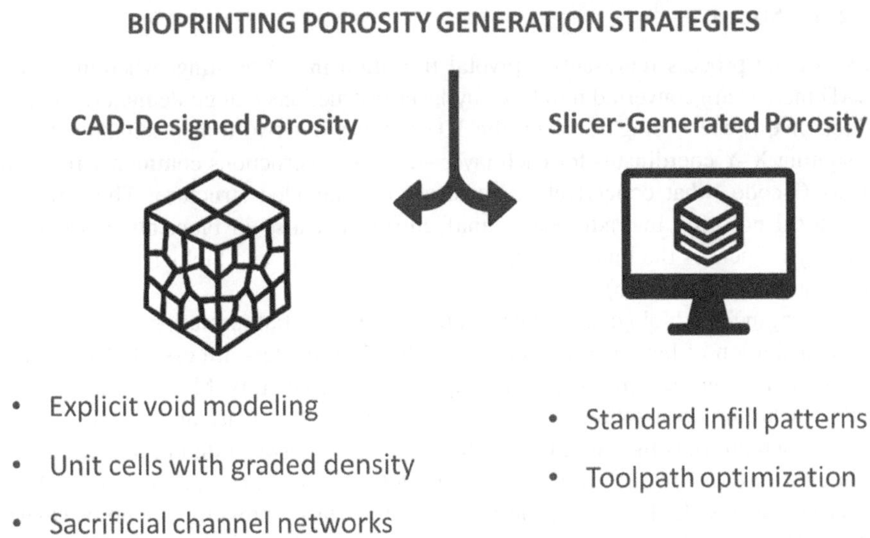

FIGURE 3.6 Complementary approaches to porosity generation in bioprinting: direct CAD modeling (a) versus slicing software parameterization (b).

the exact contribution of CAD modeling to the structural and functional outcomes of bioprinted constructs.

In scaffold design for bone tissue engineering, for example, Cox et al. (2015) developed CAD models incorporating "voids" of approximately 1 mm to replicate desired architectural features, using hydroxyapatite as the structural biomaterial. These macroporous constructs were tailored to ensure mechanical stability while supporting vascularization and osteointegration. In another study, porosity was integrated into the CAD model of auricular and nasal scaffolds as a proof of concept for fabricating soft craniofacial tissues (Zopf et al., 2015). Meanwhile, Sultan and Mathew (2018) developed a nanocellulose-based hydrogel capable of generating constructs with spatial gradients of such "voids." These gradients were engineered at a scale and orientation deemed optimal for promoting cellular interactions and guiding tissue ingrowth, demonstrating the functional relevance of CAD-driven pore architecture in directing regenerative outcomes.

Porosity is also intrinsically linked to vascularization, a critical parameter for the viability of thick or metabolically active constructs. Adequate pore interconnectivity facilitates nutrient and oxygen diffusion and can promote angiogenesis by providing physical guidance cues for endothelial cell migration. Moreover, vascular structures can be explicitly incorporated into CAD models either by importing segmented vascular trees from contrast-enhanced imaging or by embedding sacrificial materials during the design phase. These sacrificial components—such as Pluronic F127 or gelatin—can be removed postprinting to leave behind perfusable channels, which are subsequently endothelialized to form functional blood vessels (Buckley et al., 2025).

3.2.4 Slicing

The slicing process represents a pivotal transition in 3D printing, wherein digital CAD models are converted into layer-by-layer instructions that guide material deposition. In essence, slicing translates the 3D geometry into two-dimensional toolpaths, assigning X–Y coordinates for each layer—a set of instructions commonly referred to as G-code—that collectively reconstruct the intended structure. This process is critical not only in traditional manufacturing but also in bioprinting, where it directly influences the final construct's structural fidelity and biological functionality (Baumann et al., 2016).

For engineered biological tissues, slicing governs spatial resolution, porosity, and the distribution of biomaterials and cells. These parameters are essential for mimicking native microenvironments and supporting cell viability. Modern slicing software, including open-source platforms such as Ultimaker Cura and Slic3r, as well as commercial tools like Simplify3D, bridge the gap between digital modeling and fabrication. These platforms allow users to define critical print parameters such as layer height, nozzle diameter, print speed, and extrusion pressure (Webb & Doyle, 2017). However, these tools were originally developed for non-biological printing applications and are consequently limited in their ability to generate internal structures optimized for tissue engineering. Most rely on predefined infill patterns (e.g., grid and honeycomb) applied uniformly across the object, often creating a solid outer shell and a repetitive internal lattice that lacks biological relevance.

To address these limitations, some research groups have pursued "brute-force" design approaches by manually incorporating pore networks and strut geometries directly within the CAD model prior to slicing. This method allows full control over porosity and architecture but can be time-consuming and computationally demanding. Alternatively, advances in custom slicing software tailored to bioprinting have enabled the generation of user-defined gradients, anisotropic features, and porous microarchitectures that mimic the complexity of native tissues (Nyberg et al., 2019). Open-source frameworks and parametric coding environments—such as Grasshopper plugins or Python-based slicers—have been instrumental in this evolution.

In practice, two main strategies can be employed to introduce porosity into bioprinted constructs: (1) explicitly designing the pores within the CAD model itself, or (2) using slicing software capable of generating porosity during the toolpath generation phase. The latter approach leverages infill parameters—often overlooked in non-biological printing—to fine-tune structural resolution, mechanical stability, and nutrient diffusion pathways, all of which are crucial for ensuring postprinting cell survival and tissue development.

3.2.5 Bioprinting

The transition from the processed CAD model to a physical construct involves conversion to machine instructions through slicing software, which translates the 3D geometry into layer-by-layer toolpaths (G-code). This stage introduces additional considerations specific to bioprinting modalities, such as nozzle diameter constraints in extrusion-based systems or laser spot size limitations in laser-assisted platforms.

General-purpose software tools for printer control are often suboptimal for bioprinting applications, as they typically lack native support for cell-laden materials, temperature-sensitive components, and synchronized multi-material deposition (Gulyas et al., 2018). Recent advances in multi-material printing further complicate this translation, demanding sophisticated material assignment strategies within the digital model.

The conversion of these 3D models into printable instructions occurs through slicing algorithms and toolpath generation, processes that have grown increasingly sophisticated to meet bioprinting demands. Modern slicing software must account for numerous biological variables, including bioink viscosity, cell viability parameters, and the need for removable support structures. Toolpath generation algorithms now often incorporate fluid dynamics simulations to optimize printing parameters—such as nozzle speed, pressure, and layer deposition patterns—thereby minimizing shear stress on delicate biological materials. Specialized bioprinting slicers like BioSlicer and Slic3r for Bioprinting have emerged, offering features such as temperature control for thermoresponsive bioinks and the ability to alternate between different cell-laden materials within a single bioconstruct. These advancements in software and file formats enable the precise translation of complex biological designs into physical realities, pushing the boundaries of tissue engineering and regenerative medicine.

As the field progresses, automated workflows combining AI-assisted segmentation with generative design principles promise to streamline this intricate pipeline. This could enable real-time model adaptation based on intraoperative imaging or cellular self-organization patterns. Ongoing development focuses on creating more intelligent systems that can automatically adjust printing parameters using real-time feedback, potentially integrating machine learning algorithms to predict and compensate for biological variability during printing. The anticipated emergence of fully integrated Bio-CAD environments—combining design, simulation, and printing preparation into seamless workflows—will further narrow the gap between digital models and functional living tissues. The continued refinement of these image processing and printing techniques remains paramount for bridging medical imaging's diagnostic capabilities with the precision required for functional tissue biofabrication.

3.3 CHALLENGES IN CAD FOR BIOPRINTING

The development of CAD models for bioprinting presents unique challenges that stem from the need to reconcile engineering precision with biological complexity. Unlike conventional 3D printing, where designs primarily focus on geometric and mechanical requirements, bioprinting demands that digital models account for living cellular components and dynamic biological processes. This dual requirement introduces significant hurdles in model creation, particularly in balancing structural integrity with cell viability, achieving high resolution within the constraints of bioink printability, and accommodating the limitations of biomaterial properties (Figure 3.7). These challenges become even more pronounced when designing multi-material constructs that aim to replicate the intricate heterogeneity of native tissues.

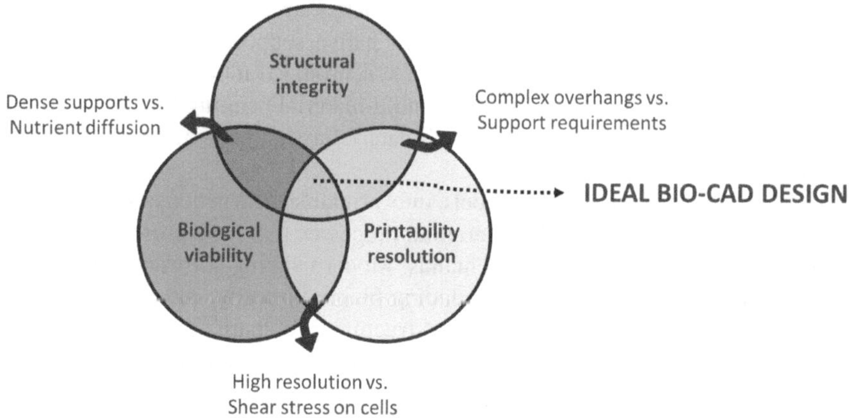

FIGURE 3.7 The inevitable compromise in Bio-CAD: the loss of microarchitectural detail from the digital model to the physical construct due to bioink rheology and printer resolution limits.

3.3.1 Balancing Structural Integrity and Biological Viability

A fundamental challenge in Bio-CAD design lies in maintaining structural stability while preserving cell viability and function. CAD models must specify geometries that provide sufficient mechanical support during and after printing, yet avoid designs that could compromise cellular viability. For instance, overhanging structures may require support materials that can be difficult to remove without damaging delicate cell-laden matrices. Similarly, the density of internal pores must be carefully calibrated—too sparse, and the construct lacks mechanical strength; too dense, and nutrient diffusion becomes inadequate for cell survival. This balance becomes particularly critical for load-bearing tissues like bone or cartilage, where the CAD design must simultaneously satisfy biomechanical performance criteria and biological requirements. The challenge extends to the microscale, where features like pore interconnectivity must be designed to facilitate cell migration and tissue integration while maintaining structural stability under physiological conditions.

3.3.2 Addressing Resolution and Printability Constraints

The resolution capabilities of bioprinting technologies impose relevant constraints on CAD designs. While medical imaging data can reveal intricate tissue features at micron-scale resolution, most bioprinters cannot faithfully reproduce these details—especially when using viscous bioinks that spread upon deposition. CAD models must therefore be optimized to accommodate the printer's capabilities, often requiring simplification of delicate features like capillary networks or thin tissue membranes. This resolution gap is particularly problematic when attempting to recreate the complex microarchitectures found in native tissues, such as lobular patterns in liver tissue or alveolar structures in lungs. Furthermore, maintaining cell viability during printing often requires compromises in resolution, as higher precision typically involves slower deposition speeds or smaller nozzles that increase shear stress on cells. These constraints force designers to prioritize which anatomical features are essential to preserve and which can be approximated without significantly compromising tissue function.

3.3.3 Material Constraints and Multi-Material Design

The limited range of printable biomaterials presents another major challenge for CAD in bioprinting. Unlike traditional 3D printing with its wide selection of engineering materials, bioinks must satisfy stringent biocompatibility requirements while providing appropriate rheological properties for printing. This restricted material palette limits the design space available to engineers, often forcing compromises between printability, mechanical properties, and biological functionality. The challenge intensifies with multi-material constructs that aim to replicate graded interfaces found in natural tissues, such as the tendon-to-bone transition or the layered structure of skin. CAD models must account for the distinct properties of each material—including their crosslinking mechanisms, shrinkage rates, and mechanical behaviors—while ensuring seamless integration between different bioinks during the printing. Additionally, the sequence of material deposition must be carefully planned to prevent contamination or unintended mixing that could compromise the final construct's functionality. These material-related challenges necessitate close collaboration between CAD designers, biomaterial scientists, and biologists to develop models that can be successfully translated into viable biological constructs.

The intersection of these challenges highlights the need for advanced CAD solutions that can simultaneously address structural, biological, and material constraints. Future developments in Bio-CAD software may incorporate predictive algorithms to simulate cell behavior within designed structures, or optimization routines that automatically adjust designs to balance competing requirements. As the field progresses, overcoming these challenges will be crucial for advancing from simple tissue analogs to complex, functional organs suitable for clinical applications.

3.4 FUTURE DIRECTIONS IN BIO-CAD

As bioprinting technology evolves, the role of CAD systems is shifting from static geometric modeling to dynamic, data-driven frameworks capable of supporting biological complexity and adaptivity. Emerging paradigms such as 4D bioprinting, AI, generative design, and *in vivo* maturation are transforming how digital models are conceived, optimized, and integrated into regenerative medicine workflows.

3.4.1 Incorporating Time and Responsiveness as a Variable: CAD and 4D Bioprinting

While traditional CAD models in bioprinting focus on the spatial configuration of biomaterials and cellular components, 4D bioprinting introduces time as a fourth dimension. This allows constructs to transform their shape, function, or mechanical properties in response to external stimuli after printing, such as temperature, pH, hydration, light, or magnetic fields (An et al., 2016; Silva, 2019). To accommodate these dynamic behaviors, CAD modeling must evolve beyond static representations to incorporate simulation-based tools that predict how the bioprinted construct will evolve over time under biological or physicochemical triggers, allowing the designer to encode dynamic behaviors directly into the construct's blueprint.

In this context, CAD environments are being integrated with computational modeling approaches—such as finite computational fluid dynamics, and multiphysics simulations (dos Santos et al., 2022)—to forecast how bioinks or smart materials will respond to variations in temperature, hydration, pH, magnetic fields, or mechanical stress. These simulations can guide the design of constructs that undergo programmed deformations, folding, swelling, or functional activation postprinting. For example, hydrogels with anisotropic swelling properties (Díaz-Payno et al., 2023) can be digitally patterned to bend or twist in specific directions when exposed to moisture, enabling self-assembly of tubular structures or dynamic drug-release systems.

The CAD tools used in 4D bioprinting must therefore support not only geometric modeling but also material behavior modeling, accounting for time-dependent changes in volume, stiffness, degradation, or interfacial interactions. Simulation-driven CAD design allows researchers to iteratively test and refine a structure's responsiveness before committing to physical fabrication, minimizing trial and error during experimental stages.

By integrating stimulus-responsive materials—such as shape-memory polymers, swellable hydrogels, or magneto-responsive composites—CAD models evolve from static geometries into programmed devices that fold, assemble, or activate on demand. This dynamic capability holds promise for minimally invasive implantation, smart drug delivery systems, and bioactuators that mimic the adaptability of living tissues. Importantly, 4D modeling workflows must also account for the kinetics of biological processes—such as cell migration, proliferation, and matrix remodeling—thereby bridging the gap between bioengineered structure and biological function.

Furthermore, data from time-lapse imaging—such as live-cell microscopy (Poologasundarampillai et al., 2021) or real-time deformation studies (Gugliandolo et al., 2022)—can be incorporated into the feedback loop, enabling the refinement of both material models and actuation protocols embedded within the CAD design. This workflow transforms the CAD model into a predictive tool for morphological programming, where the construct replicates not only biological form but also biological behavior.

By embedding time-responsive design principles into the modeling process, 4D bioprinting represents a paradigm shift toward adaptive and functional biofabrication, with broad implications for regenerative medicine, soft robotics, and *in situ* tissue engineering.

3.4.2 AI and Generative Design in Bioprinting

AI can redefine design methodologies in Bio-CAD by enabling generative design—a process where algorithms autonomously explore design permutations based on biological goals, material constraints, and manufacturing capabilities, as has been discussed in general CAD designs (Koul, 2024; Byrne et al., 2025). Unlike traditional CAD modeling, which relies on user-driven geometry, generative approaches harness optimization algorithms (e.g., genetic algorithms, topology optimization, and reinforcement learning) to propose scaffold architectures that maximize properties such as mechanical strength, nutrient diffusion, or cell attachment.

Machine learning techniques are also being employed to automate segmentation of medical images, predict bioink behavior, or anticipate postprinting structural deformations. Deep learning models trained on extensive imaging datasets can identify anatomical features with high accuracy, reducing the time and subjectivity associated with manual delineation. Additionally, AI-driven inverse design allows users to define desired functional outcomes—such as stiffness gradients (Abu-Mualla & Huang, 2023, Liu et al., 2023) or vascular perfusion—and receive optimized scaffold geometries that satisfy those conditions.

These tools are essential for managing the growing complexity of bioprinted constructs, particularly when combining heterogeneous cell types, biomaterials, and functionalities within a single design. As CAD continues to evolve through the integration of AI—such as generative adversarial networks used to propose optimal trabecular bone scaffold geometries—and the potential use of quantum computing for multidomain biological simulations, its role as a universal design language becomes increasingly pervasive (Siegkas, 2022; Shen & Buehler, 2022). One promising frontier is the development of so-called "4D Bio-CAD," where digital models not only describe static structures but also predict dynamic biological processes, including tissue remodeling over time. This progression blurs the boundary between bioengineered constructs and living systems.

3.4.3 Integration with Bioreactors and *In Vivo* Growth

The future of Bio-CAD lies in its seamless integration with bioreactors and *in vivo* environments, where constructs are not only printed but also matured under physiological or biomimetic conditions. This integration demands CAD platforms capable of simulating dynamic microenvironments, including nutrient gradients, mechanical loading, and fluid flow, which are essential for tissue maturation and vascularization.

Digital models may eventually incorporate adaptive feedback loops, where sensor data from bioreactors—such as pH, oxygen tension, or mechanical strain—are fed back into the CAD system to adjust design parameters in real time. Such closed-loop systems would allow bioprinted tissues to evolve adaptively, mimicking the homeostatic responses of living organisms. Furthermore, as bioprinting advances toward *in situ* applications (e.g., direct printing onto wounds or internal organs), Bio-CAD systems will need to integrate real-time imaging, robotic control, and tissue deformation prediction to guide accurate deposition on dynamic biological surfaces (Figure 3.8).

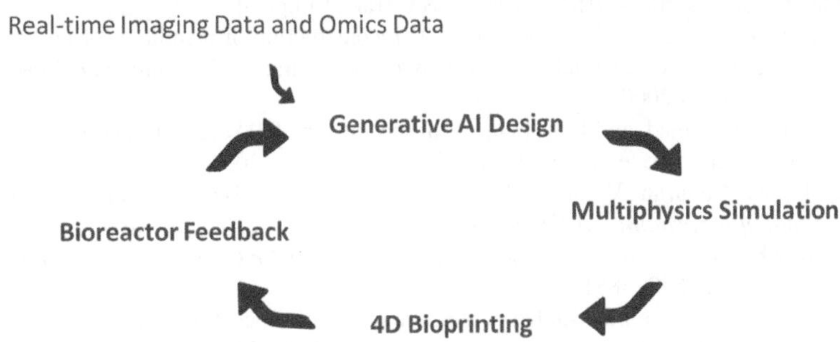

FIGURE 3.8 The future integrated Bio-CAD workflow: a closed-loop system where AI-generated designs are validated through multiphysics simulation, physically realized via 4D bioprinting, and iteratively refined using real-time biosensor data from bioreactors.

3.5 CONCLUSION

The journey from digital models to functional living tissues underscores a fundamental paradigm shift in tissue engineering, where CAD has evolved from a static visualization tool into a dynamic, biologically informed platform. By integrating anatomical data from medical imaging with computational modeling strategies—ranging from parametric unit cells to implicit surface microarchitectures—CAD enables the precise specification of scaffolds and bioconstructs. In 3D bioprinting terms, this means that CAD models must balance printing feasibility, structural integrity, and biological viability. This synergy between digital precision and biological complexity has positioned CAD as an indispensable component of the bioprinting workflow, facilitating the translation of patient-specific anatomical data into functional tissue analogs.

Despite these advances, several challenges remain in reconciling engineering design principles with the dynamic nature of organs. Issues such as printability constraints, bioink rheology, and the integration of multi-material gradients highlight the ongoing tension between geometric fidelity and cellular functionality. Moreover, the inherent limitations of current imaging and modeling techniques often result in a loss of microarchitectural detail, emphasizing the need for more sophisticated specific Bio-CAD tools capable of simulating not only shape but also function—including nutrient diffusion, mechanical stimuli, and cellular self-organization.

Looking ahead, the future of Bio-CAD lies in its integration with emerging technologies such as AI, generative design, and 4D bioprinting. These innovations promise to transform CAD from a passive modeling environment into an adaptive, predictive system that can anticipate tissue maturation and remodeling over time. By closing the loop among digital design, physical fabrication, and biological response, next-generation Bio-CAD platforms will not only narrow the gap between synthetic constructs and living tissues but also accelerate the transition of bioprinting from laboratory research to clinical reality.

REFERENCES

3D Systems, 2023. FDA clearance of EXT 220 MED system enables patient-specific PEEK cranial implants. https://www.3dsystems.com/press-releases/3d-systems-announces-fda-clearance-worlds-first-3d-printed-peek-cranial-implants

Abdullah, Johari Yap, et al. "Comparison of 3D reconstruction of mandible for pre-operative planning using commercial and open-source software." *AIP Conference Proceedings* 1791.1 (2016): 020001.

Abu-Mualla, Mohammad, and Jida Huang. "Inverse design of 3D cellular materials with physics-guided machine learning." *Materials & Design* 232 (2023): 112103.

An, Jia, Chee Kai Chua, and Vladimir Mironov. "A perspective on 4D bioprinting." *International Journal of Bioprinting* 2.1 (2016): 3–5.

Au, Anthony K., et al. "3D-printed microfluidics." *Angewandte Chemie International Edition* 55.12 (2016): 3862–3881.

Ballit, Abbass, et al. "Computer-aided parametric prosthetic socket design based on real-time soft tissue deformation and an inverse approach." *The Visual Computer* 38.3 (2022): 919–937.

Barr, Ronald E., and Davor Juricic. "From drafting to modern design representation: The evolution of engineering design graphics." *Journal of Engineering Education* 83.3 (1994): 263–270.

Baumann, Felix, et al. "Influence of slicing tools on quality of 3D printed parts." *Computer-Aided Design and Applications* 13.1 (2016): 14–31.

Bertoldi, Serena, Silvia Farè, and Maria Cristina Tanzi. "Assessment of scaffold porosity: the new route of micro-CT." *Journal of Applied Biomaterials and Biomechanics* 9.3 (2011): 165–175.

Bouxsein, Mary L., et al. "Guidelines for assessment of bone microstructure in rodents using micro–computed tomography." *Journal of Bone and Mineral Research* 25.7 (2010): 1468–1486.

Bücking, Thore M., et al. "From medical imaging data to 3D printed anatomical models." *PloS One* 12.5 (2017): e0178540.

Buckley, Christian, et al. "Sacrificial strategy towards the formation of vascular-like networks in volumetric tissue constructs." *BMEMat* 3.2 (2025): e12118.

Byrne, Daniel, Vincent Hargaden, and Nikolaos Papakostas. "Application of generative AI technologies to engineering design." *Procedia CIRP* 132 (2025): 147–152.

Cao, Zheng, et al. "Cascaded SE-ResUnet for segmentation of thoracic organs at risk." *Neurocomputing* 453 (2021): 357–368.

Choi, Kyung-Hee. "3D dynamic fashion design development using digital technology and its potential in online platforms." *Fashion and Textiles* 9.1 (2022): 9.

Cox, Sophie C., et al. "3D printing of porous hydroxyapatite scaffolds intended for use in bone tissue engineering applications." *Materials Science and Engineering: C* 47 (2015): 237–247.

Cutting, Court, et al. "Three-dimensional computer-aided design of craniofacial surgical procedures." *Craniofacial Surgery: Proceedings of the First International Congress of The International Society of Cranio-Maxillo-Facial Surgery President: Paul Tessier Cannes-La Napoule, 1985*, Daniel Marchac (ed.). Berlin, Heidelberg: Springer Berlin Heidelberg, 1987.

Díaz-Payno, Pedro J., et al. "Swelling-dependent shape-based transformation of a human mesenchymal stromal cells-laden 4D bioprinted construct for cartilage tissue engineering." *Advanced Healthcare Materials* 12.2 (2023): 2201891.

dos Santos, Bianca Cristina, et al. "Biological multiscale computational modeling: A promising tool for 3D bioprinting and tissue engineering." *Bioprinting* 28 (2022): e00234.

Elanchezhian, C., and G. Shanmuga Sundar. *Computer Aided Manufacturing*. Firewall Media, 2007.

Fay, Cormac D. "Computer-aided design and manufacturing (CAD/CAM) for bioprinting." *3D Bioprinting: Principles and Protocols*, Jeremy M. Crook (ed.). New York: Springer US, 2020. 27–41.

Fedorov, Andriy, et al. "3D Slicer as an image computing platform for the Quantitative Imaging Network." *Magnetic Resonance Imaging* 30.9 (2012): 1323–1341.

Ghosh, Reena M., et al. "Clinical 3D modeling to guide pediatric cardiothoracic surgery and intervention using 3D printed anatomic models, computer aided design and virtual reality." *3D Printing in Medicine* 8.1 (2022): 11.

Giannitelli, Sara Maria, et al. "Current trends in the design of scaffolds for computer-aided tissue engineering." *Acta Biomaterialia* 10.2 (2014): 580–594.

Groll, Juergen, et al. "A definition of bioinks and their distinction from biomaterial inks." *Biofabrication* 11.1 (2018): 013001.

Groover, Mikell P., and Emory W. Zimmers, Jr. *CAD/CAM: Computer-aided Design and Manufacturing*. Upper Saddle River, NJ: Pearson Education, 1983.

Gugliandolo, Simone Giovanni, et al. "In-situ monitoring of defects in extrusion-based bioprinting processes using visible light imaging." *Procedia CIRP* 110 (2022): 219–224.

Gulyas, Marton, et al. "Software tools for cell culture-related 3D printed structures." *PLoS One* 13.9 (2018): e0203203.

Harrysson, Ola LA, Yasser A. Hosni, and Jamal F. Nayfeh. "Custom-designed orthopedic implants evaluated using finite element analysis of patient-specific computed tomography data: femoral-component case study." *BMC Musculoskeletal Disorders* 8 (2007): 1–10.

Hollister, Scott J. "Porous scaffold design for tissue engineering." *Nature Materials* 4.7 (2005): 518–524.

Hollister, Scott J., et al. "An image-based approach for designing and manufacturing craniofacial scaffolds." *International Journal of Oral & Maxillofacial Surgery* 29.1 (2000): 67–71.

Hounsfield, Godfrey N. "Computerized transverse axial scanning (tomography): Part 1. Description of system." *The British Journal of Radiology* 46.552 (1973): 1016–1022.

Hull, Charles W. "Apparatus for production of three-dimensional objects by stereolithography." *United States Patent, Appl., No. 638905, Filed* (1984).

Ilesanmi, Ademola E., et al. "Organ segmentation from computed tomography images using the 3D convolutional neural network: a systematic review." *International Journal of Multimedia Information Retrieval* 11.3 (2022): 315–331.

Jeznach, O., Tabakoglu, S., Zaszczyńska, A. et al. Review on machine learning application in tissue engineering: What has been done so far? Application areas, challenges, and perspectives. *Journal of Materials Science* 59 (2024), 21222–21250.

Kanwar, Susheem, Oraib Al-Ketan, and Sanjairaj Vijayavenkataraman. "A novel method to design biomimetic, 3D printable stochastic scaffolds with controlled porosity for bone tissue engineering." *Materials & Design* 220 (2022): 110857.

Keklikoglou, Kleoniki, et al. "Micro-computed tomography for natural history specimens: a handbook of best practice protocols." *European Journal of Taxonomy* 522 (2019): 1–55.

Kikinis, Ron, Steve D. Pieper, and Kirby G. Vosburgh. "3D Slicer: a platform for subject-specific image analysis, visualization, and clinical support." *Intraoperative Imaging and Image-guided Therapy*, Ferenc A. Jolesz (ed.). New York, NY: Springer New York, 2013. 277–289.

Kim, Seong-Gi, and Peter A. Bandettini. "Principles of functional MRI." *BOLD fMRI: A Guide to Functional Imaging for Neuroscientists*, Scott H. Faro, Feroze B. Mohamed (eds.). New York, NY: Springer New York, 2010. 3–22.

Koul, Parankush. "A review of generative design using machine learning for additive manufacturing." *Advances in Mechanical and Materials Engineering* 41.1 (2024): 145–159.

Landers, R., et al. "Fabrication of soft tissue engineering scaffolds by means of rapid prototyping techniques." *Journal of Materials Science* 37.15 (2002): 3107–3116.

Lee, Ming-Yih, et al. "Custom implant design for patients with cranial defects." *IEEE Engineering in Medicine and Biology Magazine* 21.2 (2002): 38–44.

Liu, Wenhang, et al. "Inverse design of anisotropic bone scaffold based on machine learning and regenerative genetic algorithm." *Frontiers in Bioengineering and Biotechnology* 11 (2023): 1241151.

Lundervold, Alexander Selvikvåg, and Arvid Lundervold. "An overview of deep learning in medical imaging focusing on MRI." *Zeitschrift fuer Medizinische Physik* 29.2 (2019): 102–127.

Mangrulkar, Amol, Santosh Rane, and Vivek Sunnapwar. "Image-based bio-cad modeling: overview, scope, and challenges." *Journal of Physics: Conference Series* 1706.1 (2020): 012189.

Mankovich, Nicholas J., et al. "Surgical planning using three-dimensional imaging and computer modeling." *Otolaryngologic Clinics of North America* 27.5 (1994): 875–889.

Maricevich, Juan Pablo Borges Rodrigues, et al. "Functional and aesthetic evaluation after cranial reconstruction with polymethyl methacrylate prostheses using low-cost 3D printing templates in patients with cranial defects secondary to decompressive craniectomies: a prospective study." *Surgical Neurology International* 10 (2019): 1.

Mehta, Bhavin V., Sailesh Rajani, and Guatam Sinha. "Comparison of image processing techniques (magnetic resonance imaging, computed tomography scan and ultrasound) for 3D modeling and analysis of the human bones." *Journal of Digital Imaging* 10.Suppl 1 (1997): 203–206.

Mironov, Vladimir, et al. "Organ printing: computer-aided jet-based 3D tissue engineering." *Trends in Biotechnology* 21.4 (2003): 157–161.

Mobbs, Ralph J., et al. "The utility of 3D printing for surgical planning and patient-specific implant design for complex spinal pathologies: case report." *Journal of Neurosurgery: Spine* 26.4 (2017): 513–518.

Mondy, William Lafayette, et al. "Micro-CT of corrosion casts for use in the computer-aided design of microvasculature." *Tissue Engineering Part C: Methods* 15.4 (2009): 729–738.

Murphy, Sean V., and Anthony Atala. "3D bioprinting of tissues and organs." *Nature Biotechnology* 32.8 (2014): 773–785.

Nizamuddin, Mohammed Khaja, and S. Kirthana. "Reconstruction of human femur bone from CT scan images using CAD techniques." *IOP Conference Series: Materials Science and Engineering* 455.1 (2018): 012103.

Nyberg, Ethan, Aine O'Sullivan, and Warren Grayson. "scafSLICR: A MATLAB-based slicing algorithm to enable 3D-printing of tissue engineering scaffolds with heterogeneous porous microarchitecture." *PLoS One* 14.11 (2019): e0225007.

Ozbolat, Ibrahim, and Hemanth Gudapati. "A review on design for bioprinting." *Bioprinting* 3 (2016): 1–14.

Papachrıstou, Evridiki, and Nikolaos Bılalıs. "How to integrate recent development in technology with Digital Prototype textile and apparel applications." *Marmara Fen Bilimleri Dergisi* 27 (2015): 32–39.

Parthasarathy, Jayanthi. "3D modeling, custom implants and its future perspectives in craniofacial surgery." *Annals of Maxillofacial Surgery* 4.1 (2014): 9–18.

Peachavanish, Ratchata, et al. "An ontological engineering approach for integrating CAD and GIS in support of infrastructure management." *Advanced Engineering Informatics* 20.1 (2006): 71–88.

Poologasundarampillai, Gowsihan, et al. "Real-time imaging and analysis of cell-hydrogel interplay within an extrusion-bioprinting capillary." *Bioprinting* 23 (2021): e00144.

Ramin, Ettore, and Russell A. Harris. "Advanced computer-aided design for bone tissue-engineering scaffolds." *Proceedings of the Institution of Mechanical Engineers, Part H: Journal of Engineering in Medicine* 223.3 (2009): 289–301.

Ren, Xin, et al. "A simple auxetic tubular structure with tuneable mechanical properties." *Smart Materials and Structures* 25.6 (2016): 065012.

Ripley, Beth, et al. "3D printing from MRI data: harnessing strengths and minimizing weaknesses." *Journal of Magnetic Resonance Imaging* 45.3 (2017): 635–645.

Ritman, Erik L. "Micro-computed tomography—current status and developments." *Annual Review of Biomedical Engineering* 6.1 (2004): 185–208.

Saunders, C. G., et al. "Computer aided design of prosthetic sockets for below-knee amputees." *Prosthetics and Orthotics International* 9.1 (1985): 17–22.

Schroeder, Craig, et al. "Computer-aided design of porous artifacts." *Computer-aided Design* 37.3 (2005): 339–353.

Schulz, Adriana, et al. "Interactive design space exploration and optimization for CAD models." *ACM Transactions on Graphics (TOG)* 36.4 (2017): 1–14.

Shapi'i, Azrulhizam, et al. "Applications of computer aided design (CAD) in medical image technology." *International Journal on Advanced Science Engineering and Information Technology* 1.6 (2011): 698–701.

Shen, Sabrina Chin-yun, and Markus J. Buehler. "Nature-inspired architected materials using unsupervised deep learning." *Communications Engineering* 1.1 (2022): 37.

Siegkas, Petros. "Generating 3D porous structures using machine learning and additive manufacturing." *Materials & Design* 220 (2022): 110858.

Silva, Luciano P. "Current trends and challenges in biofabrication using biomaterials and nanomaterials: future perspectives for 3D/4D bioprinting." *3D and 4D Printing in Biomedical Applications: Process Engineering and Additive Manufacturing*, Mohammed Maniruzzaman (ed.). Hoboken, NJ: Wiley-VCH Verlag GmbH & Co. KGaA, 2019. 373–421.

Soellner, Uliana, et al. "Simulation of micro-CT acquired geometry of additively manufactured open porosities." *Procedia CIRP* 126 (2024): 680–685.

Son, Seokbae, et al. "Collaborative design environment between ECAD and MCAD engineers in high-tech products development." *International Journal of Production Research* 52.20 (2014): 6161–6174.

Starly, Binil, et al. "Three-dimensional reconstruction for medical-CAD modeling." *Computer-Aided Design and Applications* 2.1-4 (2005): 431–438.

Sultan, Sahar, and Aji P. Mathew. "3D printed scaffolds with gradient porosity based on a cellulose nanocrystal hydrogel." *Nanoscale* 10.9 (2018): 4421–4431.

Sun, Wei, et al. "Computer-aided tissue engineering: overview, scope and challenges." *Biotechnology and Applied Biochemistry* 39.1 (2004a): 29–47.

Sun, Wei, et al. "Computer-aided tissue engineering: application to biomimetic modelling and design of tissue scaffolds." *Biotechnology and Applied Biochemistry* 39.1 (2004b): 49–58.

Sun, Wei, et al. "Bio-CAD modeling and its applications in computer-aided tissue engineering." *Computer-Aided Design* 37.11 (2005): 1097–1114.

Sun, Wei, et al. "The bioprinting roadmap." *Biofabrication* 12.2 (2020): 022002.

Tate, Jess, Brett Burton, and Ayla Khan. "Seg3d basic functionality." https://www.sci.utah.edu/devbuilds/seg3d_docs/Seg3DBasicFunctionality.pdf [accessed 18 April 2017] (2016).

Teizer, Jochen, et al. "BIM for 3D printing in construction." *Building Information Modeling: Technology Foundations and Industry Practice*, André Borrmann, Markus König, Christian Koch, Jakob Beetz (eds.). Cham: Springer International Publishing, 2018. 421–446.

Tellis, Brandi C., et al. "Trabecular scaffolds created using micro CT guided fused deposition modeling." *Materials Science and Engineering: C* 28.1 (2008): 171–178.

Trifonov, Alexander, et al. "Reasoning on pore terminology in 3D bioprinting." *Gels* 10.2 (2024): 153.

Tuan, Ho Saey, and Dietmar W. Hutmacher. "Application of micro CT and computation modeling in bone tissue engineering." *Computer-Aided Design* 37.11 (2005): 1151–1161.

Vannier, Michael W., et al. "Three-dimensional cranial surface reconstructions using high-resolution computed tomography." *American Journal of Physical Anthropology* 67.4 (1985): 299–311.

Waldbaur, Ansgar, et al. "Computer-aided microfluidics (CAMF): from digital 3D-CAD models to physical structures within a day." *Microfluidics and Nanofluidics* 15 (2013): 625–635.

Webb, Braeden, and Barry J. Doyle. "Parameter optimization for 3D bioprinting of hydrogels." *Bioprinting* 8 (2017): 8–12.

Weisberg, David E. "The engineering design revolution: the people, companies and computer systems that changed forever the practice of engineering." *Cyon Research Corporation* 1 (2008): 1–26.

Witowski, Jan, et al. "Investigating accuracy of 3D printed liver models with computed tomography." *Quantitative Imaging in Medicine and Surgery* 9.1 (2019): 43.

Xu, Lin, et al. "Clinical study of 3D printed personalized prosthesis in the treatment of bone defect after pelvic tumor resection." *Journal of Orthopaedic Translation* 29 (2021): 163–169.

Zhang, Zheyuan, et al. "Large-scale multi-center CT and MRI segmentation of pancreas with deep learning." *Medical Image Analysis* 99 (2025): 103382.

Zhao, Wenshuai, et al. "MSS U-Net: 3D segmentation of kidneys and tumors from CT images with a multi-scale supervised U-Net." *Informatics in Medicine Unlocked* 19 (2020): 100357.

Zhou, Yufeng. "The application of ultrasound in 3D bio-printing." *Molecules* 21.5 (2016): 590.

Zopf, David A., et al. "Computer aided–designed, 3-dimensionally printed porous tissue bioscaffolds for craniofacial soft tissue reconstruction." *Otolaryngology–Head and Neck Surgery* 152.1 (2015): 57–62.

4 Current Bioprinting Techniques and Tools

Hemant Singh, Mohammed Aldhuhoori, Muath Tuffaha, Judy Bassaleh, Rukshana Veettil, Shahd Alshehhi, Fawzi Banat, and Shabir Hassan

4.1 INTRODUCTION

Bioprinting is an advanced marvel of engineering that utilizes the concept of 3D printing to fabricate functional biological constructs naturally mimicking complex structures and functionality of biological tissues using biomaterials, living cells, and bioactive substances that can be used for tissue engineering, regenerative medicine, drug development, and disease modeling [1,2]. Bioprinting has the efficacy to precisely place different cell types in predetermined patterns, permitting scientists to reconstruct the complex structures and functionalities of native tissues or organs. Significant benefits of bioprinting include the fabrication of custom shapes and designs, the potential for high throughput, and low costs compared to traditional tissue engineering techniques [3,4].

The process of bioprinting technology mainly depends upon the many tools and techniques required pre- and post-bioprinting process, as demonstrated in Figure 4.1.

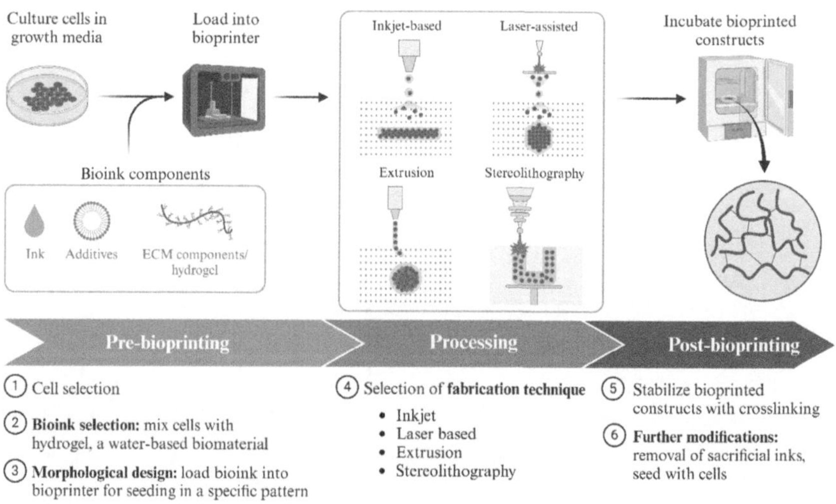

FIGURE 4.1 Schematic illustration of the basic need for bioprinting from pre-bioprinting to post-bioprinting process. (Prepared in BioRender.com.)

DOI: 10.1201/9781032638164-4

The key bioprinting techniques, including extrusion-based printing, inkjet printing, and laser-induced bioprinting, have been extensively exploited in the fabrication of tissues and organs. Each of the bioprinting techniques has an exclusive benefit and some disadvantages, depending on the desired application, such as speed, print resolution, and material compatibility [1,5]. The versatility of extrusion-based bioprinting allows for the continuous deposition of bioink at high throughput to print large constructs [6]. On the other hand, inkjet bioprinting accurately controls the droplet size with high-resolution prints [7,8].

Simultaneously, the development of bioinks is an equally important parameter that can support cell growth during and after the bioprinting process. Various types of bioinks have been introduced in the market, utilizing natural materials (e.g., gelatin and alginate) to synthetic materials (such as polyethylene glycol and polycaprolactone) [9]. Nowadays, nanomaterials and herbal compounds have also been utilized in the development of the bioinks to improve the properties such as mechanical stability, biocompatibility, expediting processing time, and bioactivity [10,11]. Anyhow, natural origin biomaterials are gaining attention in developing the bioinks due to their inherent biocompatibility and potential to promote cellular growth to tissue regeneration [12].

However, one of the most important tasks is to achieve optimal bioprintability, which leads to the essential tool of the bioprinting being the nozzles, from where bioink comes out without disrupting cell viability and maintaining the fidelity of the printed structure [13]. As the complication of bioprinted constructs increases, the requirements for precise control over cell positioning and distribution within the printed scaffold have also increased. Recent research explains the role of computational modeling and machine learning in improving printability and predicting the outcomes of bioprinting processes [3]. Therefore, interdisciplinary efforts are crucial for refining bioprinting techniques and optimizing formulations to enhance the overall effectiveness and applicability of the technology. Moreover, advancements in bioprinting have also led to the exploration of the design of smart materials. These materials can undergo programmed changes in response to environmental stimuli, allowing for dynamic modifications in shape and function post-printing [12]. This innovation holds tremendous potential for the development of self-assembling tissue constructs that could autonomously adapt to their biological environment. Despite the rapid advancements in bioprinting technology, significant hurdles remain before broader clinical application can be realized. The translation of bioprinted constructs from the laboratory to the clinic requires rigorous validation of functional outcomes, long-term stability, and regulatory compliance [2,4,9]. The complexities of scaling up bioprinting processes for commercial applications and ensuring reproducibility also pose challenges that researchers are actively addressing.

Therefore, this chapter gives an overview of bioprinting from history to current techniques and tools employed in the field today.

4.2 HISTORY OF BIOPRINTING

The history of bioprinting is marked by the invention of 3D printing (stereolithography (SLA)) technology by Charles Hull in 1984, which enabled the fabrication of 3D objects from digital data [2,4]. In the healthcare field, SLA found its initial application in crafting models for reconstructive head surgery, allowing researchers to generate exact and intricate cranium models [4]. In the same year, a student at a Texas university created an alternative technology called selective laser sintering (SLS), which utilized lasers to bond powder particles together [1]. The first demonstration of bioprinting occurred in 1988 when scientists utilized a conventional Hewlett-Packard inkjet printer to apply cells employing cytoscribing technology [4]. In 1989, another technique was patented for fused deposition modeling at the company Stratasys. This technique entailed heating and extruding plastic or metal through a nozzle. Also, in the same year, the Massachusetts Institute of Technology introduced 3D printing techniques, which involved applying a binding solution extruded onto a powder bed by modifying an inkjet printer. This technique later became known as the binder jetting method [1]. In 1999, laser-assisted bioprinting for placing living cells for the development of analogs with complicated anatomy was introduced [4].

The practical origin of bioprinting can be attributed to Thomas Boland's team in 2000 at Clemson University, which pioneered the development of the initial bioprinter. Subsequent enhancements in both the equipment and the formulation of bioinks enabled the placement of cells within denser biological hydrogels, facilitating the creation of 3D structures. Likewise, the University of Missouri devised an alternative bioprinting technique by arranging individual cell spheroids in specific patterns. Once the spheroids were positioned, they underwent fusion during cultivation, leading to the formation of denser tissues [14]. In 2001, the direct printing of a scaffold resembling a bladder shape and the subsequent seeding of human cells occurred. The year after, in 2002, scientists introduced the first extrusion-based bioprinting technology, which later became known commercially as the 3D Bioplotter [3]. In 2003, Thomas Boland and his team pioneered the development of the first inkjet bioprinter by modifying a standard HP inkjet printer. In the following year, 2004, Thomas Boland and possibly Landers' team advanced to cell-loaded bioprinting using a commercial SLA printer. Concurrently, they also achieved the development of 3D tissue consisting solely of cells without any scaffold [4,13].

Furthermore, laser-assisted bioprinting is another type of bioprinting that relies on either laser direct-write or laser-induced forward transfer mechanisms. The initial use of laser-assisted bioprinting in tissue engineering was documented in 2007, detailing the bioprinting of a microarray of droplets. In the same year, Organovo, California, USA, was the first company to bring 3D bioprinting to the commercial market. Their bioprinter, known as NovoGen, utilizes piston-based extrusion for material deposition. This milestone paved the way for the establishment of several other companies, significantly increasing the availability of 3D bioprinting for commercial use [2]. Furthermore, RegenHu, established in Switzerland in 2007, specializes in extrusion-based 3D bioprinter systems known as the Biofactory. Similarly, Envision-Tec, traditionally a manufacturer of standard 3D printers, has developed its 3D-Bioplotter system. EnvisionTec and RegenHu offer advanced bioprinter systems to researchers, empowering them to fabricate their tissue constructs [14]. In 2009, Norotte et al. utilized bioprinting to engineer vascular tissue without the need for scaffolds [4]. In Japan in 2011, Cyfuse utilized the Kenzen method, which involves supporting spheroids with a needle array, to assemble 3D structures [14]. In 2014, advancements were made in tissue integration with the circulatory system. In 2015, researchers employed coaxial technology to fabricate tubular structures. In 2016, scientists utilized rapid continuous optical 3D printing and in the same year, created a cartilage model using an integrated tissue-organ printer [4]. In 2019, researchers developed a miniature perfusable heart model. After that, bioprinted human hearts made of collagen at different scales were produced using the freeform reversible embedding of suspended hydrogels (FRESH) technology [4]. In 2020, 3D printers were employed to manufacture personalized medications tailored to individual patients' needs [1].

Recently, scientists have initiated the creation of bioinks that exhibit greater dynamism post-bioprinting. These bioinks belong to a distinct category of biomaterials termed 4D biomaterials, which alter their properties over time or in response to stimuli. Primarily, these 4D materials can undergo folding or shape alteration triggered by environmental factors like pH, light, or osmotic pressure. This advancement holds significance in tissue engineering by enabling scaffold materials to interact dynamically with the enclosed cells without requiring external intervention [14]. Since then, advancements in bioprinting have expanded significantly, leading to a wide range of applications within the healthcare field. A brief overview of some important historical timelines of bioprinting technology is provided concisely in Figure 4.2.

4.3 BIOPRINTING TOOLS

4.3.1 Bioinks

Bioinks are materials used in the fabrication of engineered tissue constructs through 3D bioprinting. They are mainly comprised synthetic or naturally derived biopolymer hydrogels, termed biomaterials, and cells. The biomaterials act as carriers that envelope the cells along with other bioink components—growth factors (GFs) and other bioactive molecules—which work to ensure cell survival and proliferation [15]. The precise physicochemical properties of bioinks—their chemical composition and mechanical properties—dictate the printability, cell viability, biocompatibility, and structural integrity of the resulting construct. Printability defines the ink's compatibility with the decided printing method while maintaining acceptable print fidelity, the material's accuracy in portraying in the lab, and the intended design of the computer-aided design (CAD) model [7,16,17]. Cell viability is a material's conduciveness to cell growth and proliferation. Biocompatibility refers to a material's lack of adverse reactions with normal tissues, i.e., low cytotoxicity and immunogenicity as well as its biodegradability under physiological conditions. Structural integrity is the material's resistance to deformation and collapse after printing. Additionally, in the context of implants, this comprises the material being a "mechanical match" to the target tissue, allowing it to assimilate into the tissue seamlessly [7,16–20]. The mechanical aspects of biomaterials will be further elaborated upon in later sections. The chosen biomaterial forms the base of the bioink to be printed. Thus, several factors must be considered, such as concentration, intended printing method, crosslinker and crosslinking behavior, swelling behavior, and application. However, the prerequisite information to all these considerations is the material's chemical composition and source [8,21–23].

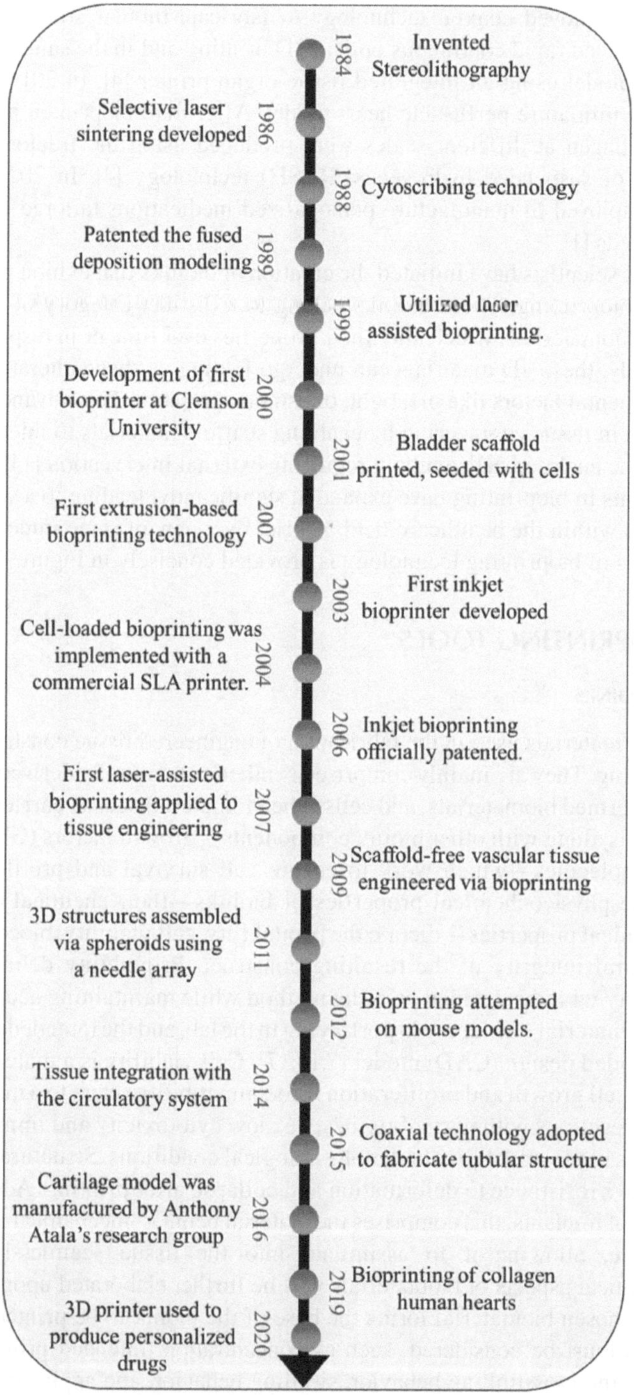

FIGURE 4.2 Some important historical timeline of bioprinting technology.

Natural bioinks are those derived from natural polymers such as collagen, gelatin, or alginate. They are typically polysaccharide or polypeptide polymers or mixtures extracted from organisms, including alginate, chitosan, gelatin, silk, and decellularized extracellular matrix (dECM) based materials [24–26]. They are advantageous in that they possess low immunogenicity, have better cell interaction and attachment due to their inherent bioactivity and their preexisting groups designed for cell–polymer interaction [1,2,5,14]. They also offer a more similar environment to the typical *in vivo* extracellular matrix (ECM), allowing their more effective integration into tissues. For example, due to the chemical similarity between dECM-based bioinks and true *in vivo* ECM, the embedded cells as well as those in the organism can modulate their interactions with the construct and even modify its composition in a similar manner to physiological ECM. This greatly improves cell–cell and cell–ECM interactions. However, natural polymer-derived bioinks are not without their disadvantages, mainly their hydrophilicity, high costs of production, and batch-to-batch inconsistencies. Furthermore, many natural polymers require crosslinkers to alleviate their lack of mechanical strength, and such crosslinkers may be cytotoxic or cause materials' properties to deviate from normal ECM behavior or composition [6,10,12].

Synthetic bioinks are, as the name suggests, made through processes of chemical synthesis. This allows greater tunability and process flexibility in these materials. Additionally, they often possess greater mechanical strength and batch consistency than natural biomaterials. Examples of synthetic polymers used in biological applications include polyethylene glycol, poly-lactic acid and polyurethane. These materials also possess greater interparticle interactions than natural materials, which imbue them with impressive print fidelity and stability against degradation. This also means that for soft tissue applications, these materials are less reliant on crosslinking [9,27–30]. However, these materials inherently lack cell adhesion sites and bioactivity, and cells need to proliferate within the interstitial spaces of these structures, limiting cell–cell communication. Furthermore, synthetic materials are typically less biodegradable, and the products of their degradation may prove toxic to cells. Due to these factors, synthetic materials are still only 10% of the polymers used in bioprinting. However, some papers have exploited the addition of Arg–Gly–Asp cell adhesion residues to improve these materials' biocompatibility. So, these materials remain relatively unexplored and have yet great growth potential in future applications [31–34].

GFs play a key role in functionalizing bioinks, influencing cellular behavior, promoting tissue regeneration, and integrating constructs with biological systems. These signaling molecules—such as fibroblast GF, vascular endothelial GF, and transforming GF-beta—are essential for controlling key cellular processes like proliferation, differentiation, vascularization, and migration. GFs enhance the bioactivity of the engineered tissue construct, promoting cellular organization and improving both structural and functional integration of the 3D-printed tissues [1,4,8,35,36].

While GFs are important for the embedded cells of the construct, another application of great importance is their controlled release into the surrounding ECM, influencing the growth of the target tissue. Their release is governed by various factors, including the bioink's degradation rate, mechanical properties, and polymer network architecture. GFs are often encapsulated within the bioink matrix, and their release can be sustained or gradual, mimicking the natural delivery of signals needed for tissue regeneration. The key to effective GF delivery lies in balancing the bioink's properties, ensuring that GFs remain bioavailable and effective over time [3,12]. For instance, bioinks made from hydrogels, such as alginate or gelatin, allow controlled release of GFs as the material gradually degrades or swells. This provides a continuous supply of growth signals to the embedded cells and surrounding tissues [4,13].

Despite their benefits, the inclusion of GFs in bioinks also poses significant challenges. These molecules are often sensitive to degradation and may lose functionality during the printing process, requiring optimized conditions to maintain their stability. Additionally, improper dosages or release profiles can lead to adverse effects such as uncontrolled tissue growth or fibrosis. To address these issues, researchers should advance biofabrication techniques, including the use of bioactive nanoparticles or encapsulation strategies should be explored [6,9,28,29].

After that, crosslinking biomaterial polymers is another critical step in bioink development. This process holds together chains of polymers to imbue the material with enhanced structural and functional properties. Crosslinking may be achieved through several modalities, including physical, chemical, thermal, and enzymatic means [21,37].

Physical crosslinking is achieved via non-covalent interactions, most commonly ionic linkages. A good example of this is the crosslinking of alginate with calcium chloride. As previously mentioned, the Ca^{2+} cations form bivalent electrostatic interactions with alginate's anionic components. This method is often used in cell encapsulation due to its high cytocompatibility. Physical crosslinking avoids the use of harsh chemicals and thus exhibits low cytotoxicity. Furthermore, this method is usually reversible under physiological conditions, allowing post-printing modifications to the construct. On the other hand, this method is often lacking in mechanical strength as electrostatic attractions and nonionic interactions in water are quite weak. While this method's low strength and reversibility may be useful for soft tissue-like constructs, those same properties may also result in uncontrolled degradation of the material [7,21,23,38].

Chemical crosslinking involves the formation of covalent bonds between polymer chains, leading to stronger and more permanent networks. A prime example is the ultraviolet (UV)-initiated crosslinking of methacrylated gelatin. In this process, a photoinitiator is activated upon exposure to UV light, catalyzing the formation of covalent bonds between methacrylate groups. This method offers high mechanical strength and is particularly useful for creating robust, load-bearing constructs [7,36,39]. This is hence often called photocrosslinking. It is worth mentioning that this is a very kinetically rapid process, which aids in print fidelity. However, the use of chemical agents like glutaraldehyde, methacrylic acid, or UV light can introduce cytotoxicity—by way of collagen calcification and reactive oxygen species (ROS) generation, respectively—especially in the case of sensitive cell-laden bioinks. While chemical crosslinking provides excellent structural integrity, its irreversibility makes post-printing adjustments challenging. Additionally, the presence of residual crosslinkers may pose biocompatibility issues if not properly removed [2,4,6,40,41].

Thermal crosslinking utilizes temperature changes to induce gelation in thermo-sensitive biomaterials. An example is collagen biomaterials; this ECM component is liquid at low temperatures (4°C) but gels at physiological temperature. This property makes collagen bioinks suitable for printing constructs that need to solidify quickly under physiological conditions. Thermal crosslinking is advantageous due to its non-toxic, reagent-free nature, which preserves cell viability. However, a major limitation is that thermally crosslinked hydrogels often lack mechanical stability, as their structures can degrade or melt when exposed to fluctuating temperatures. This makes them unsuitable for applications requiring long-term structural integrity [30–32,41].

Enzymatic crosslinking relies on specific enzymes to catalyze the formation of bonds between biopolymer chains. A common example is the use of thrombin to crosslink fibrin, forming a stable gel (thrombin converts fibrinogen to fibrin). Enzymatic crosslinking occurs under mild, physiological conditions, making it particularly biocompatible and suitable for cell-laden bioinks. This method allows for highly specific interactions, leading to precise control over the microstructure of the biomaterial. However, the resulting hydrogels tend to have lower mechanical strength compared to those formed by chemical crosslinking, which may limit their use in mechanically demanding applications. Additionally, the slower kinetics of enzymatic reactions can extend the bioprinting process and reduce print fidelity due to the risk of construct collapse during printing [34,42,43].

Dual crosslinking methods are also sometimes used when balancing cell viability and mechanical strength, such as the use of alginate–gelatin methacryloyl (GelMA) hybrids, which undergo ionic crosslinking for alginate, then UV crosslinking for GelMA. However, this approach is more complex to implement as it introduces multiple parameters to consider, which may increase the technicality and cost of bioprinting in this way [42,44,45]. After crosslinking strategies, the mechanical behavior of the fabricated bioink is the most important parameter. Rheology is the study of a material's flow properties under conditions that lead to plastic flow rather than elastic deformation. It is fundamental to bioink design in 3D bioprinting. For bioinks to be suitable for printing and use, they must exhibit specific rheological properties to ensure both print fidelity and cell viability. The key rheological parameter is viscosity, which must be optimized to balance printability and biological functionality [42,44–47]. Highly viscous bioinks provide better structural support post-printing but may lead to clogging during extrusion and reduced cell viability due to shear stress. Conversely, low-viscosity bioinks are easier to extrude but often result in poor shape fidelity and collapse after deposition. Additionally, bioinks should exhibit rapid gelation post-extrusion to maintain structural integrity. Balancing these properties is crucial for creating constructs with precise architecture and functionality [7,22,23,48].

Thixotropy, the time-dependent viscosity reduction under shear, can also play a role by allowing the bioink to flow easily during printing but to solidify quickly after extrusion, maintaining the desired shape. Thus, rheology directly impacts both the mechanical and biological outcomes of the printed constructs [7,22,23,48].

Shear thinning is a thixotropic behavior where a material's viscosity decreases as shear stress increases. This property is particularly advantageous in extrusion-based bioprinting as it allows bioinks to flow easily through the printer's nozzle under shear forces but to recover their viscosity upon deposition, providing structural stability. This flow behavior minimizes the shear forces experienced by cells, improving their survival rate during the printing process [7,22,23,48]. Hydrogels like alginate and GelMA are popular choices due to their shear-thinning properties. Moreover, shear-thinning bioinks can be precisely extruded, enhancing the resolution and accuracy of printed constructs. However, the degree of shear thinning must be carefully controlled. Excessive shear thinning can result in low mechanical stability post-printing, while insufficient shear thinning can cause nozzle clogging and print inconsistencies. A well-optimized shear-thinning profile ensures that the bioink is viscous enough to maintain its structure post-deposition while minimizing cell damage during extrusion [7,22,23,48].

Furthermore, the swelling behavior refers to a bioink's ability to absorb water or biological fluids, which can impact the mechanical stability and cell viability of the printed construct. It is critical for bioinks to maintain a balance between swelling capacity and structural integrity. Excessive swelling can compromise the mechanical properties of the scaffold, causing it to lose its intended shape and functional properties. On the other hand, controlled swelling is beneficial in applications like drug delivery or tissue engineering, where it allows for the gradual release of GFs, nutrients, or cells [7,8,23,39]. Furthermore, the loading capacity of bioinks refers to their ability to incorporate and retain biologically active molecules, such as GFs or drugs, without compromising the bioink's structural integrity. Effective loading and controlled release of these molecules can significantly enhance tissue regeneration [7,8,23,39]. However, poor control over swelling or loading may result in premature release or insufficient mechanical support, compromising the construct's functionality.

Now, the most critical parameter for a bioink is biocompatibility, which ensures bioinks support cell survival and functionality. The bioactivity of bioinks is essential for promoting cell proliferation and ensuring that printed constructs can develop into functional tissues. Bioinks must provide both biochemical cues and appropriate mechanical properties to support cell viability and proliferation. From a biochemical standpoint, bioinks must closely mimic the ECM to support cell adhesion, proliferation, and differentiation [1,2,36,40]. Furthermore, natural hydrogels such as alginate and fibrin offer bioactive cues that facilitate cell growth, while dECM-based bioinks provide essential proteins and signaling molecules for enhanced bioactivity. Additionally, incorporating GFs or peptides can further stimulate cellular activity and promote angiogenesis. Furthermore, some biomaterials may be imbued with other favorable chemical properties, such as the addition of hyaluronic acid as an antioxidant to scavenge ROS which is favorable for anti-inflammatory and wound healing applications [1,2,36,40].

Lastly, an equally important parameter is the mechanical environment provided by the bioink. The mechanical properties, particularly the viscoelastic behavior of bioinks, directly influence the cells during and after printing. Bioinks must balance between viscosity, which is crucial for printability, and elasticity, which helps maintain the structure without collapsing under its weight. For instance, hydrogels with shear-thinning properties reduce the mechanical stress on cells during extrusion, preserving their viability. However, bioinks that are too rigid may inhibit cell migration and proliferation, while excessively soft materials may fail to provide the structural support needed for tissue development [1,2,36,40].

4.3.2 Needles and Nozzles in Bioprinting

Needles and nozzles are critical components in bioprinting systems, governing the precision, resolution, and material flow during the printing process. These elements guide the deposition of bioinks, ensuring that cells, scaffolds, and biomaterials are accurately placed to form complex tissue structures. The choice of needle or nozzle significantly impacts the print fidelity, cell viability, and structural integrity of the bioprinted construct. This chapter explores the various types of needles and nozzles used in bioprinting, emphasizing their advantages and limitations [21,38,49].

Pneumatic nozzles operate by using compressed air to drive the bioink through the nozzle, making them a common choice in extrusion-based bioprinting. One of the key advantages of pneumatic nozzles is their ability to handle a wide range of bio-ink viscosities, from low-viscosity hydrogels to more viscous polymer solutions. The flexibility in viscosity range, typically between 30 and 6×10^7 mPa·s [3,13], allows for the printing of diverse bioinks with varying mechanical properties. This makes pneumatic nozzles particularly useful in applications that require both structural and bioactive components in a single construct. However, pneumatic nozzles present challenges in terms of print precision and resolution. The reliance on air pressure can lead to inconsistent extrusion rates, especially for highly viscous bioinks, resulting in poor print fidelity. Additionally, the need to carefully control air pressure introduces a degree of complexity in ensuring uniform layer deposition. While pneumatic nozzles are well-suited for large-scale bioprinting, their lower resolution limits their application in microscale tissue engineering [13,16,23]. Some of the aforementioned issues may be resolved by using mechanical (piston and screw) nozzles. These offer greater control over extrusion as the flow rate is more consistent since the variable of air compressibility is eliminated. This also allows for higher extrusion pressures, making this method ideal for printing high-viscosity bioinks, such as thermoplastic polymers and dense cell-laden hydrogels. Mechanical nozzles also allow for better modularity, with the option to employ multiple nozzles simultaneously, enabling the creation of more complex, multi-material structures. However, this system can be slower than pneumatic nozzles, and the mechanical force exerted on the bioink may cause cell damage, reducing viability in cell-laden bioinks [49,50].

Inkjet-based nozzles, a form of droplet-based bioprinting, function by ejecting small volumes of bioink in a controlled, drop-on-demand manner. These nozzles are especially useful for low-viscosity bioinks, such as hydrogels and cell suspensions, where precise deposition of small droplets is required. The main advantage of inkjet-based nozzles is their high resolution, making them ideal for printing delicate tissues and structures with intricate geometries [49,50]. Despite their high precision, inkjet-based nozzles are limited by the viscosity of bioinks they can handle. The requirement for low-viscosity bioinks (3–30 mPa·s) means that constructs printed with this method often lack mechanical strength and stability. Moreover, frequent clogging and the potential for mechanical or thermal stress on the cells during droplet ejection are common challenges associated with this method. These limitations restrict the use of inkjet nozzles in applications that require more robust or high-viscosity materials [8].

Coaxial nozzles are designed for printing multi-material constructs, allowing for the simultaneous extrusion of different bioinks through concentric nozzles.

This method is particularly advantageous for creating core–shell structures, where one bioink forms the core and the other forms the outer shell, mimicking the natural layering found in many biological tissues. Coaxial nozzles are frequently used in applications requiring complex tissue constructs, such as vascularized tissues or drug delivery systems [8]. The ability to print multiple materials at once is a significant advantage of coaxial nozzles. However, the system's complexity, particularly in balancing the flow rates and viscosities of the different bioinks, can make the process difficult to control. Additionally, as with other extrusion methods, maintaining cell viability during the extrusion of dense or highly viscous bioinks remains a challenge [8].

The size of the needle or nozzle used in bioprinting has a direct impact on print resolution, bioink flow, and cell viability. Smaller nozzles allow for higher-resolution prints, but they also increase the risk of cell damage due to higher shear stress. Larger nozzles, while reducing shear stress and enhancing cell viability, often compromise resolution and precision. Selecting the appropriate needle gauge or nozzle size requires balancing these factors based on the specific application and bioink used [21,49,50].

Bioink viscosity and flow rate are critical parameters in determining the success of a bioprinting process. High-viscosity bioinks provide structural integrity but require higher pressures or mechanical force to extrude, which can lead to nozzle clogging or cell damage. On the other hand, low-viscosity bioinks are easier to extrude but may not provide sufficient mechanical support for the printed construct. Adjusting the flow rate and extrusion pressure is essential to achieving consistent and precise prints [21,49,50].

The use of multiple nozzles allows for the simultaneous extrusion of different bioinks, enabling the creation of complex, multi-material tissue constructs. This modularity is particularly useful in applications such as organ printing or drug delivery systems, where different materials and cell types must be printed in proximity. However, synchronizing the flow rates and deposition patterns of multiple nozzles can be technically challenging, and improper coordination can lead to printing errors or compromised tissue functionality [49–51].

Most importantly, the printing resolution and precision are essential for bioprinting, and they highly depend on the choice of nozzle type, needle gauge, and bioink viscosity, all of which influence the final print resolution and precision. Inkjet-based nozzles offer the highest resolution, making them suitable for applications requiring fine detail. Pneumatic and mechanical nozzles, while less precise, are better suited for applications requiring high-viscosity bioinks and larger, more robust constructs. Optimizing resolution and precision is key to achieving a functional, biocompatible tissue construct [49–5150].

But, overall, some common challenges associated with bioprinting, like nozzle clogging, cell damage, and inconsistent extrusion, are common challenges encountered in bioprinting. Pneumatic and mechanical nozzles are prone to clogging when using high-viscosity bioinks, while inkjet nozzles may experience mechanical stress that impacts cell viability. Optimizing bioink composition, adjusting nozzle size, and carefully controlling extrusion pressure can mitigate these issues, improving the overall quality and viability of the printed constructs.

4.3.3 Software in Bioprinting

CAD software serves as a foundational tool in the bioprinting workflow, enabling the design and visualization of intricate three-dimensional models of tissues and organs [17,51]. An overview of the various software tools and their applications is shown in Figure 4.3. These advanced applications facilitate the creation of complex geometries that are essential for accurately representing the desired tissue constructs [13]. The ability to manipulate various design parameters—such as dimensions, shapes, and spatial arrangements—ensures that the final printed product meets specific structural and functional criteria. Popular CAD tools, such as AutoCAD, SolidWorks, and Blender, offer robust functionalities that allow researchers and engineers to create highly detailed models tailored for bioprinting [17,50,51]. These models not only depict the physical structure of tissues but also accommodate various bioinks and cell types, which is crucial for developing heterogeneous constructs that replicate the complexity of natural tissues. The output from CAD software acts as the blueprint for the bioprinting process, defining critical parameters that guide subsequent stages of tissue fabrication [13]. The integration of CAD software with other bioprinting systems enhances the overall efficiency of the workflow. For instance, some software packages offer features that facilitate the generation of G-code directly from the CAD model, streamlining the transition from design to printing. As tissue engineering demands grow increasingly sophisticated, the capabilities of CAD software will continue to evolve, potentially incorporating features like parametric design and real-time feedback to optimize the printing process further [1,2,36,40].

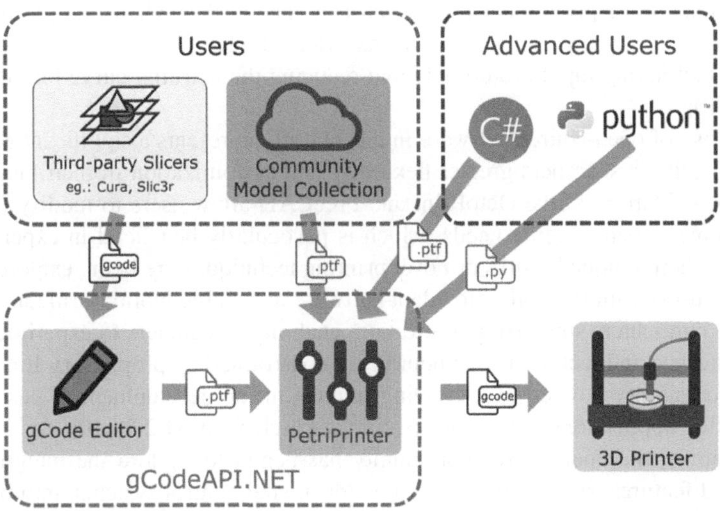

FIGURE 4.3 Overview of the various software tools and their applications. Geometrical objects can be encoded as Python or C# files, as the general use of Standard Triangle Language (.stl) files, or as a sequence of machine-specific commands (G-code). Internally, extrusion and movement commands are represented as binarized gCodeCollection objects (.ptf) that can be edited and distributed into a number of parallel Petri dishes. (From Naghieh and Chen [13].)

Following the design phase, slicing software becomes instrumental in preparing the 3D models for printing. This software converts the CAD-generated 3D models into layers and generates the G-code necessary for instructing bioprinters on how to print each layer sequentially. The precision of this conversion is critical, as it affects the mechanical properties and overall fidelity of the printed construct. Slicing software plays a vital role in defining various parameters, such as layer height, print speed, nozzle path, and temperature settings, all of which are crucial for achieving the desired structural and functional properties of the printed tissues. Widely utilized slicing tools like Cura, Repetier-Host, and Slic3r provide user-friendly interfaces that allow researchers to optimize these settings according to specific bioink characteristics and tissue requirements [1,2,36,40]. A primary challenge in using slicing software is the management of bioink deposition, particularly for materials with varying viscosities and properties. Effective slicing software must accommodate these differences, ensuring that the print settings are suitable for each specific bioink type. Advanced features such as support generation and infill strategies can also enhance the mechanical integrity of the final printed construct, ensuring that it meets the functional requirements of the intended application [1,2,36,40].

In addition to general CAD and slicing software, many bioprinter manufacturers provide proprietary software tailored to their specific machines. These manufacturer-specific platforms, such as Allevi Bioprint Online, Cellink's BioCAD, and Organovo's NovoGen Bioprinter software, come equipped with preloaded settings optimized for bioinks and cell types, streamlining the printing process for users. Such software enhances usability by integrating directly with the bioprinter's hardware, allowing for real-time monitoring and adjustments during the printing process. This capability is crucial for maintaining optimal conditions for cell viability, ensuring that bioinks are deposited accurately and consistently throughout the printing process. Moreover, many of these platforms offer templates for common tissue constructs, facilitating rapid prototyping and reducing the learning curve for new users [1,2,36,40].

The rise of open-source software in bioprinting represents a significant advancement, offering researchers greater flexibility and customization in their bioprinting workflows. Platforms like OctoPrint and FreeCAD allow users to modify the software to meet their specific needs, which is particularly beneficial in experimental settings where unique bioinks or novel printing techniques are being explored. This provides users with the ability to adapt software to specific bioink formulations and printing parameters supporting innovation, enabling researchers to experiment with new materials and techniques without being constrained by proprietary limitations. This accessibility has led to a growing interest in the development of customized bioprinting applications tailored to specific research needs [1,2,36,40].

Moreover, the open-source community has begun to explore the integration of advanced features, such as real-time monitoring and control systems, into bioprinting software. These features can provide valuable feedback during the printing process, allowing for more dynamic adjustments to optimize print quality. As the field of bioprinting continues to expand, open-source software is likely to play an increasingly crucial role in democratizing access to bioprinting technologies and fostering innovation across diverse research disciplines [17,23,51].

Despite the advancements in bioprinting software, several challenges persist. Interoperability issues between different software platforms can complicate workflows, particularly when integrating new bioinks or novel printing techniques. Ensuring compatibility between various software tools and bioprinter models remains a significant hurdle that can impact the efficiency of the bioprinting process. Additionally, as bioprinting technology continues to evolve, there is an increasing demand for sophisticated software solutions that can automate various aspects of the printing process. Future research is expected to focus on incorporating artificial intelligence into bioprinting software to allow for smarter, data-driven decision-making during the printing process. By enhancing the capabilities of software used in bioprinting, the field can achieve greater precision and efficiency, leading to more successful tissue engineering applications [1,2,36,40]. Overall, the integration of advanced software tools with bioprinting technology is essential for the continued advancement of tissue engineering. As software solutions evolve, they will undoubtedly play a critical role in improving the capabilities and applications of bioprinting, paving the way for innovative solutions in regenerative medicine and other biomedical fields.

4.4 BIOPRINTING TECHNIQUES

Bioprinting techniques are the prime component of the 3D bioprinting process. These techniques are of different types (Figure 4.4), for example, extrusion, inkjet, laser-assisted, SLA, digital light processing, and fused deposition modeling

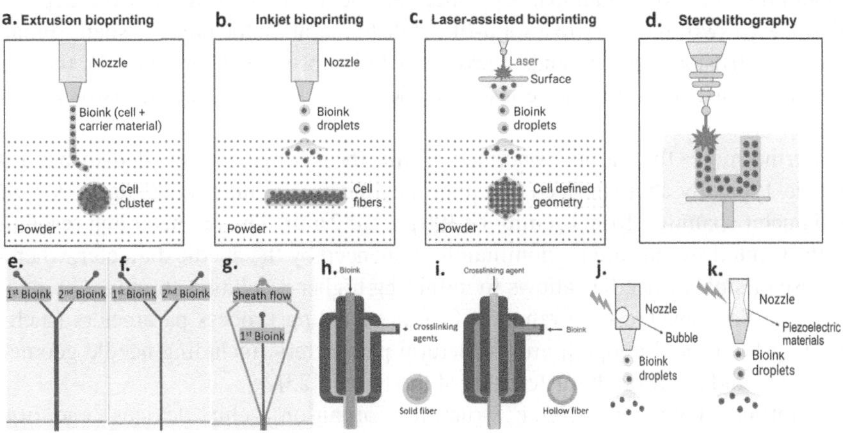

FIGURE 4.4 Basic working principles of the different bioprinters: (a) extrusion bioprinting, (b) inkjet bioprinting, (c) laser-assisted bioprinting, and (d) stereolithography. Designs of various microfluidic chips for distinct purposes: (e) parallel dispensing of bioinks, (f) quick alternate dispensing of bioinks, and (g) sheath flow surrounds the core bioink to protect the cells from shear stress; it also increases the resolution of the printed structure. Illustration of the two coaxial nozzle system arrangements: (h) printing of solid fibers by an arrangement that causes the bioink to be surrounded by the crosslinking agent, and (i) printing of hollow fibers by surrounding a crosslinking agent core with a bioink. Illustration of the two types of inkjet printing: (j) thermal inkjet printing uses heat to form bubbles that push the droplets and (k) piezoelectric printing uses a piezoelectric material that vibrates and pushes the droplets. (Made with BioRender.com.)

bioprinting, and each has unique advantageous properties and limitations that encourage its suitability for precise uses, ranging from drug delivery to tissue regeneration [1,2]. Below are some important bioprinting techniques that have been explained.

4.4.1 Extrusion Bioprinting

Extrusion bioprinting (EBP) is one of the most frequently used techniques for 3D printing. The foundation of EBP is material extrusion through a sub-millimeter aperture using syringe-driven mechanisms, air and/or pistons, as shown in Figure 4.4a, and the bioink is placed layer by layer like a filament onto a flat print surface [13,52]. An extrusion-based bioprinting system comprises a printing head, a three-axis positioning system, and a printing stage, all under the control of a computer to enable the precise deposition of materials according to 3D CAD files [3,6]. The positioning system facilitates the movement of the printing head in the X, Y, and Z directions relative to the printing stage. In contrast, the printing head dispenses the bioink loaded in the syringe onto the printing stage [23]. The selection of a bioink is often dictated by the extrusion technique employed. Currently, four distinct classes of EBP, each influencing specific design criteria for varied bioinks [16]. The first technique is direct extrusion from a nozzle, relying significantly on the non-Newtonian shear-thinning rheology of the bioink. The second technique is extrusion from a nozzle into a coagulation bath, which necessitates a rapid gelation process. The third technique is freeform reversible embedding printing, in a specialized granular or colloidal bath containing soft micro/nanoparticles that can locally fluidize around the deposited bioink with swift recovery to a solid-like state to maintain the bioink's shape. Finally, coaxial extrusion also demands a prompt gelation process. Consequently, the rheological profile and gelation kinetics of the bioinks must align with the distinct classes of EBP [16].

Furthermore, the bioink contained within the syringe is propelled through the needle, typically characterized by either a cylindrical or tapered configuration with a diameter spanning from 0.1 mm (or 100 μm) to 2 mm. The diameter and resolution of the printed strands are predominantly influenced by the needle diameter, whereby the use of smaller needles allows for attaining higher-resolution strands. The rate of flow can be impacted by a range of factors including process parameters (such as printing forces and temperature), structural parameters (including needle geometry and size), and the flow characteristics of the bioink [23].

Printing living cells, tissue structures, organ-on-a-chip devices, and organ modules have all been accomplished using this technology [16]. Extrusion 3D bioprinting offers several unique benefits, including high-cell-density bioink printing, the creation of complex three-dimensional structures with various cell types and materials, a variety of commercially accessible hardware and inks, and high cell viability [16,23].

The drawbacks of EBP include the extended time required for the printing of substantial constructs and the intricate rheological demands imposed on materials to ensure both shape fidelity and optimal cell viability. Printability represents a significant challenge in EBP. Specifically, in the bioprinting process, the bioinks, once dispensed, remain in a solution or semi-solution state, potentially leading to flow or spreading on the print bed. Consequently, the printed structure may deviate from its intended design [16,23].

There are two primary categories of EBP mechanisms distinguished by the driving force: pneumatic force (pressure-driven) systems and mechanical force (displacement-driven) systems. Pneumatic systems rely on the force generated by compressed air, utilizing pressurized air to extrude the bioink from the syringe. Conversely, mechanical systems employ pistons or auger screws to dispense the bioink directly from the material cartridge [16].

Initially, in the stages of EBP, the bioink experiences a static phase within a cylinder or syringe before extrusion (holding time), during which the embedded cells should neither sediment nor aggregate. Subsequently, the bioink must be extruded through a small orifice without subjecting the suspended cells to excessive shear, which could compromise their viability. Lastly, upon deposition, the material must promptly regain some solid-like properties to support the successive printing of layers, ensuring the preservation of macropores in the scaffold and preventing collapse under gravitational forces [22].

Crosslinking methods are crucial for retaining the material's shape after printing and promoting high cell viability. Physical crosslinking involves reversible interactions between polymer chains, while chemical crosslinking forms permanent, typically irreversible covalent bonds between polymer chains. Combinations of these strategies are also employed to leverage the advantageous properties of both approaches [22]. A study by Lee et al. used extrusion-based 3D bioprinting to print complex biological structures, such as models of human hearts at the neonatal scale, cardiac ventricles, coronary arteries, and heart valves, precisely and highly resolved. This was accomplished by utilizing the FRESH technique, which involves embedding the printed structure within a support bath [48].

4.4.2 Microfluidic Bioprinting

Microfluidic bioprinting, rather than being a distinct type of bioprinting, is better described as an enhancement of classical bioprinting techniques through the incorporation of microfluidic systems. Such inclusions facilitate an increase in the precision of printed biostructures and the easier manipulation of the bioink's flow and composition. Microfluidics is the field of technology that deals with fluids on the micron scale [53–56]. This field aims to understand how the behavior of fluids at the micron scale differs from that of normal-scale fluids and applies this knowledge in various applications such as tissue engineering (i.e., bioprinting), molecular biology (i.e., organ-on-a-chip systems), and synthetic chemistry. These differences in behavior stem from the diminished effect of gravity on fluids at this scale and the increased influence of surface tension, capillary forces, and many other factors [53–56].

The normal human tissue is governed by complex patterns involving various cell types arranged in a manner essential for the tissue's viability and function [53]. Taking human brain tissue as an example, the complexity of functional neural tissue includes, but is not limited to, interactions between two major neuronal subtypes: gamma-aminobutyric acid (GABA) interneurons and glutamatergic neurons. These subtypes need to be present in a certain ratio (in this case, 1:4) for proper function. Additionally, other cell types, such as glial cells, should be present in their proper ratios as well. Furthermore, for certain tissues, biomolecules and nutrients are present in specific gradients that are crucial for the tissue's function [53]. Therefore, printed tissue must incorporate all the complexity and specific arrangements of native tissue for optimum mimicry. However, traditional bioprinting techniques are limited in their capability to allow printing on such a scale. This limitation highlights the advantage of integrating microfluidic systems, as handling fluids on the micron scale allows increased control over the placement and organization of cells in the printed tissue [53,55].

Microfluidic systems come in a variety of forms, with the most heavily used variations in tissue engineering being microfluidic chips or coaxial nozzle systems. Microfluidic chips are structures containing a set of microchannels through which fluids flow; the advantage of this design is that multiple bioinks can flow through the chip while still having the same exit nozzle (outlet). Moreover, different purposes can be achieved based on the chip's design [53–56]. Meanwhile, a coaxial nozzle system consists of concentric needles that allow the simultaneous and separate flow of two fluids, meeting only at the extrusion point. Such a design enables the printing of fibrous structures [53–56].

The integration of microfluidic chips allows the application of various functions based on the chip's design. For example, chips with multiple fluid microchannels enable the extrusion of multiple bioinks through the same nozzle; this feature allows the printing of heterogeneous tissue structures that better mimic the native tissue's structure (Figure 4.4e and f). Additionally, other chip designs demonstrate that the advantages this technology brings to bioprinting are not just limited to the final product but also extend to the printing process itself [53–56]. A notable case arises when considering the issue of induced cell death due to the shear stress that cells experience during the printing procedure of classical bioprinting techniques. Microfluidic bioprinting can solve this problem by using a chip design that controls the fluid flow of the bioink to concentrate the cells in the middle, thus avoiding shear stress, as it mainly affects the edges of the fluid, thereby increasing cell viability (Figure 4.4g).

Furthermore, coaxial nozzle-enhanced bioprinting is mainly utilized for the production of fibrous structures. Based on the arrangement of the system's components, two types of fibers can be manufactured: solid fibers or hollow fibers [54–56]. Solid fibers are printed when the needle containing the bioink is the innermost one, while the outermost needle contains the crosslinking agent. In this way, the bioink is crosslinked from the outside inward (Figure 4.4h). Hollow fibers are printed by placing the bioink-containing needle as the outermost one and the crosslinking agent needle as the innermost one. This way, at the extrusion point, the bioink comes out surrounding a core of the crosslinking agent and starts crosslinking, resulting in a hollow fiber (Figure 4.4i). Moreover, multiple concentric needles can also be used to print fibers with multiple layers [53–56].

4.4.3 Inkjet Bioprinting

Based on the traditional technique of inkjet printing, the variant inkjet bioprinting incorporates many of its predecessor's mechanisms but replaces traditional ink with injectable biomaterials (cells, ECM, etc.) [8,35]. Specifically, among the two types of inkjet printing—continuous and drop-on-demand printing—inkjet bioprinting primarily derives from the latter. Praised for its affordability, scalability, and high resolution, inkjet bioprinting has gained momentum to become one of the most popular bioprinting techniques [8,35].

The predecessor of inkjet bioprinting, drop-on-demand inkjet printing, is one of the two types of inkjet printing [8,10,11]. The first type is known as continuous inkjet printing; as the name suggests, this type produces a continuous stream of ink droplets. Due to its operational principle, it cannot be used in a bioprinting setting, as 3D tissue models require precise placement of cells to create the heterogeneous aspect of natural tissue, which continuous inkjet printing does not provide. On the other hand, drop-on-demand inkjet printing operates by placing droplets precisely as needed, making it optimal for use in bioprinting applications [8,35]. Based on the method used to control the production of the droplets, two main versions of drop-on-demand inkjet printing exist. The first is thermal drop-on-demand (Figure 4.4j). This method uses a small printhead that is heated electrically by a resistor within a range of 200°C–300°C. The instantaneous increase in temperature causes bubbles to form, resulting in the release of a droplet from the ink. It is worth noting that the temperature increase does not cause significant damage to the cells, as it lasts for a very short period; the overall increase in temperature is only 4°C–10°C [1,8,14,35]. However, due to the small printhead, this method encounters nozzle clogs, and cells experience shear stress as they pass through. Additionally, the droplets created using this method are not uniform in size, which affects the precision of the final model [8].

The second method of drop-on-demand printing is piezoelectric printing (Figure 4.4k). This method employs a piezoelectric material lining the walls of the printhead. These materials vibrate when a voltage is applied, and the pressure from the vibration causes the droplet to be released. Furthermore, the degree of vibration is controllable based on the characteristics of the voltage pulse applied. Due to the controllable nature of the vibrations, this method allows for adjustable, precise, and uniform droplet sizes. However, if the vibrations reach a frequency between 15 and 25 kHz, the cells may experience damage to the cell wall and lysis [1,2,8].

Inkjet bioprinting is praised for its precision, effectiveness, and high resolution. These features have been demonstrated and improved multiple times in the literature. The primary goal of bioprinting is to manufacture models that are physiologically and structurally relevant to actual human tissue. Subsequently, these models can be used in pharmacology, transplantation, and other relevant applications [8]. In their paper, Madiedo-Podvrsan et al. printed a heterogeneous skin model using patterned bioprinting [57]. The study aimed to create skin lesion models similar to those seen in atopic dermatitis and ichthyosis vulgaris. The first step was to establish a proof of concept for their design by printing two groups of keratinocytes: one with green fluorescent protein (GFP) and the other without GFP. With the proof of concept showing success, they moved on to construct the skin model relevant to the aforementioned diseases by printing two subpopulations of cells—normal cells and cells with downregulated filaggrin.

Microfluidic technology encompasses the control of fluids at the microscale. The incorporation of this technology with inkjet bioprinting allows for the production of highly controlled and precise models. A study conducted by Kim et al. demonstrated the use of inkjet bioprinting in the construction of an organ-on-a-chip model [58]. The study explains that traditional lung-on-a-chip models have been limited in their ability to create thin cell layers and spatial arrangements of cells that are physiologically relevant. By using inkjet bioprinting, they successfully manufactured a micron-thick, spatially relevant lung-on-a-chip model of the alveolar membrane. The paper validated the functionality of their model by demonstrating the upregulation of genes associated with alveolar function and the presence of tight junctions.

The need for methods to achieve detailed and complex structures is ever-increasing. The development of such methods is integral to the advancement of bioprinting. To better mimic native tissue, it is necessary to use multiple bioinks (carrying different cells, extracellular matrices, etc.) in multiple printheads that work together to replicate the heterogeneity of native tissue with in vitro models. However, synchronizing the deposition of the bioinks is challenging due to inherent characteristics such as viscosity and surface tension [7]. To address this issue, Negro et al. implemented a systematic approach that focuses on optimizing printing parameters [7]. These parameters include nozzle alignment, printability of the bioink, droplet diameter, and droplet ejection speed. The study validated their concept by printing 3D models containing different bioinks.

Another challenge arises from the composition of the bioink itself. In some cases, the authenticity of the tissue model necessitates the use of reactive biomaterials [35]. These biomaterials can lose their printability and/or cytocompatibility if mixed with other components, a required step for bioink preparation in traditional bioprinting. In their paper, Christensen et al. described a method to circumvent this issue by using two intersecting printheads that release two droplets at the same location—one containing the reactive biomaterial and the other containing the remaining components. This method is referred to as printing-then-mixing. Using the same setup, they described a technique to create gradient materials by adjusting the dispensing frequencies of the printheads. One printhead (printhead A) consistently ejects its bioink, while the ejection from the other printhead (printhead B) varies based on the layer. For example, in the first layer, printhead B's ejection is high, and for each subsequent layer, the dispensing decreases; thus, the first layer has the highest concentration of the bioink from printhead B, gradually lowering in concentration with each subsequent layer.

4.4.4 Stereolithography Bioprinting

One of the earliest forms of additive manufacturing (3D printing) is the SLA printing technique, which utilizes the liquid resin polymerization to construct 3D models. When SLA is adapted for bioprinting applications, the resin is replaced by a polymerizable bioink, which contains the components needed for the tissue model (cells, ECM, etc.) along with the polymerizable components [36,40,59]. Over time, four main generations of SLA printing have developed. The first and earliest generation is laser-scanning SLA, which focuses a laser on a liquid resin to polymerize it. After polymerization, the liquid becomes solid in a specific pattern; the platform moves in the Z-axis to build additional layers, and the final construct is separated from the uncured resin [40,60]. A disadvantage of laser-scanning SLA is that the laser is used to draw the pattern needed for each layer, which can be time-consuming [60]. The second-generation, projection SLA was developed to address this issue. In this technique, a mask is added before the light hits the resin; the mask creates a specific light pattern, which is projected into the resin to create a complete layer in that pattern. The third generation is continuous SLA. The previous two generations required moving the building platform in the Z-axis and repositioning to create the construct layer by layer, which took considerable time and extended the construct's building time [59,60]. Continuous SLA was developed to build the layers continuously; this was achieved by creating a dead zone that inhibits polymerization so that the positioning of the construct can be adjusted while still exposed to the light source. The fourth generation is volumetric SLA. Instead of manufacturing constructs layer by layer, it creates 3D structures as a single unit. To achieve this, the resin is subjected to a light pattern at different angles that signify the final shape of the construct [60]. Due to its high efficiency and precision, SLA bioprinting has been used in diverse experiments. As one of the earliest methods adapted to biological settings, it has been extensively developed for various applications [40]. Ongoing research continues to explore the development of this technique. For example, Amier et al. used an SLA bioprinting approach to construct a model of the human jawbone [59,60]. The constructs were designed to consist of jawbone-derived osteoblasts and vasculature-like channels. After some time following the printing of the constructs, the cells were confirmed to express RNA- and protein-specific markers. Furthermore, the constructs demonstrated mineralization and suggested differentiation into an osteocyte phenotype.

An important factor for the authenticity of tissue models is the inclusion of vasculature-like channels [36]. Thomas et al. presented an enzymatically degradable sacrificial photoink to create these channels. The study described multiple formulations for the photoink and selected the one that exhibited optimal printing properties, degradation rates, and the production of a strong hydrogel. This research demonstrated the successful printing of a vascular model [36].

One more challenge facing SLA bioprinting is UV light as the agent for bioink polymerization, as UV irradiation has been shown to cause DNA damage [39]. To address this issue, Wang et al. developed a gelatin methacryloyl-based bioink that is crosslinkable under visible light. The fabricated bioink exhibited good cell proliferation and the formation of a 3D cellular network [39].

Since multi-material bioprinting using an SLA approach requires switching between bioinks, unwanted material mixing can occur, limiting the application of SLA in constructing heterogeneous tissues [36]. Grigoryan et al. developed a multi-material SLA approach that allows for controlled material selection and minimizes bioink mixing [61]. This was achieved by constructing a semiautomated stage containing multiple bioinks. Specifically, the bioprinting system is based on a continuous SLA setup, where the switching of bioinks occurs by lifting the building platform containing a construct made from one bioink. The construct is washed. The stage then moves along the X-axis to a different bioink, and the building platform descends into the bioink. New materials are polymerized from the selected bioink into the construct.

4.5 CONCLUSION

Bioprinting represents a transformative approach within the fields of regenerative medicine and bioengineering, using 3D printing technology with living cells to fabricate intricate biomimetic biological structures. Various studies have highlighted the potential for bioprinting to produce complex tissue constructs or organs that can be utilized for transplantation, drug testing, and disease modeling. However, the process of bioprinting mainly depends upon the many tools and techniques required in pre- and post-bioprinting processes. Each of the bioprinting techniques has an exclusive benefit and some disadvantages, such as speed, print resolution, and material compatibility, depending on the desired application. Concurrently, the development of bioinks is an equally imperative parameter that can support cell growth during and after the bioprinting process. But, one of the most important tasks is to achieve optimal bioprintability, which leads to the essential tool of the bioprinting being the nozzles from where bioink comes out without disrupting cell viability and maintaining the fidelity of the printed structure. As the complication of bioprinted constructs increases, the requirements for precise control over cell positioning and distribution within the printed scaffold have also increased. Recent research explains the role of computational modeling and machine learning in improving printability and predicting the outcomes of bioprinting processes. Therefore, interdisciplinary efforts are crucial in refining bioprinting techniques and optimizing formulations to enhance the overall effectiveness and applicability of the technology. The complexities of scaling up bioprinting processes for commercial applications and ensuring reproducibility also pose challenges that researchers need to be actively working on it addressing the challenges. For this purpose, researchers continuously explore improved materials for bioink development, technologies and methodologies, and machine learning and artificial intelligence to enhance printability, biocompatibility, and tissue function for commercialization.

ACKNOWLEDGMENTS

This work was supported by Grant Nos.: 8474000442, 8474000679, and 8474000591, from Khalifa University, Abu Dhabi, United Arab Emirates. The authors also acknowledge the kind of support from the Center for Biotechnology and Food Security and the Technology Center, Khalifa University, Abu Dhabi, United Arab Emirates. BioRender.com was used to design some of the schematics, and Grammarly software was used for proofreading of this manuscript.

ETHICS DECLARATIONS

The authors declare no competing interests.

REFERENCES

[1] V. M. Vaz and L. Kumar, "3D Printing as a Promising Tool in Personalized Medicine," *AAPS PharmSciTech*, vol. 22, no. 1, p. 49, 2021, doi: 10.1208/s12249-020-01905-8.

[2] M. A. Heinrich et al., "3D Bioprinting: from Benches to Translational Applications," *Small*, vol. 15, no. 23, p. 1805510, Jun. 2019, doi: 10.1002/smll.201805510.

[3] A. Malekpour and D. Chen, "Printability and Cell Viability in Extrusion-Based Bioprinting From Experimental, Computational, and Machine Learning Views," *J Funct Biomater*, vol. 13, no. 2, p. 40, 2022, doi: 10.3390/jfb13020040.

[4] Z. Gu, J. Fu, H. Lin, and Y. He, "Development of 3D bioprinting: From printing methods to biomedical applications," *Asian J Pharm Sci*, vol. 15, no. 5, pp. 529–557, 2020, doi: 10.1016/j.ajps.2019.11.004.

[5] H. Singh et al., "3D Printed Metamaterials: Properties, Fabrication, and Drug Delivery Applications," *Adv Drug Deliv Rev*, vol. 224, p. 115636, 2025, doi: 10.1016/j.addr.2025.115636.

[6] M. Askari, M. A. Naniz, M. Kouhi, A. Saberi, A. Zolfagharian, and M. Bodaghi, "Recent Progress in Extrusion 3D Bioprinting of Hydrogel Biomaterials for Tissue Regeneration: A Comprehensive Review With Focus on Advanced Fabrication Techniques," *Biomater Sci*, vol. 9, no. 3, pp. 535–573, 2021, doi: 10.1039/d0bm00973c.

[7] A. Negro, T. Cherbuin, and M. P. Lutolf, "3D Inkjet Printing of Complex, Cell-Laden Hydrogel Structures," *Sci Rep*, vol. 8, no. 1, p. 17099, 2018, doi: 10.1038/s41598-018-35504-2.

[8] X. Li et al., "Inkjet Bioprinting of Biomaterials," *Chem Rev*, vol. 120, no. 19, pp. 10793–10833, Oct. 2020, doi: 10.1021/acs.chemrev.0c00008.

[9] S. Liu et al., "The Cutting-edge Progress in Bioprinting for Biomedicine: Principles, Applications, and Future Perspectives," *MedComm (Beijing)*, vol. 5, no. 10, 2024, doi: 10.1002/mco2.754.

[10] X. Wang, Q. Wang, and C. Xu, "Nanocellulose-Based Inks for 3D Bioprinting: Key Aspects in Research Development and Challenging Perspectives in Applications—A Mini Review," *Bioengineering*, vol. 7, no. 2, p. 40, 2020, doi: 10.3390/bioengineering7020040.

[11] D. Yunsheng et al., "Sustained Release Ailicon from 3D Bioprinting Scaffold Using Silk/Gelatin Inks to Promote Osteogenesis," *Int J Biol Macromol*, vol. 234, p. 123659, 2023, doi: 10.1016/j.ijbiomac.2024.123659.

[12] P. D. C. Costa, D. C. S. Costa, T. R. Correia, V. M. Gaspar, and J. F. Mano, "Natural Origin Biomaterials for 4D Bioprinting Tissue-Like Constructs," *Adv Mater Technol*, vol. 6, no. 10, 2021, doi: 10.1002/admt.202100168.

[13] S. Naghieh and D. Chen, "Printability–A Key Issue in Extrusion-Based Bioprinting," *J Pharm Anal*, vol. 11, no. 5, pp. 564–579, 2021, doi: 10.1016/j.jpha.2021.02.001.

[14] P. Thayer, H. Martinez, and E. Gatenholm, "History and Trends of 3D Bioprinting," in *3D Bioprinting: Principles and Protocols*, J. M. Crook, Ed., New York, NY: Springer US, 2020, pp. 3–18. doi: 10.1007/978-1-0716-0520-2_1.

[15] P. Kumar et al., "Advances in Bioink-Based 3D Printed Scaffolds: Optimizing Biocompatibility and Mechanical Properties for Bone Regeneration," *Biomater Sci*, vol. 13, no. 10, pp. 2556–2579, 2025, doi: 10.1039/D4BM01606H.

[16] X. Cui et al., "Advances in Extrusion 3D Bioprinting: A Focus on Multicomponent Hydrogel-Based Bioinks," *Adv Healthc Mater*, vol. 9, no. 15, p. 1901648, Aug. 2020, doi: 10.1002/adhm.201901648.

[17] M. Gulyas, M. Csiszer, E. Mehes, and A. Czirok, "Software Tools for Cell Culture-Related 3D Printed Structures," *PLoS One*, vol. 13, no. 9, pp. e0203203-, Sep. 2018, doi: 10.1371/journal.pone.0203203

[18] H. Singh et al., "Technological Interventions Enhancing Curcumin Bioavailability in Wound-Healing Therapeutics," *Tissue Eng Part B Rev*, vol. 30, no. 2, pp. 230–253, 2024.

[19] H. Singh et al., "Dual Cross-Linked Gellan Gum/Gelatin-Based Multifunctional Nanocomposite Hydrogel Scaffold for Full-Thickness Wound Healing," *Int J Biol Macromol*, vol. 251, p. 126349, 2024.

[20] H. Singh et al., "Multicomponent Decellularized Extracellular Matrix of Caprine Small Intestine Submucosa Based Bioactive Hydrogel Promoting Full-Thickness Burn Wound Healing in Rabbits," *Int J Biol Macromol*, vol. 255, p. 127810, 2024.
[21] Y. B. Pottathara and V. Kokol, "Effect of Nozzle Diameter and Cross-linking on the Micro-structure, Compressive and Biodegradation Properties of 3D Printed Gelatin/Collagen/Hydroxyapatite Hydrogel," *Bioprinting*, vol. 31, Jun. 2023, doi: 10.1016/j.bprint.2023.e00266.
[22] M. E. Cooke and D. H. Rosenzweig, "The Rheology of Direct and Suspended Extrusion Bioprinting," *APL Bioeng*, vol. 5, no. 1, p. 011502, Feb. 2021, doi: 10.1063/5.0031475.
[23] X. B. Chen et al., "Biomaterials/Bioinks and Extrusion Bioprinting," *Bioact Mater*, vol. 28, pp. 511–536, 2023, doi: 10.1016/j.bioactmat.2024.06.006.
[24] H. Singh et al., "Nanoceria Laden Decellularized Extracellular Matrix-Based Curcumin Releasing Nanoemulgel System for Full-Thickness Wound Healing," *Biomater Adv*, vol. 137, p. 212806, 2022.
[25] Z. Darban et al., "β-Carotene Laden Antibacterial and Antioxidant Gelatin/Polyglyceryl Stearate Nano-Hydrogel System for Burn Wound Healing Application," *Int J Biol Macromol*, vol. 255, p. 128019, 2024.
[26] H. Singh et al., "Pathophysiology to Advanced Intra-Articular Drug Delivery Strategies: Unravelling Rheumatoid Arthritis," *Biomaterials*, vol. 303, p. 122390, 2024.
[27] Y. Ren, "3D Bioprinting for Engineering Organoids and Organ-on-a-Chip: Developments and Applications," *Med Res Rev*, 2025, doi: 10.1002/med.22121.
[28] E. M. Sánchez et al., "Hydrogels for Bioprinting: A Systematic Review of Hydrogels Synthesis, Bioprinting Parameters, and Bioprinted Structures Behavior," *Front Bioeng Biotechnol*, vol. 8, 2020, doi: 10.3389/fbioe.2020.00776.
[29] T. Genova, I. Roato, M. Carossa, C. Motta, D. Cavagnetto, and F. Mussano, "Advances on Bone Substitutes Through 3D Bioprinting," *Int J Mol Sci*, vol. 21, no. 19, p. 7012, 2020, doi: 10.3390/ijms21197012.
[30] Y. Wu, M. Qin, and X. Yang, "Organ Bioprinting: Progress, Challenges and Outlook," *J Mater Chem B*, vol. 11, no. 43, pp. 10263–10287, 2023, doi: 10.1039/d3tb01630g.
[31] L. Mendoza-Cerezo, J. M. Rodríguez-Rego, A. Macías-García, A. C. Marcos-Romero, and A. Díaz-Parralejo, "Evolution of Bioprinting and Current Applications," *Int J Bioprint*, vol. 9, no. 4, p. 742, 2023, doi: 10.18063/ijb.742.
[32] Q. Ramadan and M. Zourob, "3D Bioprinting at the Frontier of Regenerative Medicine, Pharmaceutical, and Food Industries," *Front Med Technol*, vol. 2, 2021, doi: 10.3389/fmedt.2020.607648.
[33] M. Rea et al., "Establishing a Bioink Assessment Protocol: GelMA and Collagen in the Bioprinting of a Potential *In Vitro* Intestinal Model," *ACS Biomater Sci Eng*, vol. 11, no. 4, pp. 2456–2467, 2025, doi: 10.1021/acsbiomaterials.5c00034.
[34] C. Mota, S. Camarero-Espinosa, M. B. Baker, P. Wieringa, and L. Moroni, "Bioprinting: From Tissue and Organ Development to *in Vitro* Models," *Chem Rev*, vol. 120, no. 19, pp. 10547–10607, 2020, doi: 10.1021/acs.chemrev.9b00789.
[35] K. Christensen, A. Compaan, W. Chai, G. Xia, and Y. Huang, "In Situ Printing-then-Mixing for Biological Structure Fabrication Using Intersecting Jets," *ACS Biomater Sci Eng*, vol. 3, no. 12, pp. 3687–3694, Dec. 2017, doi: 10.1021/acsbiomaterials.7b00752.
[36] A. Thomas et al., "Vascular Bioprinting with Enzymatically Degradable Bioinks via Multi-material Projection-Based Stereolithography," *Acta Biomater*, vol. 117, pp. 121–132, 2020, doi: 10.1016/j.actbio.2020.09.034.
[37] L. B. Bebiano, R. Presa, L. Fernandes, B. N. Lourenço, O. Chaudhuri, and R. F. Pereira, "Bioinks with Varying Densities of Physical and Chemical Crosslinks Modulate Cellular Responses in 3D by Altering the Viscoelasticity of the Cell Microenvironment," *Materials Today*, vol. 86, pp. 146–161, 2025, doi: 10.1016/j.mattod.2025.03.019.

[38] S. Jentsch, R. Nasehi, C. Kuckelkorn, B. Gundert, S. Aveic, and H. Fischer, "Multiscale 3D Bioprinting by Nozzle-Free Acoustic Droplet Ejection," *Small Methods*, vol. 5, no. 6, Jun. 2021, doi: 10.1002/smtd.202000971.

[39] Z. Wang et al., "Visible Light Photoinitiation of Cell-Adhesive Gelatin Methacryloyl Hydrogels for Stereolithography 3D Bioprinting," *ACS Appl Mater Interfaces*, vol. 10, no. 32, pp. 26859–26869, Aug. 2018, doi: 10.1021/acsami.8b06607.

[40] H. K. Park, M. Shin, B. Kim, J. W. Park, and H. Lee, "A Visible Light-Curable yet Visible Wavelength-Transparent Resin for Stereolithography 3D Printing," *NPG Asia Mater*, vol. 10, no. 4, pp. 82–89, 2018, doi: 10.1038/s41427-018-0021-x.

[41] M. Yeo, A. Sarkar, Y. P. Singh, İ. D. Derman, P. Datta, and İ. T. Özbolat, "Synergistic Coupling Between 3D Bioprinting and Vascularization Strategies," *Biofabrication*, vol. 16, no. 1, p. 012003, 2023, doi: 10.1088/1758-5090/ad0b3f.

[42] M. Palo, H. Jenny, S. Jaakko, Y. Jouko, and N. and Sandler, "3D Printed Drug Delivery Devices: Perspectives and Technical Challenges," *Expert Rev Med Devices*, vol. 14, no. 9, pp. 685–696, Sep. 2017, doi: 10.1080/17434440.2017.1363647.

[43] R. Levato, J. Visser, J. A. Planell, E. Engel, J. Malda, and M. A. Mateos-Timoneda, "Biofabrication of Tissue Constructs by 3D Bioprinting of Cell-Laden Microcarriers," *Biofabrication*, vol. 6, no. 3, p. 035020, 2014, doi: 10.1088/1758-5082/6/3/035020.

[44] H.-G. Yi, H. Kim, J. Kwon, Y.-J. Choi, J. Jang, and D.-W. Cho, "Application of 3D Bioprinting in the Prevention and the Therapy for Human Diseases," *Signal Transduct Target Ther*, vol. 6, no. 1, p. 177, 2021, doi: 10.1038/s41392-021-00566-8.

[45] Y. Jiang and Y. Li, "3D Printed Auxetic Mechanical Metamaterial with Chiral Cells and Re-entrant Cores," *Sci Rep*, vol. 8, no. 1, p. 2397, 2018, doi: 10.1038/s41598-018-20795-2.

[46] J. Chen et al., "3D Bioprinted Multiscale Composite Scaffolds Based on Gelatin Methacryloyl (GelMA)/Chitosan Microspheres as a Modular Bioink for Enhancing 3D Neurite Outgrowth and Elongation," *J Colloid Interface Sci*, vol. 574, pp. 162–173, 2020, doi: 10.1016/j.jcis.2020.04.040.

[47] Y. Yang et al., "Photocrosslinkable Nanocomposite Ink for Printing Strong, Biodegradable and Bioactive Bone Graft," *Biomaterials*, vol. 263, p. 120378, 2020, doi: 10.1016/j.biomaterials.2020.120378.

[48] A. Lee et al., "3D Bioprinting of Collagen to Rebuild Components of the Human Heart," *Science*, vol. 365, no. 6452, pp. 482–487, Aug. 2019, doi: 10.1126/science.aav9051.

[49] K. Yao, K. Guo, H. Wang, and X. Zheng, "Multi-Nozzles 3D Bioprinting Collagen/Thermoplastic Elasto-Mer Scaffold with Interconnect Pores," *Micromachines*, vol. 16, no. 4, Apr. 2025, doi: 10.3390/mi16040429.

[50] J. C. G. Blanco et al., "Optimising Bioprinting Nozzles through Computational Modelling and Design of Experiments," *Biomimetics*, vol. 9, no. 8, p. 460, Aug. 01, 2024, doi: 10.3390/biomimetics9080460.

[51] R. Chand, B. S. Muhire, and S. Vijayavenkataraman, "Computational Fluid Dynamics Assessment of the Effect of Bioprinting Parameters in Extrusion Bioprinting," *Int J Bioprint*, vol. 8, no. 2, pp. 45–60, 2022, doi: 10.18063/ijb.v8i2.545.

[52] W. Liu et al., "Rapid Continuous Multimaterial Extrusion Bioprinting," *Adv Mater*, vol. 29, no. 3, p. 1604630, Jan. 2017, doi: 10.1002/adma.201604630.

[53] E. Davoodi et al., "Extrusion and Microfluidic-Based Bioprinting to Fabricate Biomimetic Tissues and Organs," *Adv Mater Technol*, vol. 5, no. 8, p. 1901044, Aug. 01, 2020, doi: 10.1002/admt.201901044.

[54] Y. S. Zhang et al., "3D Extrusion Bioprinting," *Nat Rev Methods Primers*, vol. 1, no. 1, p. 75, Dec. 01, 2021, doi: 10.1038/s43586-021-00073-8.

[55] D. N. du Chatinier, K. P. Figler, P. Agrawal, W. Liu, and Y. S. Zhang, "The Potential of Microfluidics-Enhanced Extrusion Bioprinting," *Biomicrofluidics*, vol. 15, no. 4, p. 041304, Jul. 01, 2021, doi: 10.1063/5.0033280.

[56] M. Filippi, T. Buchner, O. Yasa, S. Weirich, and R. K. Katzschmann, "Microfluidic Tissue Engineering and Bio-Actuation," *Adv Mater*, vol. 34, no. 23, p. e2108427, Jun. 01, 2022, doi: 10.1002/adma.202108427.
[57] S. Madiedo-Podvrsan et al., "Utilization of Patterned Bioprinting for Heterogeneous and Physiologically Representative Reconstructed Epidermal Skin Models," *Sci Rep*, vol. 11, no. 1, p. 6217, 2021, doi: 10.1038/s41598-021-85553-3.
[58] W. Kim, Y. Lee, D. Kang, T. Kwak, H.-R. Lee, and S. Jung, "3D Inkjet-Bioprinted Lung-on-a-Chip," *ACS Biomater Sci Eng*, vol. 9, no. 5, pp. 2806–2815, May 2023, doi: 10.1021/acsbiomaterials.3c00089.
[59] W. Li, M. Wang, H. Ma, F. A. Chapa-Villarreal, A. O. Lobo, and Y. S. Zhang, "Stereolithography Apparatus and Digital Light Processing-Based 3D Bioprinting for Tissue Fabrication," *iScience*, vol. 26, no. 2, p. 106039, 2023, doi: 10.1016/j.isci.2023.106039.
[60] J. Huang, Q. Qin, and J. Wang, "A Review of Stereolithography: Processes and Systems," *Processes*, vol. 8, no. 9, p. 1138, Sep. 01, 2020, doi: 10.3390/PR8091138.
[61] B. Grigoryan et al., "Development, Characterization, and Applications of Multi-Material Stereolithography Bioprinting," *Sci Rep*, vol. 11, no. 1, p. 3171, 2021, doi: 10.1038/s41598-021-82102-w.

5 Information Technology toward Bioprinting

Juliano Marcello,
Paulo Henrique Junqueira Amorim,
Arthur Schimith,
Leonardo Mendes Ribeiro Machado,
Paula Midori Kaneko, Marcília Valéria Guimarães,
Pedro Yoshito Noritomi,
and Rodrigo Alvarenga Rezende

5.1 INTRODUCTION

With the evolution of additive manufacturing (AM) processes—meaning the development of new manufacturing techniques, biomaterials, and IT as a whole—new ideas have emerged, such as the bioprinting of human tissues and organs, or simply 3D bioprinting.

3D bioprinting, also widely known in its early days as "Organ Printing," emerged at the beginning of this century from bold ideas by scientists who adapted paper (2D) printers into a mechanism that "gained" the third dimension, thus enabling the possibility of three-dimensional constructions.

The term "organ printing," on the other hand, first appeared in 2003 and was defined as "a rapid prototyping computer-aided 3D printing technology, based on using layer-by-layer deposition of cells and/or cell aggregates into a 3D gel with sequential maturation of the printed construct into perfused and vascularized living tissue or organs" (Mironov et al., 2003).

One of the pioneers of bioprinting, scientist Thomas Boland from the University of Texas at El Paso, United States, together with his team, began developing the first known bioprinting technique, called "inkjet printing," in which cells could be robotically manipulated for tissue engineering (Wilson and Boland, 2003; Boland et al., 2003). Boland et al. (2006) demonstrated how modified inkjet printers could deposit living cells with high spatial precision, preserving their viability. Boland's advances laid the foundation for research lines and the development of commercial bioprinters that still use inkjet principles or derivatives of the technique today.

In all developments in bioprinting, information technology (IT) has always been directly or indirectly associated. A 3D (bio)printer only operates automatically if there are well-established and embedded algorithms, codes, programs, and firmware—in other words, software—that control the hardware for proper operation. Other software is constantly used, for example, in the processing of medical images,

DOI: 10.1201/9781032638164-5

in the generation of an anatomical design, in process optimization, and in computational simulations.

The concept of IT is very broad. The National Institute of Standards and Technology (NIST, 2025) defines IT as "any equipment or interconnected system or subsystem of equipment that is used in the automatic acquisition, storage, manipulation, management, movement, control, display, switching, interchange, transmission, or reception of data or information by the executive agency."

Murphy and Atala (2014) defined IT in bioengineering as "the use of computational systems, mathematical modeling, simulations, medical image processing, and digital control to design, optimize, and manage complex biomedical processes, such as 3D bioprinting." Rezende et al. (2015) stated that IT is an integral part of bioprinting and that IT gradually transforms many fields related to 3D bioprinting.

Bioprinting is defined as computer-aided, additive, layer-by-layer robotic biofabrication of functional 3D organ constructs using tissue spheroids and based on a digital model (Rezende et al., 2015).

According to Moroni et al. (2018a), bioprinting is "the use of computer-aided transfer processes for patterning and assembly of living and non-living materials with a prescribed 2D or 3D organization to produce bioengineered structures."

3D bioprinting involves the precise, layer-by-layer deposition of biological and biochemical materials and living cells to fabricate 3D biological structures with multiple components and functional, structural, and mechanical properties (Lam et al., 2023).

3D bioprinting offers repeatability, reproducibility, controllability, and high-throughput, enabling the production of personalized devices with continuous and stable biological patterns (Wu et al., 2023).

Printing conditions—such as nozzle orifice, print speed, temperature, and layer thickness—can vary and significantly impact cell survival and construct fidelity, requiring parameter optimization (Wu et al., 2023), which can be addressed through techniques such as genetic algorithms, particle swarm optimization, ant colony optimization, and machine learning (ML), among others.

The relationship between IT and bioprinting unfolds along multiple dimensions, including the planning, operation, and control of equipment (bioprinters, bioreactors, sensors, digital scanners, and devices in general); prototype design; digital modeling; structural geometry optimization; process optimization (encompassing materials, techniques, and cells); data storage and security; computational simulations; and AI-driven sophistication. IT transforms bioprinting from an experimental technique into a precise, personalized, and integrated technology that links data, modeling, printing, and clinical validation in a single digital chain.

5.1.1 Biofabrication and Bioprinting: Concepts

Biofabrication is an umbrella term encompassing a set of advanced technologies for producing complex biological structures, from tissues and organs to biomedical devices. This may involve a variety of processes, such as cellular self-assembly, additive manufacturing (e.g., bioprinting), and tissue-culture techniques in bioreactors. Its primary objective is to replicate the complexity and functionality of biological systems for research, drug testing, and ultimately therapeutic applications (Murphy and Atala, 2014; Groll et al., 2018).

The International Society for Biofabrication (ISBF) published an article intended as a reference guide for the biofabrication community, comprising terminology across different technologies (Moroni et al., 2018b). In this guide, the term "Biofabrication" was defined as "the automated generation of biologically functional products with structural organization from living cells, bioactive molecules, biomaterials, cell aggregates such as microtissues, or hybrid cell-material constructs, through bioprinting or bio assembly and subsequent tissue maturation processes."

Biofabrication and bioprinting represent a quantum leap in the human ability to create and repair biological tissues. Although often used interchangeably, these two disciplines have important nuances. Within biofabrication, bioprinting stands out as an additive manufacturing technology rooted in conventional 3D printing but with a fundamental distinction: it employs biological materials—such as living cells and biomaterials (hydrogels, biocompatible polymers)—to build three-dimensional structures layer by layer. The process involves the precise deposition of "bioinks"—a mixture of cells and biomaterials—according to a digital design, resulting in biological constructs that mimic the architecture and physiology of natural tissues and organs. Bioprinting offers unprecedented control over cellular deposition and structure geometry, paving the way for personalized tissue engineering and more accurate disease models (Mandrycky et al., 2016; Ozbolat and Hospodiuk, 2016).

5.1.2 IT for Biofabrication and Bioprinting

According to the Gartner report, IT comprises a myriad of information-processing technologies, including software, hardware, communications technologies, and related services, excluding embedded technologies that do not generate data for general use. The same consultancy explicitly classifies 3D printing and bioprinting as branches of IT (Gartner, 2025).

IT is not merely an auxiliary tool in biofabrication and bioprinting; it is a fundamental, transversal pillar permeating all phases of the process, propelling biomedical innovation to new heights. From design and conception to optimization and validation, IT empowers scientists and engineers to translate complex ideas into biological reality (Gu et al., 2020).

First, the design and modeling of complex biological structures would be impossible without advanced Computer-Aided Design (CAD) and Computer-Aided Engineering software (Dernowsek et al., 2017a). These systems enable the creation of detailed 3D models of tissues and organs, incorporating precise anatomical and physiological information. The ability to simulate the behavior of cells and biomaterials prior to printing saves considerable time and resources (Melchiorri and Fischer, 2018).

IT is equally crucial for the management and analysis of massive datasets. Biofabrication generates huge amounts of data, from high-resolution microscopy images to process parameters and functional test results. The use of Big Data analytics and artificial intelligence (AI), including ML, enables pattern identification, protocol optimization, prediction of the viability of biological constructs, and even treatment personalization based on patient data (Jung et al., 2020; Ribas and Morais, 2022).

Process automation and control are also driven by IT. Bioprinters and bioreactors are complex systems that require precise control of temperature, pH, nutrient flow, and material deposition. Integrated control software ensures reproducibility and consistency, minimizes human error, and optimizes production efficiency (Hospodiuk and Ozbolat, 2017).

Therefore, IT is very important for knowledge dissemination. Online platforms, shared databases, and data-visualization tools facilitate interaction among researchers from different disciplines and institutions, accelerating discovery and innovation in biofabrication and bioprinting (Gu et al., 2020).

The next sections present some important topics about the relationship between bioprinting and IT.

5.2 MEDICAL IMAGES

Medical imaging technologies can be employed to customize implants according to the dimensions and shapes of the patient's defect site (Wu et al., 2023) and to provide fundamental support for developing a blueprint for bioprinting.

5.2.1 Acquisition

To enable the bioprinting of an anatomical part, it is first necessary to obtain the geometry of the tissue to be replicated. Since most tissues are internal to the body, three-dimensional medical imaging techniques must be used, such as computed tomography (CT), magnetic resonance imaging (MRI), and ultrasound (US) (Dernowesk et al., 2017b).

CT (Withers et al., 2021) uses X-rays to differentiate anatomical regions based on each tissue's ability to attenuate X-ray beams. The CT scanner features a gantry ring containing an examination table that moves during the scan while the patient remains stationary. The gantry houses oppositely aligned X-ray emitters and detectors. As the table advances through the ring, the gantry rotates around both the table and the patient, performing a complete scan of the region of interest. The acquired signals (known as a sinogram) undergo processing through reconstruction algorithms such as filtered backprojection or iterative methods. These algorithms reconstruct the spatial distribution of attenuation coefficients, generating tomographic images in Hounsfield units (HU), a quantitative scale measuring radiodensity relative to water (0 HU) and air (−1000 HU). To create three-dimensional images, individual tomographic slices are stacked according to their acquisition spacing. CT's primary advantages include rapid acquisition speed, high anatomical resolution, and the capability for 3D reconstructions. The main disadvantages are patient exposure to ionizing radiation and limited soft tissue contrast.

MRI (Minhas and Oliver, 2022) utilizes strong magnetic fields and radiofrequency (RF) waves to generate 2D or 3D images of internal body structures. The MRI scanner features a cylindrical bore, into which the patient is advanced on a motorized examination table. This technique exploits the resonance phenomenon of hydrogen nuclei (protons) found in bodily water and fat molecules. When tissue is exposed to a powerful magnetic field, the spins of hydrogen protons align with the field. Spin is a quantum property describing a particle's angular momentum (Bass, 2005). Following alignment, targeted RF pulses disrupt this orientation. When the pulses cease, the protons return to their original state, releasing energy as electromagnetic signals. These signals are detected by specialized receiver coils and processed through computational algorithms to create grayscale images.

There are several MRI modalities available, including structural MRI with T1, T2, and FLAIR weightings that enable anatomical assessment and lesion identification, diffusion MRI which visualizes nerve fiber connections (diffusion tensor imaging, DTI) and water movement patterns (diffusion-weighted imaging, DWI), as well as functional MRI, perfusion MRI, and others. The main advantages of MRI are the absence of ionizing radiation and its excellent soft tissue contrast, particularly for the brain, muscles, and ligaments. On the other hand, its disadvantages include lengthy image acquisition times, restrictions for claustrophobic patients due to the relatively narrow bore diameter, and incompatibility for patients with pacemakers or ferromagnetic prosthetics, who cannot undergo MRI examinations (Dill, 2008).

US is an imaging technique that uses high-frequency sound waves to create images (Ortiz et al., 2012). The system includes a transducer that the technician glides and applies gentle pressure over the area of interest. Depending on the device, the transducer contains one or multiple piezoelectric crystals that are special materials that vibrate when an electrical current is applied, producing ultrasonic waves. These same materials exhibit the reverse piezoelectric effect: when mechanical vibrations occur, they generate electrical currents. The technique works by directing high-frequency sound waves toward the area of interest, where they are either absorbed or reflected. The reflected waves (echoes) are captured by the transducer and converted into electrical signals. These signals undergo noise-reduction processing before being transformed into diagnostic images. Many modern transducers incorporate Doppler mode, which analyzes frequency shifts between transmitted and returning sound waves to evaluate blood flow patterns. While most US systems produce conventional 2D images, specialized transducers can generate detailed 3D reconstructions, particularly valuable in obstetrics, cardiology, urology, musculoskeletal, and surgical guidance (Huang and Zeng, 2017). The technique offers significant advantages: it uses no ionizing radiation, and the equipment is generally more affordable and portable compared to CT or MRI systems. However, US does have limitations, including poor visualization of air-filled structures (like lungs) and bone tissue, along with greater susceptibility to image artifacts.

5.2.2 Medical Image Storage and Processing

Medical imaging exams are typically saved in the Digital Imaging and Communications in Medicine (DICOM) (NEMA, 2025) format, which enables interoperability between different equipment and software. In addition to being an image format, DICOM is also a communication protocol used for transmitting information between imaging acquisition devices and image servers, also known as Picture Archiving and Communication System (PACS). There are various PACS solutions available, ranging from proprietary systems to open-source options such as DCM4CHEE (Warnock et al., 2007) and Orthanc (Jodogne, 2018).

In the case of DICOM-format images, in addition to the visual information in the form of pixels, they also contain metadata such as the patient's name, the physician's name, the brand and model of the imaging equipment used, and information necessary for 3D image reconstruction, including pixel dimensions, slice thickness, and spatial position of the slices.

Currently, there are numerous software tools available for processing and analyzing medical images. These range from free and open-source solutions such as 3D Slicer (Fedorov et al., 2012), InVesalius (Amorim et al., 2015), and ITK-SNAP (Yushkevich et al., 2019), to proprietary software like Amira-Avizo 3D (Thermo Fisher Scientific), Analyze (Mayo Clinic), and Mimics (Materialise).

For bioprinting purposes, the most important features of these software tools are segmentation methods, as well as the generation and export of triangular meshes for 3D printing. Segmentation allows the isolation of a region of interest within an image. There are manual segmentation methods, in which the user selects the desired area pixel by pixel. There are semiautomatic methods, which require setting parameters such as growth seeds. Finally, AI-based methods, capable of performing segmentation automatically.

Once segmentation is completed, a triangular mesh can be generated typically using the marching cubes (Lorensen and Cline, 1998) algorithm, or a derivative such as marching tetrahedra (Treece et al., 1999) or dual contouring (Ju et al., 2002). The triangular mesh is then exported, usually in STL (stereolithography) format, which is the de facto standard in the 3D printing field and is widely supported by both printing equipment and software. Figure 5.1 shows the main steps for generating a 3D model from the patient's anatomy for bioprinting.

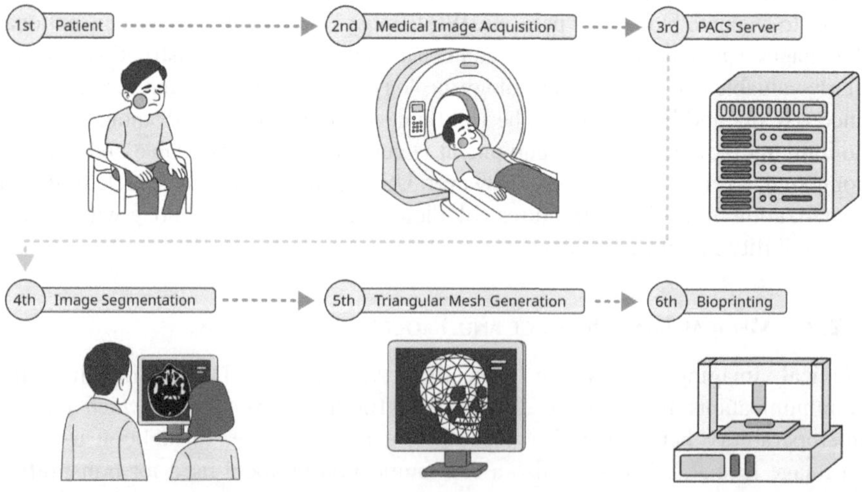

FIGURE 5.1 Model generation flow for bioprinting. (The authors.)

5.3 COMPUTER SIMULATIONS

According to Dernowesk et al. (2017b), the most logical approach to construct a complex human organ is first to specify it virtually and conduct *in silico* simulations. The use of CAD in bioprinting has revolutionized the way tissue scaffolds and anatomical 3D structures are conceived, enabling precise modeling of biological structures and facilitating the creation of constructs adapted to both anatomical and functional requirements (Mikaeeli Kangarshahi et al., 2024). Through CAD, complex scaffold architectures can be digitally designed with controlled porosity, spatial gradients, and geometrical features that support tissue regeneration (Egan, 2019). This capability is further enhanced by the incorporation of metamaterial concepts, which allow for the design of architected scaffolds with tunable mechanical responses and biomimetic behavior (Karathanasopoulos and Al-Ketan, 2022). The convergence of CAD, tissue engineering, and metamaterial science not only improves structural performance and biological integration but also paves the way for the development of advanced, multifunctional scaffolds that better replicate native tissue environments and respond dynamically to physiological conditions (Haag et al., 2022).

Importing CAD into bioprinting enables precise digital modeling of complex biological geometries, helping to translate anatomical data, often derived from medical imaging modalities such as MRI or CT, into printable, three-dimensional models that mimic the structural and functional characteristics of native tissues (Hussain et al., 2024). CAD tools also enable the integration of multiple domains, including mechanical performance, vascularization pathways, and cell-specific patterning, which are crucial for the successful engineering of functional biological constructs (Fleischer et al., 2020). Furthermore, the adaptability of CAD platforms supports iterative design modifications and the incorporation of patient-specific features, making it a fundamental component in personalized regenerative medicine workflows (Filardi, 2025).

In the engineering of tissue scaffolds, CAD cannot be ignored in designing and optimizing three-dimensional architectures that support cellular growth, differentiation, and tissue integration (Zhang et al., 2019). Through parametric design, parameters such as pore size, porosity, interconnectivity, and scaffold morphology can be controlled to improve the creation of structures (Herath et al., 2021) that closely emulate the mechanical and biological environment of native extracellular matrices, allowing fast modifications and adaptability in the design (Chen et al., 2020). This is particularly relevant in the development of load-bearing implants, where mechanical performance must be balanced with nutrient diffusion and cellular infiltration (Breish et al., 2024).

The integration of CAD with advanced computational methods, such as topology optimization and triply periodic minimal surfaces, has significantly enhanced scaffold functionality. In addition, the use of other architected materials, such as metamaterials (Figure 5.2), enables the rational design of architectures tailored to specific tissue types and clinical needs (Kalogeropoulou et al., 2024).

The integration of metamaterial design principles into CAD-based scaffold modeling has opened new possibilities for adaptable mechanical and biological properties in tissue engineering (Dogan et al., 2020). Metamaterials, defined by their architected

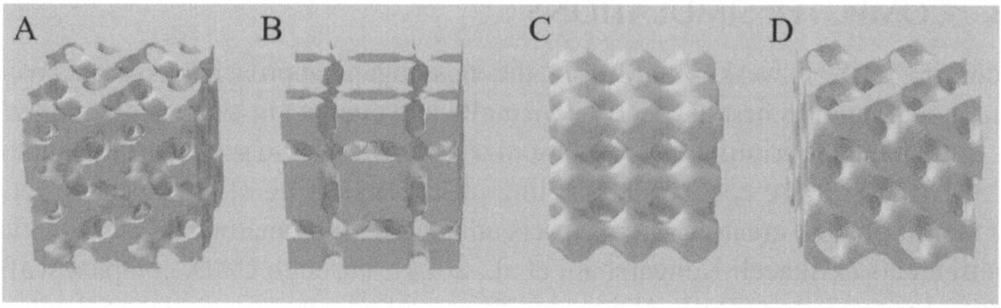

FIGURE 5.2 TPMS 3D scaffolds examples, Fisher Koch(A), Nevius(B), Schwarz P(C), and Schwarz D (D). (The authors.)

structures rather than their chemical composition, enable the creation of scaffolds with highly tunable behaviors such as anisotropic stiffness, negative Poisson's ratio, and mechanical gradients that closely replicate the biomechanical properties of native tissues (Zadpoor, 2020). By leveraging the design freedom offered by CAD platforms, researchers can implement periodic or hierarchical patterns that introduce localized mechanical cues, which are known to influence cellular behavior and tissue regeneration (Josephson and Morgan, 2023).

Architected scaffolds can improve load distribution and stiffness, while also facilitating integration with surrounding biological tissues (Entezari et al., 2020). For example, CAD-based metamaterial scaffolds may include spatial variations in porosity to support the development of osteochondral or vascularized tissues (Chen et al., 2023). This combination of metamaterial science and CAD modeling marks a significant step in scaffold design, enabling properties beyond those of conventional materials and topologies (Qin et al., 2025).

The incorporation of metamaterial concepts into bioprinted scaffold design demands sophisticated simulation tools to accurately predict their complex mechanical and fluidic behaviors (Xiao and Li, 2024).

5.3.1 FEA and CFD

Mechanical finite element analysis (FEA) and computational fluid dynamics (CFD) play a key role in advancing organ bioprinting, making it possible to use mathematical modeling and predictive simulations to better understand and optimize how bioprinted tissues fuse and mature (Rezende et al., 2015).

FEA and CFD are the main solutions to understand the performance of metamaterial-inspired scaffolds, enabling detailed evaluation of stress distribution, deformation, and structural stability under physiological loads (Bazyar and Sheidaee, 2024) as well as fluid transport and shear stresses within porous or vascularized metamaterial scaffolds (Peng et al., 2023).

Together, mechanical analysis and CFD constitute an integrated multiphysics approach that supports the rational design of advanced biomimetic scaffolds, enhancing their biological functionality and mechanical reliability before experimental validation and bioprinting (Carracciuolo and D'Amora, 2024).

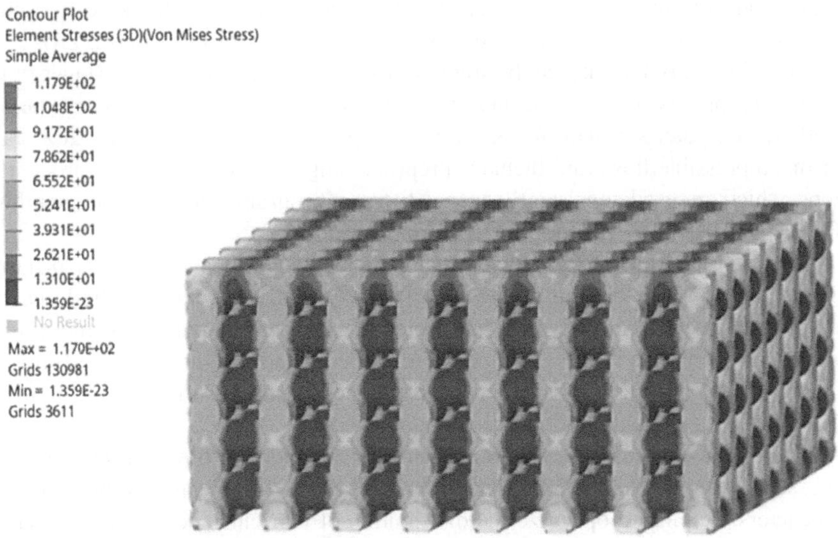

FIGURE 5.3 Von Mises stress analysis to validate scaffold stiffness under compression. (The authors.)

Besides its use in metamaterial-based scaffold design, mechanical analysis can also be applied to predict and validate complex behaviors in the bioprinting process. Typically performed using finite element analysis (FEA), this approach discretizes complex geometries into smaller finite elements, enabling the prediction of stress distribution, deformation patterns, and failure mechanisms under various physiological loading conditions. Thus, FEA serves not only as a validation method but also as a predictive design tool, reducing experimental iterations and enhancing the reliability and functional performance of bioprinted constructs (Soufivand et al., 2020). This is particularly critical in the design of scaffolds intended for load-bearing applications, such as bone (Sakthiabirami et al., 2021), cartilage (Koh et al., 2019), or intervertebral discs (Jiang et al., 2023), where mechanical integrity and biomechanical compatibility must be carefully assessed (Carluccio et al., 2020). Additionally, FEA can be used to investigate anisotropic behaviors and heterogeneous materials, reflecting the complex mechanical environments of native tissues (Teixeira and Martins, 2023), and to validate the mechanical response, as shown in Figure 5.3.

Otherwise, CFD could be applied to simulate fluid flow and mass transport phenomena within porous and vascularized structures. Helping to understand the effectiveness of nutrient delivery, waste removal, and cellular signaling in engineered tissues, due to the scaffold internal fluid dynamics, which directly influence cell viability and tissue maturation. This type of analysis makes it possible to predict shear stresses, flow velocities, and pressure distributions, and to identify potential regions of stagnation or inadequate perfusion (Zhao et al., 2019).

That insight is essential for the design of scaffolds that promote homogeneous nutrient distribution and facilitate angiogenesis (Mao et al., 2023). The predictive capability of CFD thus informs scaffold architecture refinement, contributing to the advancement of clinically relevant, biologically functional bioprinted tissues (Shi et al., 2021).

The behavior of bioinks can be studied by CFD analyses at different stages of the bioprinting process (Emmermacher et al., 2020). CFD has been used since the late 1950s in computer software for 3D transient applications (Blanco et al., 2024) and for incompressible flow, and includes preprocessing, resolution, and postprocessing steps, which are used consistently across different programs and additional methods (Fareez et al., 2024).

According to Neagu (2017) given that cells rearrange themselves after printing, understanding the evolution of the bioprinted system is essential to building tissue constructs with precise form and function. Several computational models are employed to simulate multicellular self-organization and post-printing structure formation, including Metropolis Monte Carlo, Kinetic Monte Carlo, Cellular Particle Dynamics, Phase Field, and Lattice Boltzmann.

CFD can also be used to create predictive simulations of how multicellular systems self-organize (Neagu, 2017) and to simulate blood flow in vascular branches and bioreactors, helping to optimize the distribution of nutrients and oxygen (Passamai et al., 2016).

CFD has emerged as indispensable in refining bioprinting processes. By simulating fluid flow, stress distribution, and other parameters, CFD minimizes the need for costly and time-consuming experimental iterations, optimizing factors such as bioink printability, cell viability, and nozzle design. This union between CFD and bioprinting has been critical in assessing the issues in tissue engineering due to the acceleration of the development of lab-grown tissues and organs (Fareez et al., 2024).

The most known commercial CFD software include Comsol, Multiphysics, ANSYS Workbench, ABAQUS, SolidWorks Flow Simulation, OpenFOAM, and Flow 3D.

CompuCell 3D (CC3D) is another multiscale software that is widely used and has open-source code. It allows the resolution of biocomplexity problems through integrating specific mathematical models, which help develop chemical and enzymatic reactions in biological tissues (Santos et al., 2022). It allows simulating the dynamics of multicellular systems from the implementation of regulatory signals, physical properties, and cell-specific behaviors (Hutson et al., 2017). CC3D software has been used to simulate how tissue spheroids behave, as well as processes like angiogenesis and cell aggregation, at both micro- and mesoscales (Rezende et al., 2015).

Finally, the choice of the most appropriate simulation method depends on the system of interest, the required level of detail, and the available computational power (Neagu, 2017).

5.4 EMERGING TECHNOLOGIES

5.4.1 Artificial Intelligence (AI), Machine (ML), and Deep Learning (DL)

AI is a field of computer science that has been explored for many years. In the 1950s, Alan Turing proposed the famous "Turing Test" to evaluate machine intelligence. The first programs that used AI were developed around 1951 at the University of

Manchester in the United Kingdom, one for playing checkers and another for playing chess. In 1952, IBM (International Business Machines Corporation) created a more advanced program for playing checkers. Then, in 1955, a new version of the program was developed, capable of learning from each game played, and it is considered the first practical application of AI.

During the second decade of the 2000s, AI evolved significantly with the availability of high computational power provided by graphics processing unit (GPU). Various types of deep neural networks became popular, such as convolutional neural networks (CNNs) which, although originally proposed in 1990 with the LeNet architecture, only gained widespread popularity about 20 years later. These networks are widely used in tasks such as segmentation and object detection. Additionally, there are generative neural network architectures that enable the creation of synthetic data, including images, audio, and text.

In the field of bioprinting, AI is an enabling technology that supports everything from the creation of digital models for printing to the monitoring of cell growth.

Blueprints can be generated from medical images, and in this context, algorithms based on CNNs accelerate the automatic segmentation of human organs such as the mandible, liver, and kidneys, among others.

Another application of CNNs is the monitoring of the bioprinting process. This type of equipment is primarily used in research settings, where it is common for researchers to test different materials. Until all parameters are properly configured, various printing failures may occur, highlighting the importance of monitoring during the printing process. The literature reports studies that perform this monitoring using hydrogels, especially in bioprinters that use extrusion-based technologies.

The correct size of a cellular spheroid is an important factor for various types of studies, such as drug toxicity testing and bioprinting applications. In this field, CNNs have been applied to classify the quality of spheroids, taking their size into account. Meanwhile, the work by Oncu et al. (2025) compares the use of deep neural network models for parameterizing images of scaffolds intended for bioprinting.

Generative neural networks, such as generative adversarial networks (GANs), can be used to create anatomical scaffold structure models for bioprinting applications. Although no studies have yet been found in the literature directly exploring the use of GANs in bioprinting, several works demonstrate their application in generating geometric models in other fields. For bioprinting, it would be necessary to train these networks with datasets containing models specific to bioprinting.

With the growing variety of biomaterials and printing technologies, ML has been introduced as a tool to optimize processes, fine-tune material applications, and enhance the mechanical and biological performance of bioprinted constructs. Both ML and deep learning (DL) have the potential to streamline the current bioprinting workflow (Sun et al., 2023).

Bonatti et al. (2022) proposed the use of DL as a tool to automatically optimize printing parameters and monitor the printing process in real time. In a controlled environment, they demonstrated that ML technology can be effectively applied to optimize bioprinting parameters.

Another study employed fuzzy systems to identify sets of optimized printing parameters that improve the printing accuracy of both existing and newly formulated bioinks.

Sedigh et al. (2022) found that optimization using a fuzzy system improved printing accuracy by 15% for a collagen bioink and by 68% for Pluronic F127, compared to the printing parameters recommended by the manufacturer.

The incorporation of AI into bioprinting can transform the tissue engineering industry, and thus, lead to further development in regenerative medicine and pave the road for personalized healthcare solutions (Fareez et al., 2024).

ML and AI have been utilized in the CFD and tissue engineering sectors due to the increasing need for optimization and automation in different aspects of tissue engineering. As large amounts of data are assessed by ML algorithms, trends can be identified that can optimize bioprinting parameters, which would in turn reduce the cost of protracted preliminary test runs. The precision and efficiency of bioprinting methods can be improved as well due to the predictive modeling of AI, which can produce favorable results that are more precise and reproducible (Fareez et al., 2024).

ML helps optimize the properties of biomaterials and bioinks to ensure reliable printability and shape fidelity. ML models can predict the relationship between ink formulations and printability, suggesting that printable inks should have a high elastic modulus for greater fidelity and a low yield stress for smooth extrusion (Sun et al., 2023).

Traditional ML methods (such as support vector machine (SVM), linear regression, and random forest) can be used to develop predictive models for fiber or droplet diameter, optimizing parameters such as polymer weight fraction, solvent concentration, feed rate, applied voltage, and collector distance. To maintain stability and reliability in large-scale bioprinting and long-term manufacturing, it is essential to develop *in situ* process monitoring. This enables the quality of constructs to be intelligently controlled, rather than relying solely on the operator's experience (Sun et al., 2023).

5.4.2 Digital Twins

According to the Committee on Foundational Research Gaps and Future Directions for Digital Twins, after a definition update from the American Institute of Aeronautics and Astronautics, a digital twin is a set of virtual information constructs that mimics the structure, context, and behavior of a natural, engineered, or social system (or system-of-systems), is dynamically updated with data from its physical twin, has a predictive capability, and informs decisions that realize value. The bidirectional interaction between the virtual and the physical is central to the digital twin (NAS, 2023).

Linked to the use of FEA and CFD tools in scaffold design and bioprinting, digital twin techniques offer a framework that extends beyond isolated analyses to enable real-time feedback, process control, and system-level optimization (Ahmed et al., 2024). A digital twin is a virtual, continuously updated replica of a physical or simulated system that integrates multiscale models, sensor data, and predictive analytics to reflect the behavior of a system in its life cycle (*Jia* et al., 2022). In the context of tissue engineering and scaffold fabrication, this technique serves to combine patient-specific geometries, material properties, and physiological conditions to enable iterative simulation and performance evaluation (Poletti et al., 2022). These systems enable the coupling of mechanical and fluidic simulations, not only to predict but also to adaptively guide the printing process and design preferences, reducing design uncertainty, enhancing process reliability, and improving the biological and mechanical performance of bioprinted constructs (Möller and Pörtner, 2021). This integrative approach supports the development of intelligent biofabrication systems capable of self-correction and personalization, moving toward more accurate and functional tissue analogues (Shen and Li, 2024).

ML has the potential to enable the creation of digital twins of human tissues and organs at cellular resolution and with cellular properties, paving the way for a standardized bioprinting simulation practice that balances virtual and physical experiments (Sun et al., 2023).

The design process in 3D bioprinting should be structured around the concept of digital twins of organs. Creating digital twins at the cellular level, for example, requires high-quality tissue samples along with advanced imaging and 3D reconstruction methods (An et al., 2021). Digital twins, which are virtual representations continuously updated with data from their physical counterparts, possess predictive capabilities and guide value-driven decision-making (NAS, 2023).

5.4.3 Big Data: Data Storage and Manipulation

ML cannot be applied without large volumes of data (Big Data) encompassing clinical images of organs, histology, immunohistochemistry, biomechanical properties of tissues and organs, and molecular profiles of cells, tissues, and organs (including genomics and proteomics), among others. This data may be structured, unstructured, or semistructured. Leveraging ML, Big Data, and the development of digital twins, IT is poised to be the driving force that shifts bioprinting from an empirical endeavor to a digital, predictive, and seamlessly integrated discipline—ultimately aiming to maximize resource efficiency and pave the way for personalized clinical applications (An et al., 2021).

The U.S. Human BioMolecular Atlas Program (HuBMAP, 2019), for example, aims to develop an open, global framework to create a 3D molecular and cellular atlas of the human body—an effort that could enable the construction of an integrated tissue map across multiple scales. HuBMAP makes extensive use of IT to process and integrate large volumes of molecular and spatial data at cellular resolution. Its infrastructure combines high-performance computing, interoperable databases, open APIs, and 3D visualization tools. These capabilities allow for the continuous updating of the human atlas and foster global collaborative analysis, laying the groundwork for biomedical digital twins and personalized tissue modeling. HuBMAP stands as an outstanding example of the far-reaching role of IT in healthcare—and more specifically in bioprinting—by providing a rich data foundation for designing anatomical models, whether a tissue or an organ, that serve as the starting point for sophisticated, high-precision, and data-intensive blueprints.

5.5 3D PRINTING: MATERIALIZATION

5.5.1 Bioprinters

Biopriners did not exist until the early 2000s. The evolution of these devices over the years has been remarkable. Bioprinters, designed to work with bioinks, are based on additive manufacturing techniques. The most well-known techniques are extrusion bioprinting, inkjet bioprinting and inkjet-based deposition, and laser-assisted bioprinting (Murphy and Atala, 2014).

The process is guided by computer-controlled systems and integrated computer numerical control equipment. The movements of the printing platform are governed by coordinates saved in file formats such as G-code (Wu et al., 2023).

5.5.2. Slicing and G-code Generation Software

With the three-dimensional model established (such as a file in .STL, .OBJ, or .3MF format), the object is loaded into slicing software, such as Ultimaker Cura or Prusa Slicer (open-source software) (Figure 5.4) or more sophisticated ones, where it undergoes the slicing process. In AM, the division into layers that will form the volume of the object to be printed is known as slicing. This is the most important step in AM process planning (Livesu et al., 2017), since without it, 3D printing is not possible.

This process consists of creating a set of planar cross-sections along the vertical axis of the 3D model, which are converted into sequential machine command language (commonly G-code) for additive manufacturing (Gibson et al., 2015).

The quality of bioprinting largely depends on the parameters of the materials used in the process. Changes in parameters such as temperature, time, printing speed, nozzle diameter, and dispensing pressure can affect the outcome of the bioprinting process (Bahraminasab, 2020).

Slicing algorithms seek to find the contours through the result of the intersection of the model with the layers (Livesu et al., 2017). Basically, the slicing algorithm for triangular meshes identifies the line segments resulting from the intersections of the mesh triangles with the layers, joining the endpoints of the lines to form the contour of the object (Kirschman and Jaraalmonte, 1992).

The G-code generated during slicing from the 3D model will be interpreted by the 3D printer. Each printer has embedded software called firmware. The firmware is responsible for managing all operations performed by the 3D printer's hardware. It coordinates the heaters, sensors, lights, LCD display, buttons, and everything else related to the 3D printing process (Marlin, 2025).

5.5.3 Integration of Printing Parameters with Predictive Mathematical Models

Based on the generation of G-code derived from the geometry and following parameters established by the operator, predictive mathematical models govern the algorithm that creates the "pathing" (the route traveled by the machine's extruder nozzle during printing) for the selected geometry.

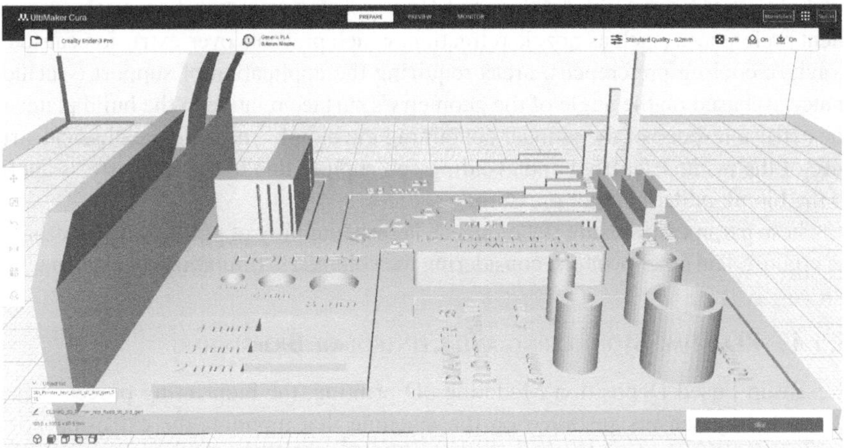

(a)

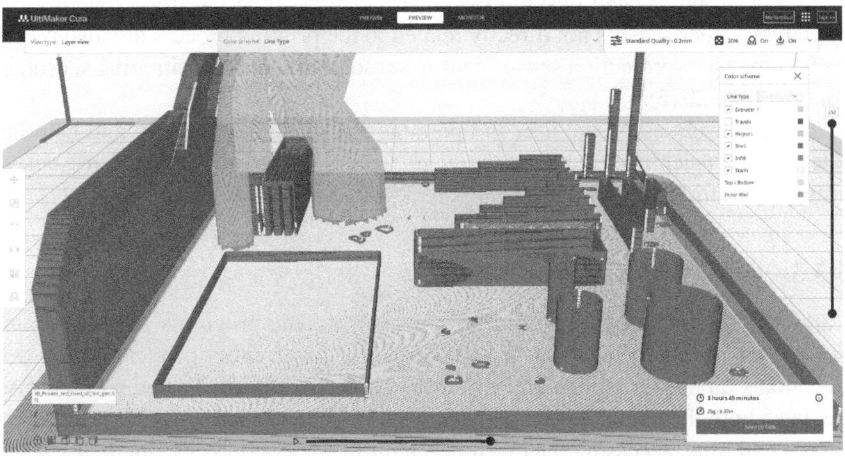

(b)

FIGURE 5.4 Home screen of Ultimaker Cura 5.10.1 software with a 3D model before slicing (a) and after slicing, showing a preview of time and material estimates and a color legend (b). (The authors.)

Those models calculate the amount of material to be used in printing and the process time, based on parameters such as: thickness and number of layers to be extruded; thickness of the internal and external walls; thickness of the top and bottom layers of the geometry; infill density (pattern of structures responsible for providing stability to the geometry while reducing material usage and distributing weight evenly); temperature and extrusion speed/pressure of the material; movement speed of the extruder head to create overhangs (printing a line of material between two separated points without the need for supports to prevent deformation); movement preferences (such as nozzle retraction, which prevents over-extrusion caused by gravity); cooling preferences; areas requiring the application of support (sacrificial material) based on the angle of the geometry's surface relative to the build plate; and the extrusion speed of the plunger containing the bioink, ensuring the physical structure of the printed scaffold and avoiding cell rupture due to the shear stress applied to the bioink under plunger pressure.

These parameters ensure the sequenced reproducibility of prints and allow them to be produced on other printers, considering the volumetric limitations of each machine.

5.5.4 Real-Time Monitoring and Control of Bioprinting

Present in Fused Deposition Modeling 3D printing, the bioprinting process can be controlled by sensors installed on the machine that monitor: the extrusion nozzle temperature (commonly between 4°C and 37°C) to regulate the viscosity of the bioink and prevent cell death; the pressure applied to the bioink to prevent clogs and irregular material flow; the positions and speeds of the motors controlling the printer's axes; and cameras for remote monitoring via a workstation or smartphone.

In more sophisticated desktop machines, such as the X1 Carbon manufactured by Bambu, other sensors not directly related to the printing process are also present, such as the open-protection sensor, fan-on sensor, build plate positioning sensor, etc. (Bambu Lab, 2025).

These sensors assist the user in operating the machine correctly and help indicate possible machine failures, speeding up repairs and improving the consistency of printing parameters.

5.5.5 Automated Control Platforms

Currently, slicing software—especially printer-specific programs such as "Bambu Studio" for Bambu printers or "Ultimaker Cura" for Creality printers—offer dedicated tools for printer monitoring and automation. Through dedicated sections, users can view both the planned print path encoded in G-code and the actual printing process in real time, accessing the machine's built-in cameras either from their workstation or remotely via a monitoring app on their smartphone (Ultimaker, 2025).

Furthermore, it is possible to modify the G-code matrix after slicing the object or to program predefined movements to be executed in every print. For example, you could set the machine to raise the extruder nozzle at the start of each print, or program it so that, once a print is finished, the nozzle "pushes" the printed object out of the way, allowing the next one to be printed without requiring the operator to restart the process.

5.6 APPLICATIONS

5.6.1 Virtual Surgical Planning and Applications

Virtual Surgical Planning (VSP) represents a significant advancement in oral, maxillofacial, and cranial surgery, integrating computational technologies, medical imaging, and 3D modeling to enhance surgical precision and clinical outcomes

(Zoabi et al., 2022). By utilizing patient-specific imaging data, VSP enables highly accurate anatomical representation, thereby improving surgical decision-making and offering notable clinical benefits, such as reduced operating time (Imahiyerobo et al., 2024), cost optimization (Maricevich and Campolina, 2017), and more efficient allocation and coordination of the surgical team (Jang et al., 2019; Kim et al., 2023).

An essential component of VSP is its integration with additive manufacturing, which enables the creation of biomodels and surgical guides tailored to individual patients (Borbon et al., 2025). These models support surgical simulation and aid in communication with both medical teams and patients (Imahiyerobo et al., 2024).

This process is summarized in Figure 5.5, which illustrates the main steps of the VSP workflow: acquisition of medical images (CT and MRI), segmentation using tools such as InVesalius (Amorim et al., 2011), 3D reconstruction of the region of

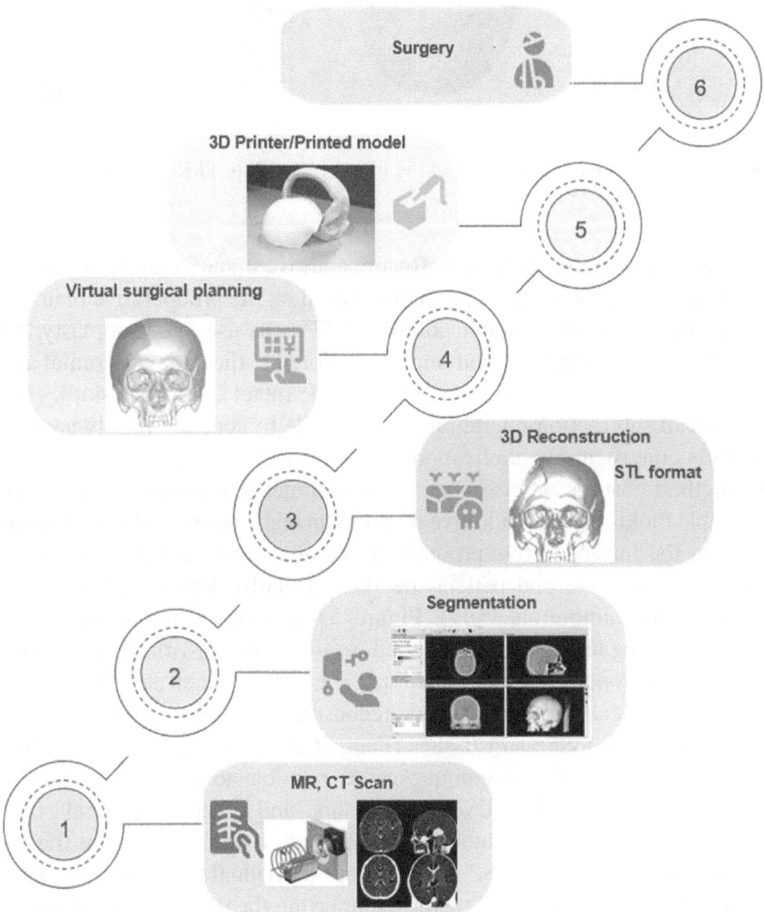

FIGURE 5.5 VSP steps: (1) medical images from MRI and CT scans, (2) segmentation of the region of interest, (3) reconstruction of the 3D biomodel in STL format, (4) VSP using 3D modeling software, (5) 3D printing of the virtual biomodel, and (6) surgical procedure assisted by the biomodel. (The authors.)

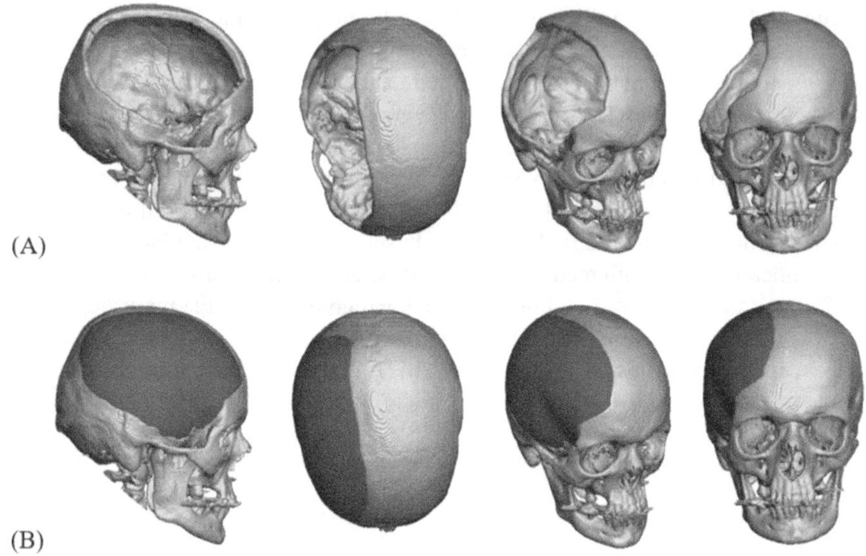

FIGURE 5.6 Cranioplasty model using the mirroring tool. (CTI Renato Archer.)

interest, surgical planning in CAD software, additive manufacturing of the biomodels, and execution of the surgical procedure based on the preoperative plan.

Among the most relevant applications of VSP is its use in cranioplasty, where it facilitates the design of customized implants tailored to the patient's cranial anatomy. By employing a mirroring technique based on the intact side of the skull, combined with a Boolean subtraction operation, it is possible to generate highly accurate and anatomically congruent prosthetic models (Amorim et al., 2025).

This method ensures precise anatomical symmetry and enables the fabrication of sterilizable molds through additive manufacturing. These molds are subsequently employed in the intraoperative production of polymethyl methacrylate prostheses, offering a cost-effective and patient-specific alternative for cranial reconstruction (Maricevich and Campolina, 2017). Figure 5.6 presents a representative case in which the mirroring technique was applied, resulting in a prosthesis with symmetrical contours and proper alignment with the patient's cranial structure.

Beyond its applications in hard tissue reconstruction, VSP has also shown promise in procedures involving soft tissues (Fang et al., 2018). By employing the same segmentation and modeling techniques, it is possible to generate virtual models that assist in identifying blood vessels, tumors, and other anatomical structures. Figure 5.7 illustrates a virtual model of conjoined twins connected at the sternum and sharing internal organs. VSP enabled both individual and collective visualization of the anatomical structures, thereby supporting the development of appropriate surgical strategies.

In summary, VSP enhances the precision and personalization of complex surgical procedures, reduces surgical time and complications, and improves communication

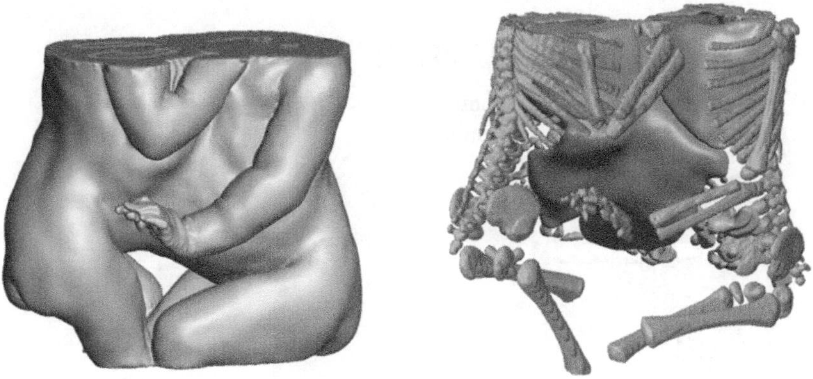

FIGURE 5.7 Virtual model of conjoined twins showing organ differentiation. Image courtesy of the State Hospital for Children and Adolescents of the State of Goiás; lead surgeon: Zacarias Calil Hamu. (CTI Renato Archer.)

between surgeons and patients. Its integration with additive manufacturing further broadens its clinical applicability and impact.

VSP combines medical imaging with computational modeling to generate precise three-dimensional representations of a patient's anatomy. Based on these models – obtained, for instance, from CT or MRI—it is possible to simulate and refine procedures before surgery. When integrated with bioprinting, such data can be exported and transformed into scaffolds, surgical guides, or customized implants. Beyond reproducing external geometry, this approach also allows for the definition of internal architecture and cellular distribution, which supports functionality and integration with surrounding tissues. By reducing intraoperative uncertainties and guiding the selection of materials and printing parameters, VSP becomes a digital bridge between medical imaging diagnosis and personalized biofabrication, enhancing the likelihood of clinical and regenerative success.

5.6.2 *In Situ* Biofabrication

The *in situ* bioprinting – also known as intraoperative bioprinting – enables the direct deposition of biomaterials and cells at the site of an injury or defect, removing the need for prefabricated implants. The *in situ* bioprinting is based on computer-assisted scanning results of the defect site and is able to print cells directly at this site with biomaterials, bioactive factors, and other materials without the need to transfer prefabricated grafts as with traditional *in vitro* 3D bioprinting methods, and the resulting grafts can accurately adapt to the target defect site (Li et al., 2023).

Two different approaches (Figure 5.8) have been developed which include (1) fixed robotic bioprinters, which operate with assisted movement and enhanced precision, including versions designed for use at clinical bedsides (Mahmoudi et al., 2023), and (2) hand-held portable devices that offer flexibility, easy sterilization, and quick deployment in the field or at the patient's bedside (MacAdam et al., 2022).

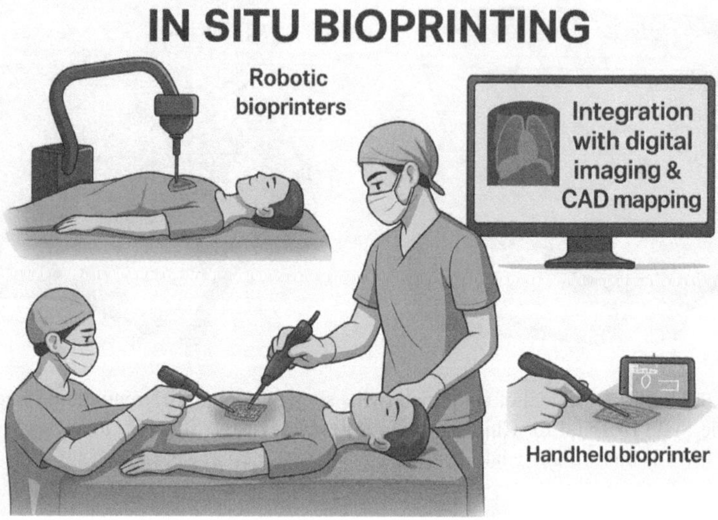

FIGURE 5.8 *In situ* bioprinting: difference between the two techniques: robotic (above) and manual (below). (The authors by Gemini.)

An automated robotic arm, controlled by sophisticated software and algorithms, translates the digital design into physical reality in real time and applied it directly onto the patient. It precisely maneuvers the bioprinter's nozzle, depositing specialized bioinks layer by layer directly onto the damaged tissue. High fidelity to the digital model, critical for replicating the complex, often gradient, structures of native tissues is ensured by the automated controls.

This field is promising but still emerging, with initial applications in cartilage, bone, and skin (Halper, 2025).

Integration with scanning technologies (medical imaging) and CAD platforms enables precise mapping of the patient's anatomy, allowing for accurate printing based on the actual defect (Li et al., 2023).

Concerning IT infrastructure, imagine a patient undergoing remote surgery in a potential in situ bioprinting scenario. Smart robotic systems would be required, which in turn demands a high-speed and uninterrupted internet connection throughout the procedure. Additionally, Big Data architectures are needed to store and retrieve information in real time, along with ultra-high processing capabilities to support the computational demands of the system.

5.7 CHALLENGES AND PERSPECTIVES

IT, whether through computerized control or, more recently, advanced ML techniques, is indispensable in driving 3D bioprinting forward. These computational tools assure high precision, optimize processes and materials by avoiding waste of time and extra costs, allow real-time monitoring, and help understand cellular interactions for applications in personalized medicine and tissue engineering.

In biofabrication, software is straightly immersed from the initial design of the model to be printed to the preparation of the biomaterials used. It also assists in controlling devices such as bioprinters and bioreactors and in handling the data produced during the process. Some authors suggest that, in the coming years, it may be possible to manage the entire organ biofabrication workflow from a single software platform, which would also control the robotic equipment involved. Achieving this will require combining established tools with new modules capable of introducing innovative functions, improving both the scope and efficiency of biofabrication.

Additionally, looking toward bioprinting evolution, this field must attract professionals from fields such as computer science, mathematical modeling, computational simulation, and ML. The development and formalization of skill sets that bridge engineering, mathematics, and the biological sciences, covering areas such as systems engineering, data analysis, ML/AI, statistical and probabilistic modeling, uncertainty quantification, computational mathematics, and decision science are fundamental.

ACKNOWLEDGMENTS

We are grateful to our agencies Capes, CNPq, Funadesp, and Fapesp for financial support. We also thank the digital designer Otávio Henrique Junqueira Amorim for creating some of the illustrations and pictures.

REFERENCES

Amorim, P. H., T. F. de Moraes, F. D. S. Azevedo, e J. V. da Silva. 2011. *InVesalius: Software Livre de Imagens Médicas*. Campinas (SP): Centro de Tecnologia da Informação Renato Archer–CTI.

Amorim, P. H. J. 2025. "Automatic Generation of Customized Cranial Implants through Deep Learning." Tese de doutorado, Universidade Estadual de Campinas (UNICAMP), Campinas (SP).

Amorim, P., et al. 2015. "InVesalius: An Interactive Rendering Framework for Health Care Support." Em *International Symposium on Visual Computing*, Las Vegas, NV, 45–54. Springer.

An, J., C. K. Chua, e V. Mironov. 2021. "Application of Machine Learning in 3D Bioprinting: Focus on Development of Big Data and Digital Twin." *International Journal of Bioprinting* 7 (1): 342. https://doi.org/10.18063/ijb.v7i1.342.

Ahmed, N., L. K. Narayanan, e R. Shirwaiker. 2024. "A Framework for Digital Twin Integration in Biofabrication and a Scaffold 3D Bioplotting Case Study." *Manufacturing Letters* 41: 1182–1191. https://doi.org/10.1016/j.mfglet.2024.09.144.

Bahraminasab, M. 2020. "Challenges on Optimization of 3D-Printed Bone Scaffolds." *BioMedical Engineering OnLine* 19 (1): 1–33.

Bambu Lab. 2025. "X1 Carbon." Bambu Lab. https://bambulab.com/pt-br/x1. Accessed July 5, 2025.

Bass, S. D. 2005. "The Spin Structure of the Proton." *Reviews of Modern Physics* 77 (4): 1257–1302.

Bazyar, P., e E. Sheidaee. 2024. "Design and Simulating Lattice Structures in the FE Analysis of the Femur Bone." *Bioprinting* 37: e00326. https://doi.org/10.1016/j.bprint.2023.e00326.

Bender, J. D., et al. 2024. "The Use of Information and Communication Technologies in Primary Health Care in Brazil – The Period of 2014 to 2018." *Ciência & Saúde Coletiva 29*: e19882022. https://www.scielo.br/j/csc/a/RMGFtwjzx55kFM4fNNZtgCy/.

Blanco, J. C. G., A. Macías-García, J. M. Rodríguez-Rego, L. Mendoza-Cerezo, F. M. Sánchez-Margallo, A. C. Marcos-Romero, e J. B. Pagador-Carrasco. 2024. "Optimising Bioprinting Nozzles through Computational Modelling and Design of Experiments." *Biomimetics* 9 (460). https://doi.org/10.3390/biomimetics9080460.

Boland, T., et al. 2003. "Cell and Organ Printing 2: Fusion of Cell Aggregates in Three-Dimensional Gels." *Anatomical Record Part A* 272A: 497–502.

Boland, T., et al. 2006. "Application of Inkjet Printing to Tissue Engineering." *Biotechnology Journal* 1: 910–917. https://doi.org/10.1002/biot.200600081.

Bonatti, A. F., et al. 2022. "A Deep Learning Quality Control Loop of the Extrusion-Based Bioprinting Process." *International Journal of Bioprinting* 8 (4).

Borbon, C., et al. 2025. "Evaluating Osteotomy Accuracy in Mandibular Reconstruction: A Preliminary Study Using Custom Cutting Guides and Virtual Reality." *Diseases* 13 (3): 81. https://doi.org/10.3390/diseases13030081.

Breish, F., C. Hamm, e S. Andresen. 2024. "Nature's Load-Bearing Design Principles and Their Application in Engineering: A Review." *Biomimetics* 9 (9): 545. https://doi.org/10.3390/biomimetics9090545.

Carluccio, D., et al. 2020. "Additively Manufactured Iron-Manganese for Biodegradable Porous Load-Bearing Bone Scaffold Applications." *Acta Biomaterialia* 103: 346–360. https://doi.org/10.1016/j.actbio.2019.12.018.

Carracciuolo, L., e U. D'Amora. 2024. "Mathematical Tools for Simulation of 3D Bioprinting Processes on High-Performance Computing Resources: The State of the Art." *Applied Sciences* 14 (14): 6110. https://doi.org/10.3390/app14146110.

Chen, A., et al. 2023. "3D/4D Printed Bio-Piezoelectric Smart Scaffolds for Next-Generation Bone Tissue Engineering." *International Journal of Extreme Manufacturing* 5 (3): 032007. https://doi.org/10.1088/2631-7990/acd88f.

Chen, H., et al. 2020. "Porous Scaffold Design for Additive Manufacturing in Orthopedics: A Review." *Frontiers in Bioengineering and Biotechnology* 8: 609. https://doi.org/10.3389/fbioe.2020.00609.

Dernowsek, J. A., Rezende, R. A., e da Silva, J. V. L. 2017a. "BioCAE: A New Strategy of Complex Biological Systems for Biofabrication of Tissues and Organs." *Journal of Tissue Science & Engineering* 8 (2): 200. https://doi.org/10.4172/2157-7552.1000200.

Dernowsek, J. A., Rezende, R. A., & da Silva, J. V. L. 2017b. "The Role of Information Technology in the Future of 3D Biofabrication." *Journal of 3D Printing in Medicine* 1 (1): 63–74. https://doi.org/10.2217/3dp-2016-0005.

Dill, T. 2008. "Contraindications to Magnetic Resonance Imaging." *Heart* 94 (7): 943–948.

Dogan, E., et al. 2020. "3D Printing Metamaterials towards Tissue Engineering." *Applied Materials Today* 20 (Setembro): 100752. https://doi.org/10.1016/j.apmt.2020.100752.

Egan, P. F. 2019. "Integrated Design Approaches for 3D Printed Tissue Scaffolds: Review and Outlook." *Materials* 12 (15): 2355. https://doi.org/10.3390/ma12152355.

Emmermacher, J., et al. 2020. "Engineering Considerations on Extrusion-Based Bioprinting: Interactions of Material Behavior, Mechanical Forces and Cells in the Printing Needle." *Biofabrication* 12: 025022.

Entezari, A., et al. 2020. "A Modular Design Strategy to Integrate Mechanotransduction Concepts in Scaffold-Based Bone Tissue Engineering." *Acta Biomaterialia* 118: 100–112. https://doi.org/10.1016/j.actbio.2020.10.012.

Fang, X., et al. 2018. "Improved Virtual Surgical Planning with 3D-Multimodality Image for Malignant Giant Pelvic Tumors." *Cancer Management and Research* 7: 6769–6777.

Fareez, U. N. M., et al. 2024. "Computational Fluid Dynamics (CFD) Analysis of Bioprinting." *Advanced Healthcare Materials* 13 (20): 2400643.

Fedorov, A., et al. 2012. "3D Slicer as an Image Computing Platform for the Quantitative Imaging Network." *Magnetic Resonance Imaging* 30 (9): 1323–1341. https://doi.org/10.1016/j.mri.2012.05.001.

Filardi, V. 2025. "The Evolution and Impact of Customized Implants with Intricate Designs." Em *Biomaterials in Orthopaedics & Trauma*, editado por R. Vaishya e S. Ghosh. Springer, Singapore. https://doi.org/10.1007/978-981-96-3017-2_17.

Fleischer, S., D. N. Tavakol, e G. Vunjak-Novakovic. 2020. "From Arteries to Capillaries: Approaches to Engineering Human Vasculature." *Advanced Functional Materials* 30 (37): 1910811. https://doi.org/10.1002/adfm.201910811.

Gartner. 2025. "2015 Hype Cycle for Emerging Technologies." https://www.gartner.com/smarterwithgartner/whats-new-in-gartners-hype-cycle-for-emerging-technologies-2015. Accessed August 13, 2025.

Gibson, I. et al. 2015. *Additive Manufacturing Technologies: 3D Printing, Rapid Prototyping, and Direct Digital Manufacturing*. 2a ed. Springer. https://doi.org/10.1007/978-1-4939-2113-3.

Groll, J., et al. 2018. "Biofabrication: Status and Future." *Biofabrication* 10 (3): 032001.

Groll, J., et al. 2016. "Biofabrication: Reappraising the Definition of an Evolving Field." *Biofabrication* 8 (1): 013001. doi:10.1088/1758-5090/8/1/013001.

Gu, X., et al. 2020. "Information Technology for Biomanufacturing: Recent Advances and Challenges." *Biofabrication* 12 (3): 032003.

Haag, H., P. D. Dalton, e V. Bloemen. 2022. "The Synergy of Biomimetic Design Strategies for Tissue Constructs." *Advanced Functional Materials* 32 (32): 2201414. https://doi.org/10.1002/adfm.202201414.

Halper, J. 2025. "Narrative Review and Guide: State of the Art and Emerging Opportunities of Bioprinting in Tissue Regeneration and Medical Instrumentation." *Bioengineering* 12: 71. https://doi.org/10.3390/bioengineering12010071.

Herath, B., et al. 2021. "Mechanical and Geometrical Study of 3D Printed Voronoi Scaffold Design for Large Bone Defects." *Materials & Design* 212: 110224. https://doi.org/10.1016/j.matdes.2021.110224.

Hospodiuk, M., e I. T. Ozbolat. 2017. "Automation and Control in Bioprinting." *Manufacturing Letters* 12: 1–6.

Huang, Q., e Z. Zeng. 2017. "A Review on Real-Time 3D Ultrasound Imaging Technology." *BioMed Research International* 2017 (1): 6027029.

HuBMAP Consortium. 2019. "The Human Body at Cellular Resolution: The NIH Human Biomolecular Atlas Program." *Nature* 574: 187–192. https://doi.org/10.1038/s41586-019-1629-x.

Hussain, C. G., et al. 2024. "Computer-Aided Modeling Principles for Anatomic Design." Em *Medical Additive Manufacturing*, editado por S. Mallakpour e C. M. Hussain, 117–152. Elsevier. https://doi.org/10.1016/B978-0-323-95383-2.00002-0.

Hutson, S., et al. 2017. "Computational Model of Secondary Palate Fusion and Disruption." *Chemical Research in Toxicology* 30: 965–979.

Imahiyerobo, T. A., et al. 2024. "The Role of Virtual Surgical Planning in Surgery for Complex Craniosynostosis." *Plastic and Reconstructive Surgery Global Open* 12 (1): e5524.

Jang, W. H., et al. 2019. "Mirror Image Based Three-Dimensional Virtual Surgical Planning and Three-Dimensional Printing Guide System for the Reconstruction of Wide Maxilla Defect Using the Deep Circumflex Iliac Artery Free Flap." *Journal of Craniofacial Surgery* 30 (6): 1829–32.

Jiang, Y., et al. 2023. "3D-Printed Auxetic-Structured Intervertebral Disc Implant for Potential Treatment of Lumbar Herniated Disc." *Bioactive Materials* 20: 528–538. https://doi.org/10.1016/j.bioactmat.2022.06.002.

Jia, W., W. Wang, e Z. Zhang. 2022. "From Simple Digital Twin to Complex Digital Twin Part I: A Novel Modeling Method for Multi-Scale and Multi-Scenario Digital Twin." *Advanced Engineering Informatics* 53: 101706. https://doi.org/10.1016/j.aei.2022.101706.

Jodogne, S. 2018. "The Orthanc Ecosystem for Medical Imaging." *Journal of Digital Imaging* 31 (3): 341–352. https://doi.org/10.1007/s10278-018-0082-y.

Josephson, T. O., e E. F. Morgan. 2023. "Harnessing Mechanical Cues in the Cellular Microenvironment for Bone Regeneration." *Frontiers in Physiology* 14: 1232698. https://doi.org/10.1002/cbic.201900686.

Ju, T., et al. 2002. "Dual Contouring of Hermite Data." Em *Proceedings of the 29th Annual Conference on Computer Graphics and Interactive Techniques*, San Antonio, Texas, 339–346.

Jung, W. S., et al. 2020. "Artificial Intelligence and Big Data in 3D Bioprinting: Prospects and Challenges." *Journal of Industrial and Engineering Chemistry* 81: 1–13.

Kalogeropoulou, M., et al. 2024. "Blueprints of Architected Materials: A Guide to Metamaterial Design for Tissue Engineering." *Advanced Materials* 36 (47): 2408082. https://doi.org/10.1002/adma.202408082.

Karathanasopoulos, N., e O. Al-Ketan. 2022. "Towards Biomimetic, Lattice-Based, Tendon and Ligament Metamaterial Designs." *Journal of the Mechanical Behavior of Biomedical Materials* 134: 105412. https://doi.org/10.1016/j.jmbbm.2022.105412.

Kim, J. Y., et al. 2023. "Advancements in Oral Maxillofacial Surgery: A Comprehensive Review on 3D Printing and Virtual Surgical Planning." *Applied Sciences* 13 (17): 9907.

Kirschman, C., e C. Jara-Almonte. 1992. "A Parallel Slicing Algorithm for Solid Freeform Fabrication Processes." Em *Solid Freeform Fabrication Symposium*, Austin, Texas, 26–33.

Koh, Y.-G., et al. 2019. "Optimal Mechanical Properties of a Scaffold for Cartilage Regeneration Using Finite Element Analysis." *Journal of Tissue Engineering* 10: 2041731419832133. https://doi.org/10.1177/2041731419832133.

Lam, E. H. Y., et al. 2023. "3D Bioprinting for Next-Generation Personalized Medicine." *International Journal of Molecular Sciences* 24: 6357. https://doi.org/10.3390/ijms24076357.

Li, R., et al. 2023. "Bioinks adapted for in situ bioprinting scenarios of defect sites: a review." *RSC Advances* 13: 7153–7167.

Livesu, M., et al. 2017. "From 3D Models to 3D Prints: An Overview of the Processing Pipeline." *Computer Graphics Forum* 36 (2): 537–564.

Lorensen, W. E., e H. E. Cline. 1998. "Marching Cubes: A High Resolution 3D Surface Construction Algorithm." Em *Seminal Graphics: Pioneering Efforts That Shaped the Field*, editado por R. Wolfe, 347–353. ACM SIGGRAPH.

MacAdam A., et al. 2022. "Development of In Situ Bioprinting: A Mini Review." *Frontiers in Bioengineering and Biotechnology* 10: 940896.

Mahmoudi, Z., et al. 2023. "In Situ 3D Bioprinting: A Promising Technique in Advanced Biofabrication Strategies." *Bioprinting* 31: e00260. https://doi.org/10.1016/j.bprint.2023.e00260.

Mandrycky, C., et al. 2016. "3D Bioprinting for Engineering Complex Tissues." *Biomaterials Science* 4 (1): 26–44.

Mao, R., et al. 2023. "Flow Channel Performance in 3D Printed Hydroxyapatite Scaffolds to Improve Metabolism and Tissue Ingrowth in Flat Bone Repair." *Composites Part B: Engineering* 259: 110727. https://doi.org/10.1016/j.compositesb.2023.110727.

Maricevich, P., e A. C. Campolina. 2017. "Reconstrução de Calota Craniana com Prótese Customizada de PMMA Após Craniectomias Descompressivas." *Revista Brasileira de Cirurgia Plástica* 32 (1): 123–27.

Marlin. 2025. "What Is Marlin?" https://marlinfw.org/docs/basics/introduction.html#how-marlin-works. Accessed August 13, 2025.

Melchiorri, A. J., e J. P. Fisher. 2018. "The Role of Computed-Aided Design and Manufacturing in Tissue Engineering." *Methods in Molecular Biology* 1826: 273–294.

Mikaeeli Kangarshahi, B., S. M. Naghib, e N. Rabiee. 2024. "3D Printing and Computer-Aided Design Techniques for Drug Delivery Scaffolds in Tissue Engineering." *Expert Opinion on Drug Delivery* 21 (11): 1615–1636. https://doi.org/10.1080/17425247.2024.2409913.

Minhas, A. S., e R. Oliver. 2022. "Magnetic Resonance Imaging Basics." Em *Electrical Properties of Tissues: Quantitative Magnetic Resonance Mapping*, editado por Rosalind Sadleir, Atul Singh Minhas, 47–82. Springer Nature.

Mironov, V., et al. 2003. "Organ Printing: Computer-Aided Jet-Based 3D Tissue Engineering." *Trends in Biotechnology* 21: 157–161.

Mironov, V., G. Prestwich, e G. Forgacs. 2007. "Bioprinting Living Structures." *Journal of Materials Chemistry* 17: 2054–2060.

Moroni, L., et al. 2018a. "Biofabrication Strategies for 3D In Vitro Models and Regenerative Medicine." *Nature Reviews Materials* 3: 21–37.

Moroni, L., et al. 2018b. "Biofabrication: A Guide to Technology and Terminology." *Trends in Biotechnology* 36 (4): 384–402. https://doi.org/10.1016/j.tibtech.2017.10.015.

Möller, J., e R. Pörtner. 2021. "Digital Twins for Tissue Culture Techniques—Concepts, Expectations, and State of the Art." *Processes* 9 (3): 447. https://doi.org/10.3390/pr9030447.

Murphy, S. V., e A. Atala. 2014. "3D Bioprinting of Tissues and Organs." *Nature Biotechnology* 32 (8): 773–85. https://doi.org/10.1038/nbt.2958.

National Academies of Sciences (NAS), Engineering, and Medicine. 2023. *Foundational Research Gaps and Future Directions for Digital Twins*. The National Academies Press. https://doi.org/10.17226/26894.

National Electrical Manufacturers Association (NEMA). 2025. *DICOM – Digital Imaging and Communications in Medicine*. https://www.dicomstandard.org/. Accessed on June 9, 2025.

Neagu, A. 2017. "Role of Computer Simulation to Predict the Outcome of 3D Bioprinting." *Journal of 3D Printing in Medicine* 1 (2): 103–121.

NIST. 2025. https://nvlpubs.nist.gov/nistpubs/SpecialPublications/NIST.SP.800-12r1.pdf. Accessed on August 8, 2025.

Oncu, E., et al. 2025. "Comparative Analysis of Deep Learning Models for Predicting Biocompatibility in Tissue Scaffold Images." *Computers in Biology and Medicine* 192: 110281.

Ortiz, S. H. C., T. Chiu, e M. D. Fox. 2012. "Ultrasound Image Enhancement: A Review." *Biomedical Signal Processing and Control* 7 (5): 419–428.

Ozbolat, I. T., e M. Hospodiuk. 2016. "Current Advances and Future Perspectives in Bioprinting." *Biomaterials* 76: 303–323.

Passamai, V. E., J. A. Dernowsek, J. Nogueira, V. Lara, F. Vilalba, V. A. Mironov, R. A. Rezende, e J. V. da Silva. 2016. "From 3D Bioprinters to a Fully Integrated Organ Biofabrication Line." *Journal of Physics: Conference Series* 705: 012010. https://doi.org/10.1088/1742-6596/705/1/012010.

Peng, X., et al. 2023. "Controlled Mechanical and Mass-Transport Properties of Porous Scaffolds through Hollow Strut." *International Journal of Mechanical Sciences* 248: 108202. https://doi.org/10.1016/j.ijmecsci.2023.108202.

Poletti, G., et al. 2022. "Towards a Digital Twin of Coronary Stenting: A Suitable and Validated Image-Based Approach for Mimicking Patient-Specific Coronary Arteries." *Electronics* 11 (3): 502. https://doi.org/10.3390/electronics11030502.

Qin, Y., et al. 2025. "A Metamaterial Scaffold Beyond Modulus Limits: Enhanced Osteogenesis and Angiogenesis of Critical Bone Defects." *Nature Communications* 16 (1): 2180. https://doi.org/10.1038/s41467-025-57609-9.

Rezende, R. A., et al. 2015. "Organ Printing as an Information Technology." *Procedia Engineering* 110: 151–158.

Ribas, R. G., e C. Morais. 2022. "Artificial Intelligence and Machine Learning in 3D Bioprinting for Tissue Engineering." *Journal of Tissue Engineering and Regenerative Medicine* 16 (5): 458–471.

Sakthiabirami, K., et al. 2021. "Three-Dimensional Zirconia-Based Scaffolds for Load-Bearing Bone-Regeneration Applications: Prospects and Challenges." *Materials* 14 (12): 3207. https://doi.org/10.3390/ma14123207.

Santos, B. C., et al. 2022. "Biological Multiscale Computational Modeling: A Promising Tool for 3D Bioprinting and Tissue Engineering." *Bioprinting* 28: e00234. https://doi.org/10.1016/j.bprint.2022.e00234.

Sedigh, A., et al. 2022. "Enhancing Precision in Bioprinting Utilizing Fuzzy Systems." *Bioprinting* 25: e00190.

Shen, T., e B. Li. 2024. "Digital Twins in Additive Manufacturing: A State-of-the-Art Review." *International Journal of Advanced Manufacturing Technology* 131: 63–92. https://doi.org/10.1007/s00170-024-13092-y.

Shi, F., et al. 2021. "The Effect of Macropore Size of Hydroxyapatite Scaffold on the Osteogenic Differentiation of Bone Mesenchymal Stem Cells under Perfusion Culture." *Regenerative Biomaterials* 8 (6): rbab050. https://doi.org/10.1093/rb/rbab050.

Soufivand, A. A., et al. 2020. "Prediction of Mechanical Behavior of 3D Bioprinted Tissue-Engineered Scaffolds Using Finite Element Method (FEM) Analysis." *Additive Manufacturing* 33: 101181. https://doi.org/10.1016/j.addma.2020.101181.

Sun, J., et al. 2023. "Machine Learning and 3D Bioprinting." *International Journal of Bioprinting* 9 (4): 717. https://doi.org/10.18063/ijb.717.

Teixeira, A. M., e P. Martins. 2023. "A Review of Bioengineering Techniques Applied to Breast Tissue: Mechanical Properties, Tissue Engineering and Finite Element Analysis." *Frontiers in Bioengineering and Biotechnology* 11: 1161815. https://doi.org/10.3389/fbioe.2023.1161815.

Treece, G. M., R. W. Prager, e A. H. Gee. 1999. "Regularised Marching Tetrahedra: Improved Iso-Surface Extraction." *Computers & Graphics* 23 (4): 583–598.

Ultimaker. 2025. "Ultimaker Cura." https://ultimaker.com/software/ultimaker-cura/. Acessado em 13 de agosto de 2025.

Warnock, M. J., et al. 2007. "Benefits of Using the DCM4CHE DICOM Archive." *Journal of Digital Imaging* 20 (S1): 125–129. https://doi.org/10.1007/s10278-018-0082-y.

Wilson, C., e T. Boland. 2003. "Cell and Organ Printing 1: Protein and Cell Printers." *Anatomical Record* 272A: 492–497.

Withers, P. J., et al. 2021. "X-ray Computed Tomography." *Nature Reviews Methods Primers* 1 (1): 18.

Wu, C. A., Y. Zhu, e Y. J. Woo. 2023. "Advances in 3D Bioprinting: Techniques, Applications, and Future Directions for Cardiac Tissue Engineering." *Bioengineering* 10: 842. https://doi.org/10.3390/bioengineering10070842.

Xiao, X., e H. Li. 2024. "Predicting Mechanical Responses of Additively Manufactured Metamaterials with Computational Efficiency." *CIRP Journal of Manufacturing Science and Technology* 52: 149–158. https://doi.org/10.1016/j.cirpj.2024.06.004.

Yushkevich, P. A., Y. Gao, e G. Gerig. 2019. "ITK-SNAP: An Interactive Tool for SemiAutomatic Segmentation of Multi-Modality Biomedical Images." Em *2019 41st Annual International Conference of the IEEE Engineering in Medicine and Biology Society (EMBC)*, Berlin, Germany. https://doi.org/10.1109/EMBC.2019.8856659.

Zadpoor, A. A. 2020. "Meta-Biomaterials." *Biomaterials Science* 8 (1): 18–38. https://doi.org/10.1039/C9BM01247H.

Zhao, F., et al. 2019. "A Multiscale Computational Fluid Dynamics Approach to Simulate the Micro-Fluidic Environment within a Tissue Engineering Scaffold with Highly Irregular Pore Geometry." *Biomechanics and Modeling in Mechanobiology* 18 (6): 1965–1977. https://doi.org/10.1007/s10237-019-01188-4.

Zoabi, A., et al. 2022. "3D Printing and Virtual Surgical Planning in Oral and Maxillofacial Surgery." *Journal of Clinical Medicine* 11 (9): 2385.

6 3D Bioprinting in Regenerative Medicine Applications

Larissa Tessaro, Maria Eduarda de Almeida Astolfo, Renan Nascimento Araújo, Samile Bezerra de Aguiar, and Bianca Chieregato Maniglia

6.1 INTRODUCTION

Research and development in the field of regenerative medicine have advanced significantly worldwide, aiming to address the limitations of conventional treatments for tissue and organ repair. Techniques such as organ transplantation are inherently constrained by donor shortages, immunological complications, and high financial costs (e.g., Ref. 1). In response, regenerative medicine emerged as a therapeutic strategy harnessing the body's intrinsic healing capacity to enhance tissue recovery, alleviate pain, and improve physiological function. The strategic use of living cells, biocompatible materials, biochemical signals (e.g., growth factors), and physical stimuli (e.g., cyclic mechanical loading), whether applied separately or in combination, enables the fabrication of constructs that mimic native tissues and support tissue regeneration or the restoration of organ function.[2,3]

These approaches can be applied to a wide range of physiological functions, including structural support (such as in bone and cartilage), barriers and transport mechanisms (such as those of the skin and blood vessels), and biochemical or secretory activities (as seen in the liver and pancreas). In addition, regenerative strategies have shown promise in pain management, being utilized in the treatment of various conditions, from musculoskeletal diseases to neuropathic pain and spinal cord injuries.[1,4,5]

Within this framework, tissue engineering emerges as a key discipline, contributing significantly to therapeutic advancements through the design of functional three-dimensional (3D) scaffolds. These scaffolds are developed using sophisticated techniques that integrate vascular engineering with advanced microtechnologies, aiming to replicate the native cellular and tissue microenvironment.[2,3] Concurrently, the development of regenerative medical products continues to advance. As of October 2023, Japan had authorized nine therapies based on somatic cells and seven derived from stem cells (SCs).[4]

Regenerative medicine has transitioned from a theoretical framework to clinical application, with several therapies already in use. Prominent examples include skin regeneration for extensive burn injuries, reconstruction of articular cartilage, myocardial regeneration postinfarction, and treatments aimed at neurodegenerative

 DOI: 10.1201/9781032638164-6

disorders. Further notable advancements involve corneal transplantation, soft tissue reconstruction, and the repair of bone defects.[5–9]

The advent of enabling technologies like 3D bioprinting, also referred to as additive manufacturing or rapid prototyping, has opened new possibilities for creating highly personalized therapeutic approaches. By combining principles from tissue engineering, cell biology, and the use of bioactive materials, this technique allows for the fabrication of functional biological constructs. Its transformative impact stems from the layer-by-layer deposition process, which permits the development of intricate, anatomically precise structures. As a result, 3D bioprinting has become increasingly significant in biomedical research, especially in the realms of regenerative medicine and tissue engineering.[10–12] Figure 6.1 illustrates the diverse applications of 3D bioprinting in tissue engineering, highlighting its potential to fabricate functional constructs for a wide range of organs and systems, from skin and bone to cardiovascular, neural, and reproductive tissues.

A variety of 3D bioprinting techniques have been developed, each tailored to specific biomedical applications. Extrusion-based bioprinting is frequently employed for

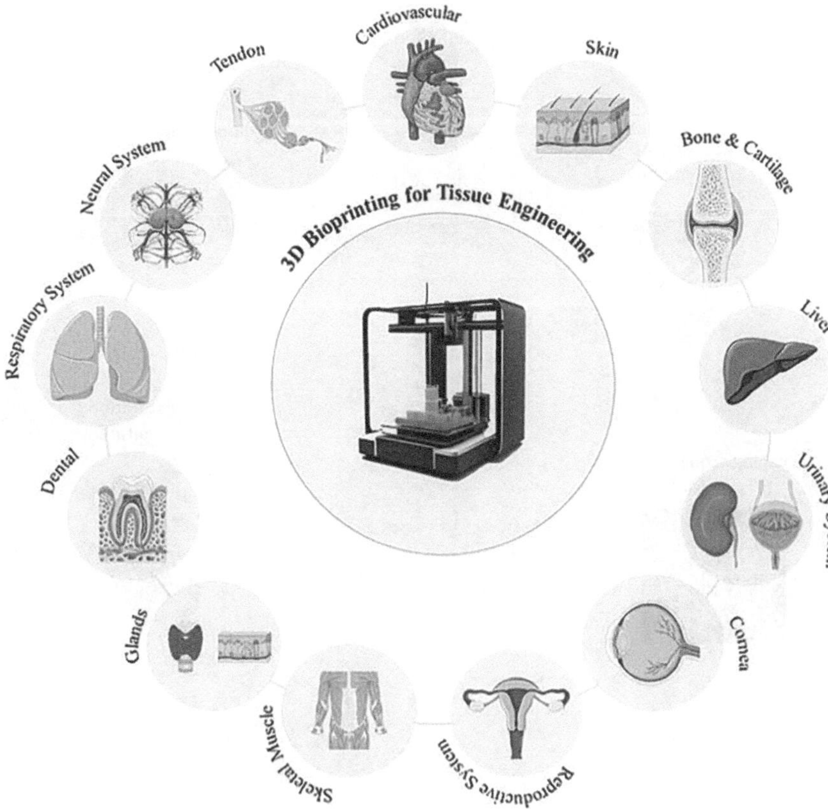

FIGURE 6.1 Overview of tissue and organ targets for 3D bioprinting in regenerative medicine, including cardiovascular, musculoskeletal, neural, and other biological systems. (From Mirshafiei et al.[13] Copyright 2024, Elsevier.)

fabricating load-bearing or structural tissues, while inkjet bioprinting offers high-resolution capabilities suitable for constructing intricate microenvironments. Laser-assisted bioprinting, on the other hand, allows for highly precise spatial arrangement of cells.[10,14] This technology marks a significant shift in therapeutic modeling and tissue fabrication, as it enables the accurate deposition of bioinks, typically aqueous hydrogel-based formulations to create 3D constructs that emulate the structural and functional characteristics of native tissues.[2] Recent developments have also led to the formulation of advanced bioinks containing SC-derived cells, bioactive molecules, and growth factors, presenting promising strategies to address the global shortage of transplantable organs.[15]

One of the primary advantages of this technique lies in its capacity for patient-specific customization of printed tissues. Imaging modalities like computed tomography (CT) and magnetic resonance imaging (MRI) provide 3D data of the affected tissue, which can be processed through computer-aided design (CAD) software to direct the bioprinting process. This integration ensures that the resulting constructs are both anatomically and functionally aligned with the individual patient's morphology.[14,16] Figure 6.2 depicts the sequential workflow of organ bioprinting, beginning with imaging

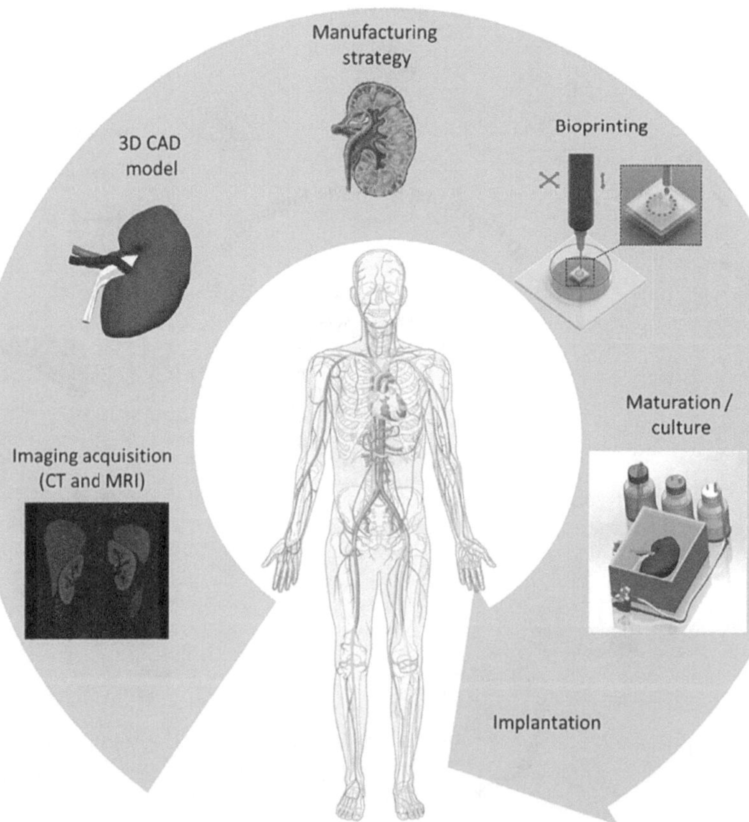

FIGURE 6.2 Schematic workflow of organ bioprinting, from imaging acquisition and digital modeling to manufacturing, maturation, and implantation. (From Mota et al.[20] Copyright 2020, ACS.)

acquisition (CT or MRI) to create a 3D CAD model, followed by the manufacturing strategy, bioprinting process, *in vitro* maturation, and culminating in implantation.

Such a degree of personalization allows the production of transplantable tissues with minimized immunogenicity, in addition to enabling the bioprinting of intricate anatomical structures like blood vessels, skin, liver, cartilage, and bones. The integration of vascular networks, suitable mechanical properties, and biochemical cues within the printed constructs significantly improves their biological integration and overall therapeutic performance.[17] Moreover, incorporating bioactive molecules into printed biomaterials has been shown to enhance their functionality, particularly through the development of bioactive scaffolds. These scaffolds have exhibited varying levels of effectiveness in facilitating tissue regeneration.[18,19]

For instance, the incorporation of specific bioactive proteins into scaffolds can modulate key cellular processes, including proliferation, migration, and differentiation.[21] In addition, scaffolds supplemented with enzymes exhibiting particular catalytic activities can engage in redox reactions that neutralize free radicals, thereby safeguarding cells from oxidative stress. By integrating these enzymes into the scaffold for localized delivery at the injury site, it is possible to offset insufficient endogenous antioxidant enzyme expression and improve the tissue's overall antioxidant defense.[11]

3D printing is compatible with diverse material types, such as filaments, powders, semisolid substances, and liquids. Various printing technologies, such as fused deposition modeling using thermoplastic filaments; extrusion-based printing with pneumatic or mechanical dispensing of solutions, gels, pastes, or composites; stereolithography using UV-curable resins; digital light processing with light-curable resins; selective laser sintering of powdered materials; and binder jetting and laminated object manufacturing, can process a broad range of biomaterials, including polymers, hydrogels, ceramics, and composites, each offering unique advantages for tailoring drug delivery systems (Figure 6.3). Through modification of the digital design and printing parameters, it is possible to obtain drugs with precise control over composition and release kinetics, thus reducing adverse effects and facilitating the creation of complex delivery systems customized for particular diseases or patient groups.[14,22] The versatility of 3D printing has facilitated its use in producing a wide variety of drug delivery devices, including solid oral formulations, liquid capsules, rectal and vaginal delivery platforms, and transdermal patches.[14,23]

In the realm of diagnostics, 3D printing allows for the precise design of surface topographies and functional gradients within microchannels, thereby optimizing fluid dynamics and improving the efficiency of diagnostic microchips. Additionally, it supports the fabrication of engineered tissue constructs for use in diagnostic screening applications.[25] These innovations improve nucleic acid separation efficiency, reduce cross contamination, and foster more effective interaction between fluids and functional components, leading to enhanced diagnostic accuracy.

A notable example is the study by Dong et al.,[26] in which 3D printing was employed to construct four functional components of a diagnostic chip: sample preparation, nucleic acid amplification, detection and analysis, and fluid regulation. These elements were assembled into a compact, portable platform for nucleic acid detection. The extracted nucleic acids were introduced into an amplification chamber, where they underwent thermal amplification in a fully sealed environment, followed by transfer to a testing chamber for colorimetric analysis. The system achieved 100%

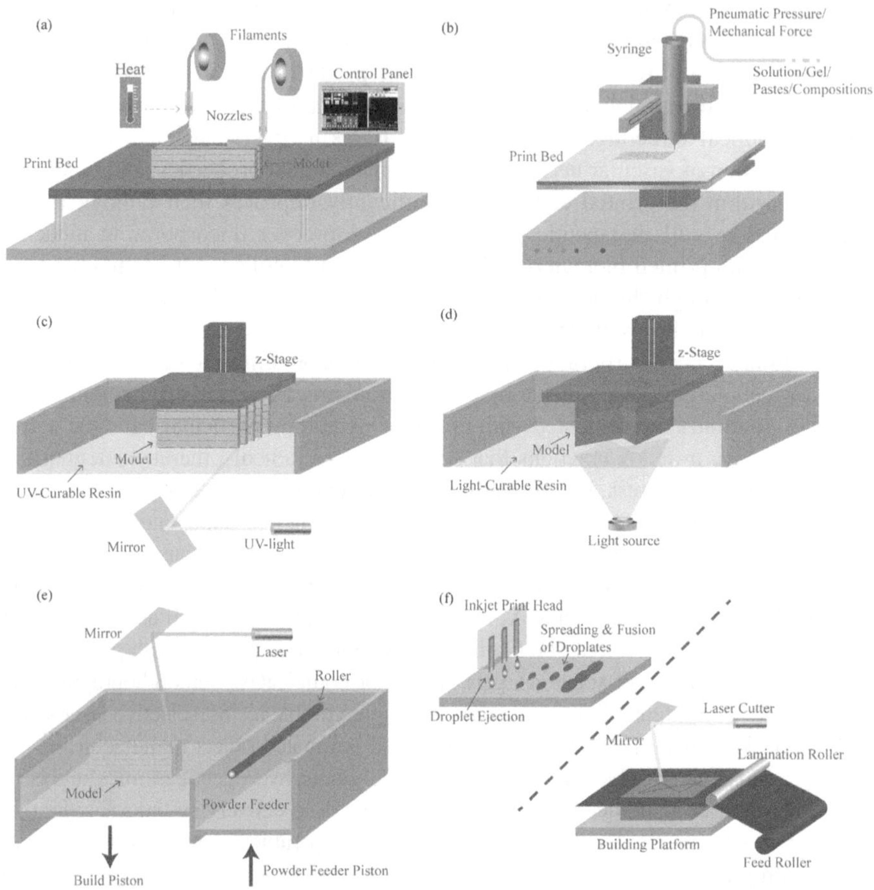

FIGURE 6.3 Schematic representation of different 3D printing technologies applied to drug delivery and biomedical applications: (a) fused deposition modeling (FDM) using thermoplastic filaments; (b) extrusion-based printing with pneumatic or mechanical dispensing of solutions, gels, pastes, or composites; (c) stereolithography (SLA) using UV-curable resins; (d) digital light processing (DLP) with light-curable resins; (e) selective laser sintering (SLS) of powdered materials; and (f) binder jetting and laminated object manufacturing (LOM) using droplet deposition, spreading, fusion, and laser cutting. (From Zhu et al.[24] Copyright 2024, Advanced HealthCare Materials.)

clinical sensitivity and specificity in tuberculosis detection, underscoring its practical utility and on-site reliability.[25,27]

Each of these applications, whether in regenerative medicine, pharmaceuticals, or diagnostics, follows unique regulatory frameworks, development timelines, and clinical goals. Pharmacological therapies prioritize long-term functionality and safety, whereas pharmacological testing systems are chiefly designed to accurately replicate biological responses.[8,14,25]

Thus, 3D bioprinting serves as a technological bridge between diagnosis, drug development, and personalized therapy, redefining the landscape of translational medicine.

The convergence of regenerative medicine, 3D bioprinting, and diversified clinical applications represents one of the most promising frontiers in modern healthcare. By uniting biotechnological innovation with individualized treatment strategies, it opens new avenues for restoring health with precision, efficiency, and reduced invasiveness.

6.2 CLINICAL NEEDS AND TARGET TISSUES

6.2.1 Major Medical Challenges: Bone Defects, Chronic Wounds, and Organ Failure

In the past several years, regenerative medicine, along with tissue engineering, has been getting more popular. The aim is to restore cellular functions as well as repair or replace damaged tissues. The ultimate purpose is to facilitate functional recovery through interventions that lead to long-lasting clinical outcomes.[28]

This field addresses a broader spectrum of important medical problems, including challenging large bone defects, stubborn chronic wounds that do not respond to traditional therapy, and vital organ failure (Figure 6.4). These conditions severely influence the quality of life and are associated with public health and healthcare expenses.[29]

Bone, an organ that is highly vascularized and dynamic in nature, has a remarkable inherent ability to heal. However, in the case of critical-size defects, which are referred to as lesions unable to heal by themselves, this ability gets reduced. These defects are mostly trauma-related due to high-energy soft tissue damage, oncologic resections, chronic osteomyelitis, and degenerative pathologies including osteoporosis.[28] Surgical reconstruction with grafts is required in these situations. Autologous and allogeneic grafts are still the most employed strategies, but both methods are limited because of clinical challenges that consist of donor site morbidity, restricted availability in cell and tissue products with an immune response, and increased hazards for infection.[29] Especially in oral and maxillofacial reconstructions, these constraints are much more significant due to the enormous complexity of anatomical and functional requirements.[30]

Cartilage injuries, similarly, are extremely difficult to manage. Articular cartilage is an avascular and relatively low cell density tissue with a very limited intrinsic ability to repair. In response to traumatic injuries, or because of progressive degeneration such as in osteoarthritis, chronic inflammation, joint dysfunction, and persistent pain can result. This tissue has practically no regenerative potential since it is not vascularized. Traditional treatments, including physical therapy, lifestyle adaptations, and pharmacological treatment with anti-inflammatory agents or analgesics, often fail when the extent of injury to tissue becomes significant.[31]

The clinical frame to treat chronic wounds is still an unanswered problem. Diabetic foot ulcers, venous leg ulcers, and pressure injuries are conditions that often have poor healing outcomes with high complication rates. The skin is the largest organ of the body and plays an essential role in protection, thermoregulation, and sensory interaction.[32] Therapeutic approaches are few when extended injuries exceed the endogenous potential for skin regeneration, as is evidenced by events such as major burns or chronic ulceration. Although autologous skin grafts have been widely

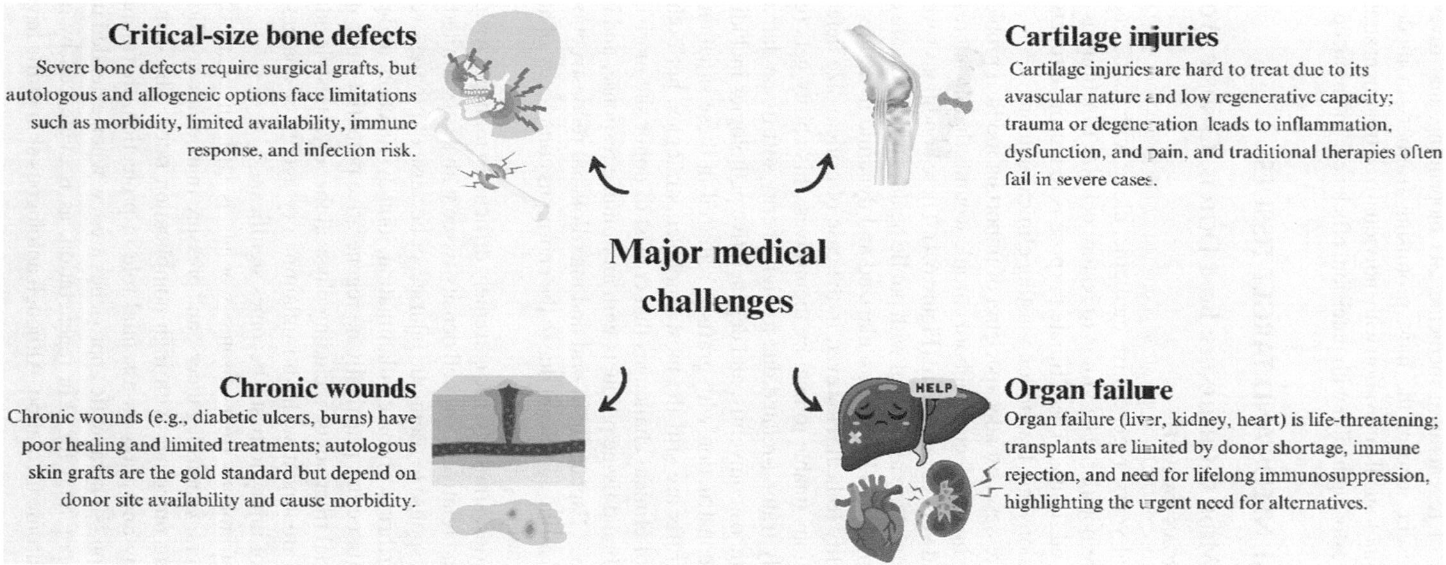

FIGURE 6.4 Current major medical challenges in regenerative medicine.

regarded as the gold standard, they are contingent upon the availability of an appropriate donor site and cause morbidity at the harvest area.[33]

In severe cases, organ failure of the liver, kidney, or heart can develop rapidly and become life-threatening. While transplant can correct these defects, transplantation is limited by the availability of suitable donors/grafts, recipient immune rejection, and lifelong dependence on immunosuppression.[34] The fact that there are global increases in chronic diseases, that innovation is severely inhibited, and that the world population continues to age only reinforces the need for alternative strategies.

In this context, 3D bioprinting has been considered a strategy with great potential. Using this tool, we can deposit living cells, biomaterials, and bioactive factors with great precision in spatial design to create constructs that mimic the architecture and function of native tissues.[28,34] Bioprinting offers promise in the context of clinical challenges, including bone and cartilage repair, chronic wound healing, or critical organ needs, due to the versatility and adaptability bioprinting can provide.

6.2.2 Examples of Tissue-Specific Applications

6.2.2.1 Bone and Cartilage: Scaffolds for Orthopedic and Dental Repair

Critical-sized bone defects are the most challenging problems in orthopedics, dentistry, as well as reconstructive surgery. Annually, about four million people need to be treated for fractures.[30] The use of 3D bioprinting offers the ability to produce extracellular matrix (ECM)-based structures, such as custom bone scaffolds with fine-tuned pore sizes, geometry, and compositions that can support both osteoinduction and osteoconduction.[28,35] This also allows spatially localized deposition of cells, biomaterials, drugs, and signaling molecules to print structures that can be custom designed for each patient.[33]

Scaffolds for bone tissue engineering should possess sufficient mechanical strength, osteoconduction, and a porous structure to maintain vascularization, cell infiltration, and proliferation.[36] Extrusion-based 3D printing is the most common strategy, which can be performed with inks containing hydrogels and ceramic materials (e.g., hydroxyapatite, which replicates the major minerals in natural bone and teeth) that can contribute to both bioactivity and increased mechanical properties.[37]

Other materials, such as tricalcium phosphate (TCP) and poly(ε-caprolactone) (PCL)-based biodegradable composites, have also been used alone or in combination with mesenchymal SCs and human bone morphogenetic protein-2 (rhBMP-2), a growth factor that enhances regeneration ability, for bone tissue engineering strategies.[37] These strategies have demonstrated great potential in bone generation/repair of preclinical models (Table 6.1), thus providing a solution for treating large, difficult-to-heal defects, mainly in the head and neck area but also in other regions such as the spine.[38,39]

3D-printed PCL/β-TCP scaffolds incorporating rhBMP-2 were successful in regenerating large (5 cm) bone defects in a sheep metatarsus model with cortical bridging and increasing the amount of bone volume after 24 weeks.[40] Another study fabricated a magnesium phosphate/PCL scaffold used for maxillofacial healing, which exhibited accelerated *in vitro* osteogenesis and significantly improved bone

TABLE 6.1
3D Bioprinting Studies About Bone and Cartilage Regeneration and *In Situ* Bioprinting and Engineered Skin Substitutes

3D Printing Technology	Ink Composition	Application	Key Results	*In Vivo* Animal Model	Reference
Extrusion	Poly(ε-caprolactone), carboxymethyl chitosan and deferoxamine	Scaffolds for bone regeneration	Increased vascular regeneration in the scaffolds, and greater bone growth and osseointegration	Rats	43
Fused deposition modeling	L-polylactic acid and nano hydroxyapatite	Scaffolds for bone regeneration	Tunable mechanical strength, biocompatibility and osteogenic induction properties	Rabbits	44
Extrusion	Hyaluronic acid methacrylate and acrylate-terminated four-armed polyethylene glycol	*In situ* 3D printing in cartilage regeneration	Rapid repair of osteochondral defects and cartilage regeneration	Rabbits	45
Extrusion	Silk fibroin, gelatin, and endogenic bone marrow stem cells (BMSCs)	Scaffolds for cartilage regeneration	Retention of BMSCs, mechanical protection, and cartilage regeneration.	Rabbits	46
Extrusion	Carboxymethyl chitosan and nanoclay	*In situ* 3D-printed diabetic wound dressing	Promoted the healing of diabetic wounds through antibacterial and proangiogenic effects.	Rats	47
Extrusion	Chitosan, alginate, and copper oxide	Amniotic membrane scaffold for skin wound dressing	Blood vessel formation and pro-regenerative gene expression, accelerating wound healing without toxicity.	Rats	48

formation following implantation into defective rabbit models,[38] illustrating its future application as highly personalized bone repair.

In the case of cartilage, there are different challenges given to the avascular nature of this tissue and the type II collagen- and proteoglycans-rich ECM.[31] As the native tissue has a zonal structure, multi-material bioprinted scaffolds provide beneficial results in promoting chondrogenic differentiation of the encapsulated cells.[41] GelMA (gelatin methacryloyl), alginate, and collagen are common hydrogel bioinks in cartilage tissue engineering to support the chondrocyte or mesenchymal SCs phenotype survival and ECM production.[42,43]

Figure 6.5 illustrates the *in vivo* evaluation of bone regeneration using different scaffolds (PCL, PCH, and PCD) implanted in rat femoral defects, with detailed micro-CT imaging and quantitative analysis of bone microarchitecture compared to a scaffold-free control group.[44]

In a recent study, the development of a biphasic, 3D-printed scaffold targeting cartilage regeneration was described using cell-laden constructs with an upper layer consisting of GelMA hydrogels containing human costal chondrocytes while the lower layer contained both pre-osteoblasts in PCL and GelMA simultaneously with

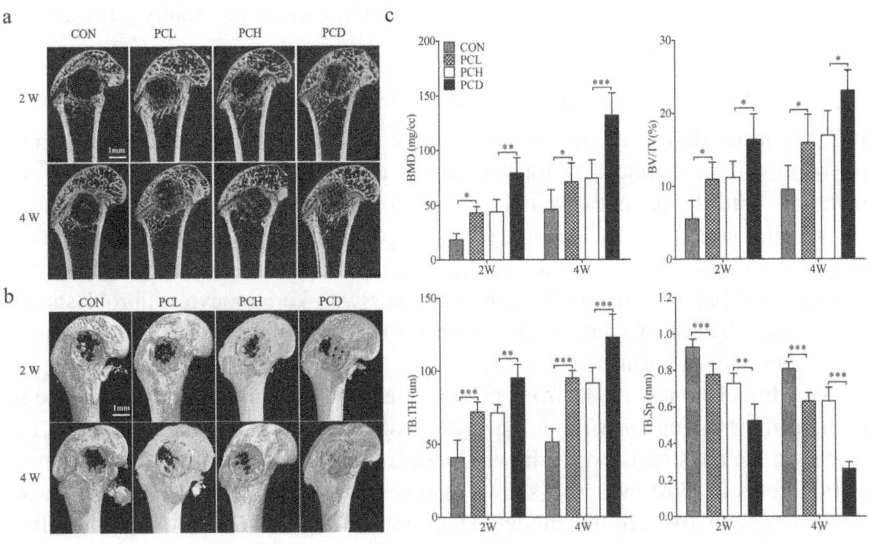

FIGURE 6.5 Micro-CT analysis of scaffold-mediated bone repair *in vivo*. Scaffolds (PCL, PCH, and PCD) were implanted into femoral defects in rats, with a scaffold-free group serving as the control (CON). (a and b) Representative two-dimensional (a) and three-dimensional reconstructed (b) micro-CT images illustrating new bone formation within the defect site for each group. The defect area is outlined with a red dashed line. (c) Quantitative analysis of micro-architectural parameters of the newly formed bone at two and four weeks, based on three-dimensional micro-CT reconstructions. Parameters include bone mineral density (BMD), bone volume fraction (BV/TV), trabecular thickness (Tb.Th), and trabecular separation (Tb.Sp). Data are expressed as mean ± SD. Statistical analysis: one-way ANOVA with Tukey's post-hoc test (*$p < 0.05$, **$p < 0.01$, ***$p < 0.001$). (From Yan et al.[45] Copyright 2019, Elsevier.)

human bone marrow-derived mesenchymal SCs.[49] Coculture of those cells, particularly in the presence of TGF-β3, facilitated chondrogenesis. In a rat model, the implants facilitated cartilage regeneration and reduced pain with mechanical properties similar to native tissue.

Osteochondral lesions can be very difficult to treat for several reasons. More recently, 3D bioprinting has been able to create biphasic or gradient scaffolds that mimic the transition from cartilage to subchondral bone, improving biomechanical performance and implant durability. Zhong et al.,[50] for instance, engineered a GelMA-based biomimetic trilayered scaffold using hydroxyethyl methacrylate-functionalized nanohydroxyapatite to model the layers of hyaline cartilage, calcified cartilage, and subchondral bone. This biphasic ceramic hydrogel construct, with bone-like mechanical strength, gradient porosity, as well as chondrogenesis and osteogenesis abilities, could be an ideal candidate for repairing critical osteochondral defects.

Although considerable progress has been made, there are several challenges in the clinical translation of these 3D bioprinted scaffolds for bone and cartilage. However, regulatory issues, bioink standardization, and production scalability prove to be significant bottlenecks. Moreover, such personalized grafts should be tested in human patients for validation in long-term clinical studies to ensure safety, efficacy, and functional integration.

6.2.2.1.1 Skin: *In Situ Bioprinting and Engineered Skin Substitutes*

In 3D printing skin, there are two main ways: *in situ* bioprinting and bioengineered (*in vitro*) skin substitutes. As for the former, this is to directly print cells and biomaterials onto the patient's wound site, which brings local regeneration adapted to the specific conditions of the injury. The approach has several advantages. It can facilitate not only the elimination of intermediate steps such as extended laboratory cultivation,[29] but also the application of bioinks with keratinocytes, fibroblasts, and even mesenchymal SCs encapsulated within biocompatible hydrogels such as collagen, alginate, or fibrin.[51]

A hydrogel bioink made from gelatin, GelMA, and fibroblasts was developed to 3D print dressings *in situ* on the surface of diabetic skin wounds in rats.[52] This biopolymeric construct, which showed biodegradability, antibacterial, and proangiogenic effects *in vitro*, was also shown to speed up wound healing effectively when integrated with live animal models. This indicates its potential for personalized chronic wound therapy. The wound healing performance of this bioink was assessed *in vivo*, as shown in Figure 6.6, which presents the macroscopic healing progression, histological evaluation, epidermal thickness measurements, and neovascularization markers in the treated wounds.

However, bioengineered skin substitutes are grown *in vitro*. This environment provides a more controlled one, allowing for the development of organized tissues that closely resemble native skin. These substitutes typically exhibit a layered structure, with a dermal component formed by fibroblasts embedded within an ECM (commonly collagen or gelatin) and an epidermal layer composed of keratinocytes cultured on the surface.[51] According to this principle, advanced model systems may also contain such elements as melanocytes, endothelial cells, and even hair follicles to enhance graft functionality.[29]

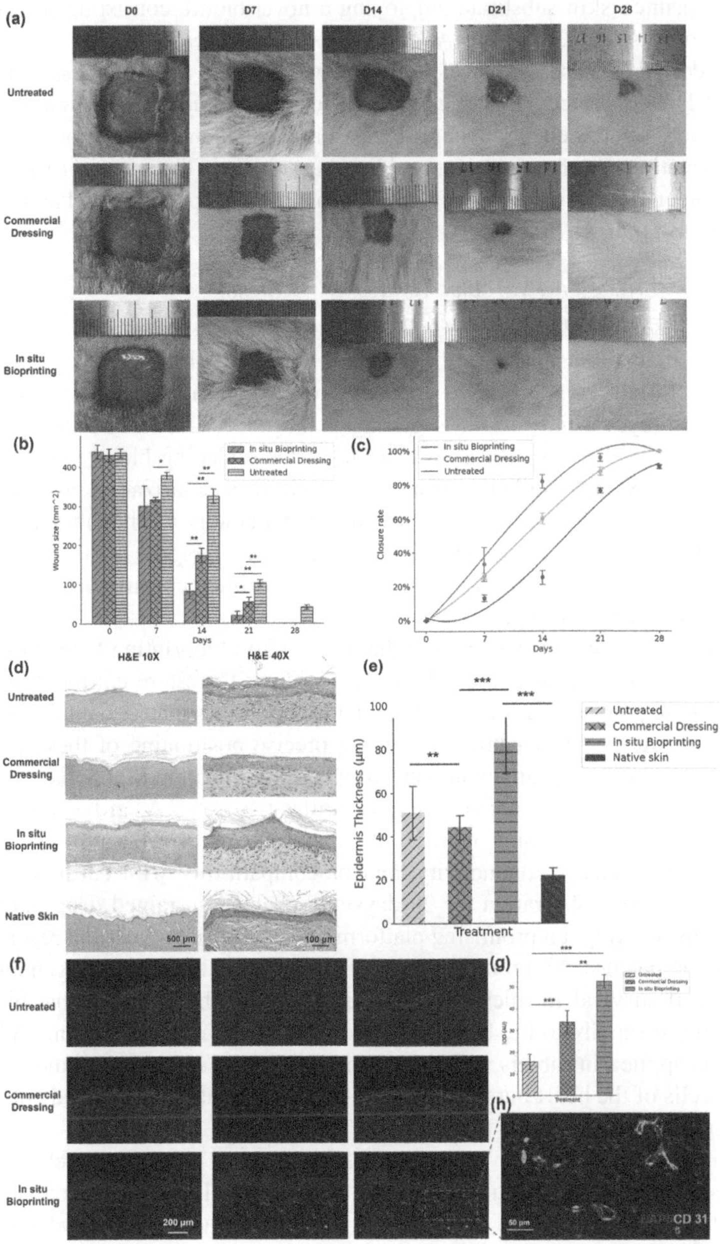

FIGURE 6.6 Repair experiments in a rat wound model. (a) Digital photographs taken at days 0, 7, 14, 21, and 28, compiled for each wound. (b) Wound size measurements for different treatments (*$p<0.05$, **$p<0.01$). (c) Wound closure curves showing accelerated healing in treated groups. (d) Hematoxylin and eosin (H&E) staining confirming epithelialization in bioprinted skin. (e) Quantification of reconstructed epidermal thickness (**$p<0.01$, ***$p<0.001$). (f) Immunohistochemical staining for endothelial cell marker CD31 and (g) corresponding fluorescence intensity, indicating neovascularization. (h) Presence of well-defined luminal structures in regenerated vessels. (From Zhou et al.[52] Copyright 2024, Springer Nature.)

A 3D-printed skin substitute employing a novel bioink consisting of decellularized adipose tissue ECM, GelMA, and methacrylated hyaluronic acid, with human adipose-derived SCs penned inside this mix, was put onto full-thickness skin wounds in rats.[53] The construct encouraged wounds to heal by cutting inflammation as well as promoting re-epithelization, angiogenesis, and collagen regeneration in a way that is significantly more favorable for residing host tissues. Therefore, *in situ* bioprinting and bioengineered skin substitutes have potential as personalized approaches to complex skin injuries (Table 6.1).

6.2.2.1.2 Cardiac and Vascular Tissues: Myocardial Patches and Vascular Conduits

Cardiovascular diseases are still the main reason behind death globally. The heart muscle has a very limited capacity for regeneration; one of the main hurdles of post-myocardial infarct is getting damaged cardiac tissue to regenerate.[54] Simultaneously, there is also a pressing need for replacing blood vessels that are damaged, for example, failed coronary arteries in revascularization procedures.[55] In this sense, 3D bioprinting has arisen as a novel technology for the fabrication of personalized myocardial patches and vascular conduits.[56,57] Figure 6.7 illustrates recent advances in the design and fabrication of these bioprinted constructs for cardiac and vascular tissue engineering.

A myocardial patch is a construct that is based on bioprinting technology for its application over the infarct area of the myocardium to restore cardiac function. In general, these patches are composed of a natural polymer matrix containing cardiac cells and/or drugs.[56] Bioprinting allows for precise positioning of these cells, promoting muscle fiber alignment and electrical communication (Table 6.2), which are key factors for coordinated contraction of cardiac tissue.[58,59] A cardiac patch printed via direct ink writing using nanocellulose, poly(glycerol sebacate), and polypyrrole showed elasticity, conductivity, and biocompatibility with cardiomyoblasts.[60] It supported cell proliferation for 28 days and enabled sustained drug release over five months, making it a promising platform for long-term myocardial regeneration.

Also, the patches can promote blood vessel invasion to supply oxygen and nutrients for cell survival in thick tissues. Animal studies have shown that bioprinted patches fused rapidly to the heart wall and improved cardiac function.[65] When the patch was applied in rabbits suffering from myocardial infarction, it did not generate new cells of the heart but induced local vessel generation, decreased collagenous fibers, and improved cardiac function.

Synthetic prostheses for vascular grafts are used in place of vessels, and these prostheses have a high failure rate, as there is no real biological compatibility.[55] Bioprinted vascular conduits, based on inks with or without endothelial and smooth muscle cells seeded in biodegradable matrices, can be manufactured in different sizes and geometries.[66] These properties can be combined in a scaffold that is able to build structures resembling the nature of blood vessels but also have excellent remodeling and anti-collapse capability. Perfusable blood vessels (~1 mm), with endothelial cells, smooth muscle cells, and fibroblasts in a biomimetic trilayered architecture, using drop-on-demand bioprinting.[67] After three weeks in the perfusion bioreactor, the constructs exhibited excellent cell viabilities and expressed critical vascular

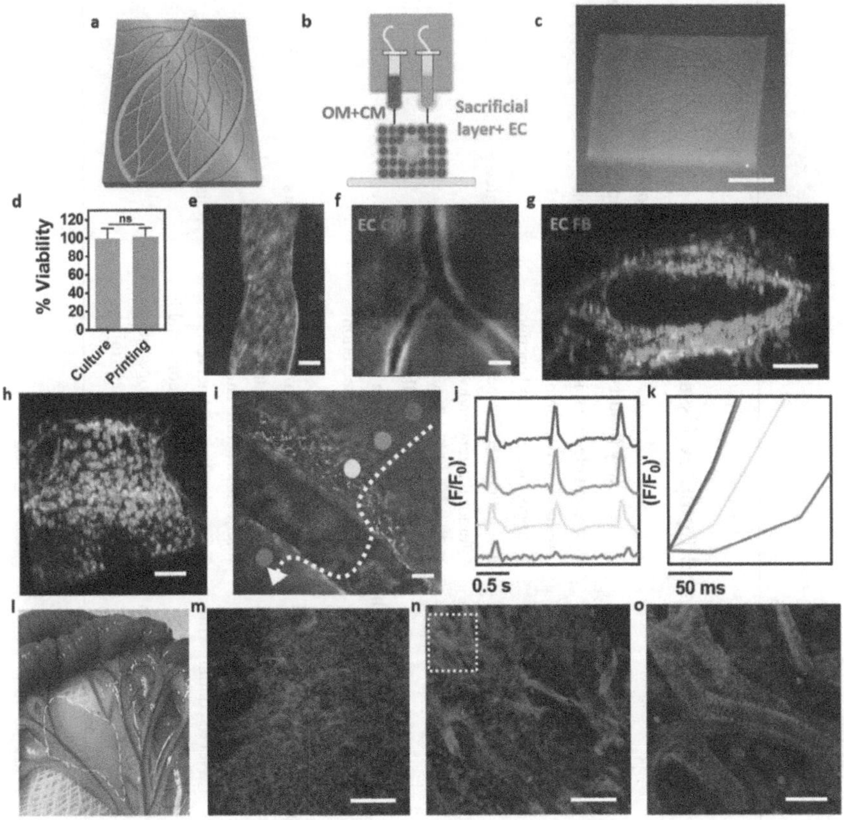

FIGURE 6.7 3D printing of personalized vascularized cardiac patches. (a) 3D model of the cardiac patch. (b) Side view of the printing concept illustrating distinct cellular bioinks. (c) Printed vascularized cardiac patch. (d) Cell viability post-printing. (e) Printed blood vessel with continuous layers of GFP-expressing endothelial cells (ECs). (f) Printed iPSC-derived cardiac patch showing blood vessels (CD31, green) interspersed between cardiac tissue (sarcomeric actinin, pink). (g and h) Cross-sections of a single lumen displaying interactions between GFP-expressing ECs and RFP-expressing fibroblasts. (i–k) Calcium imaging in the printed vascularized patch, with regions of interest shown in distinct colors; white arrow indicates signal direction. (i) Lumen of a blood vessel visible between cardiac cells. (j and k) Quantification of calcium transients across a vessel lumen. (l) Transplantation of the printed patch between two layers of rat omentum (dashed white line marks patch boundaries). (m–o) Sarcomeric actinin (red) and nuclei (blue) staining of sections from the explanted patch; (o) shows high magnification of the marked area in (n). *Scale bars*: c = 1 cm; e, g, h, l, m = 100 μm; f = 500 μm; n = 50 μm; o = 25 μm. (From Noor et al.[56], Chen et al.[57] Copyright 2019, Advanced Science.)

markers, thereby demonstrating their potential as a more realistic *in vitro* platform for drug screening and disease modeling.

The use of coaxial bioprinting has been a recent breakthrough in this area and allows the assembly of multiple-layer tubes with an inner lumen and cell walls.[68] These bioprinted conduits have demonstrated good patency in preclinical models, as well

TABLE 6.2
3D Bioprinting Studies About Myocardial Patches and Vascular Conduits and Complex Tissue Constructs

3D Printing Technology	Ink Composition	Application	Key Results	*In Vivo* Animal Model	Reference
Extrusion	Fibrinogen, mesenchymal stem cells and graphene oxide	Conductive patch for myocardial infarction repair	Improved electrical integration, reduced cell apoptosis, and support for cardiac function	Rats	60
Projection stereolithography	Poly(ethylene glycol) diacrylate	Vascular conduits	Robust connection between the femoral artery and vein, allowing blood flow for up to 6 hours without collapse.	Piglets	61
Inkjet	Sodium alginate, hyaluronic acid, peptides, hepatocytes and human umbilical cord cells	Liver organoids with biomimetic lobule structure	Liver organoids with high cell viability, albumin secretion, and urea synthesis.	*In vitro*	62
Extrusion-based tri-coaxial nozzles	Collagen, human bone marrow-derived mesenchymal stem cells, and epithelial cells	Renal tubular tissue analog	Creation of vascularized tubular renal tissue, maintaining cellular structure and function	Rats	63
Digital light processing	Gelatin methacryloyl, lithiumphenyl-2,4,6-trimethylbenzoylphosphinate, and R-NPs,	Nerve conduit with drug release for nerve regeneration	Remyelination and nerve regeneration, with comparable performance to autogenous in repairing sciatic nerve injury.	Rats	64

as promoted functional endothelial coverage and resistance to thrombus formation.[69] Although major advancements have been made, hurdles, including high-performance electrical integration with cardiac tissue, large-scale manufacturability, persistent vascularization, and long-term safety still need to be addressed.[68] In a similar fashion, we can say that 3D bioprinting also expects to find powerful and custom solutions for regeneration in cardiac and vascular pathologies benefiting the global population suffering from cardiovascular diseases, whether they are of congenital or acquired origin.

6.2.2.1.3 Liver, Kidney, and Nerve Regeneration: Complex Tissue Constructs in Development

The liver is an organ which is metabolically active and is devoted to crucial functions, including detoxification of endogenous and exogenous toxicants, production of protein, bile, as well as metabolic intermediates. One approach to hepatic bioprinting is the formation of functional liver lobules by patterning hepatocytes, endothelial cells, and Kupffer cells in microenvironments of the size and variation that mimic lobular architecture.[34,70] Liver ECM bioinks have been applied for hepatocyte differentiation and functionality.[71]

While the liver-in-a-dish (non-epigenetically modified) remains a distant prospect, it is now possible to generate transgenically engineered hepatoids, responsive with predictable physiological form and function to drugs—an extremely valuable novelty for pharmacology.[72] Another study achieved successful bioprinting of liver organoids with patient-derived bioinks, which exhibited capacitated drug metabolism similar to native liver tissue, and thus could be used for personalized toxicity tests.[73] Figure 6.8 showcases representative examples of these bioprinted hepatic models and their potential applications in drug testing and personalized medicine.

For the kidney, this is an even taller order because of the intricate and multiple structures such as nephrons, renal tubules, and glomeruli. New research has worked to achieve bioprinting of renal substructures, such as biomaterial-based approaches to facilitate proximal tubule function in isolation from the rest of the kidney.[74,75] The utilization of these self-organizing methods to generate renal organoids for selective filtration and solute reabsorption using bioprinting provides an important new tool, especially in the context of hereditary kidney disease models and as a drug toxicology platform.[75] Homan et al.[74] created a bioprinted proximal tubule model that showed evidence of functional reabsorption and responsiveness to nephrotoxic drugs, which serves as an important tool for the study of kidney disease.

3D bioprinting has also opened avenues for the challenging topic of peripheral nerve injuries that do not regenerate well in the nervous system. An important point involves the creation of guidance tracks for axonal growth where injured axons can grow along, including its promotion of local axon regeneration.[76] Generating conduits can likewise combine aligned inner channels, conductive biomaterials, and Schwann cells to advance quicker and practical regeneration.[77] However, multi-head bioprinting technologies facilitated the accurate distribution of multiple types of cells on the conduit to establish a suitable environment for nerve regeneration.[76] A 3D bioprinted nerve guide multi-functionalized with canine mesenchymal stromal cells combined with Schwann cells resulted in a pro-regenerative state after critical sciatic nerve injury in rats.[78]

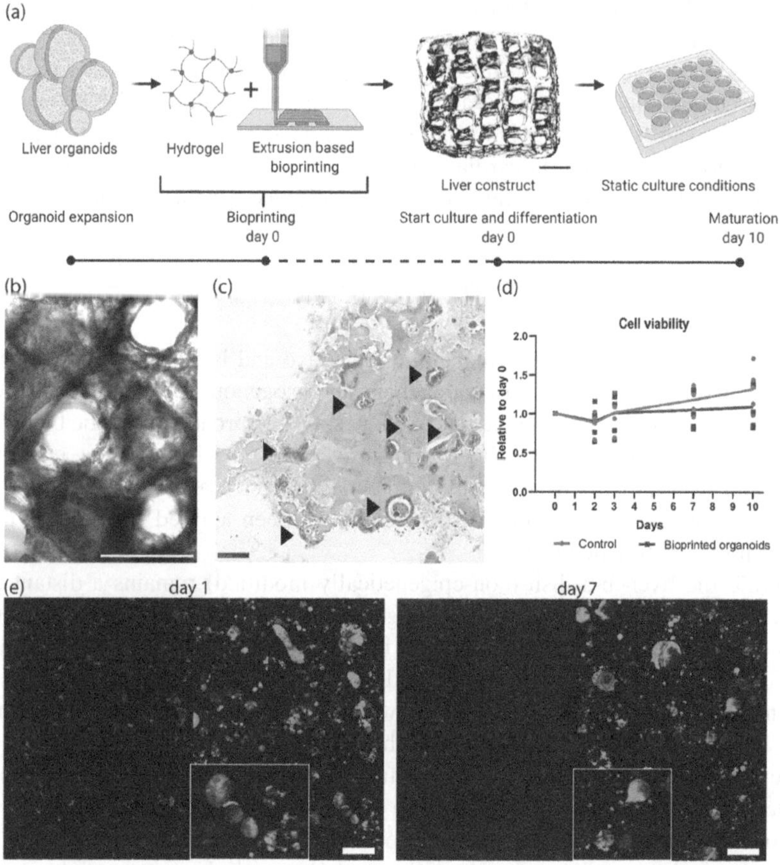

FIGURE 6.8 Bioprinting of liver constructs. (a) Schematic representation of the experimental workflow for liver construct bioprinting. Expanded liver organoids (ICOs) are encapsulated in a GelMA hydrogel, and a porous structure is fabricated via extrusion-based bioprinting of the bioink. Constructs are cultured in organoid differentiation medium to promote maturation toward a hepatocyte-like phenotype. Scale bar = 1,000 μm. Created with BioRender.com. (b) Brightfield image of a bioprinted liver construct. Scale bar = 1,000 μm. (c) H&E staining of the bioprinted construct. Arrowheads indicate cystic organoid structures within printed struts; insets show twofold magnification. Scale bar = 100 μm. (d) Viability of liver organoids in GelMA (five donors) immediately after plating (control; orange) and post-printing (blue). Each dot represents the mean of a technical triplicate from a single donor. (e) Representative live/dead staining of liver organoids at days 1 and 7 post-printing. Image shows an entire printed strut. (From Bouwmeester et al.[73] Copyright 2021, Macromolecular Bioscience.)

Nevertheless, 3D bioprinting of the liver, kidney, and nerves is moving forward quickly with technical limitations and requirements for effective vascularization being considered. These multilayered tissue constructs can be considered a breakthrough in the field of tissue engineering and hold promise to change the face of treatment for organ failure, nerve injuries, and degenerative diseases shortly.

6.3 BIOPRINTING MEETS STEM CELL THERAPY

SCs are undifferentiated cells present in multicellular organisms. These cells possess the capacity for self-renewal, multiplication, and differentiation into various specific cell types (potency).[79] In the context of cell development, these cells represent the initial stages and can be found in embryos, adult tissues, and even menstrual blood.[80] These cells have been shown to possess an inherent capacity for disease treatment, rendering them a promising candidates for applications in the domains of cell therapy,[81] regenerative medicine,[82] and 3D bioprinting.[83]

SCs can be classified into two major groups, distinguishing between cell origin and differentiation.[79] With respect to cell differentiation, the following classifications can be made: Totipotent SCs, cells that have the capacity to generate any cell type, whether from embryonic or extraembryonic tissues, such as the amniotic sac, placenta, and umbilical cord.[84] Pluripotent SCs are cells capable of differentiating into derivatives of all three germ layers (ectoderm, mesoderm, and endoderm).[84] Multipotent SCs can differentiate into a limited set of cell types belonging to a specific tissue or organ.[85] Oligopotent SCs differentiate into an even more restricted group of closely related cell types.[86]

About the origins of SCs, they can be classified as follows: Embryonic SCs, cells that are derived from the blastocyst and represent the initial stage of embryo development, exhibiting characteristics of pluripotency.[87] Mesenchymal SCs, a type of stromal cell with a high degree of plasticity and the capacity to differentiate into mesodermal cells, including myocytes (muscle cells), osteocytes (bone cells), chondrocytes (cartilage cells), and adipocytes (fat cells).[88] Fetal SCs, a cell obtained from the developing fetus during pregnancy, exhibits pluripotency.[89] Adult SCs, a specialized cell category present in mature tissues such as bone marrow, blood vessels, and adipose tissue, represent a distinct entity. It has the capacity to differentiate into particular cell types (multipotency).[90] Amniotic SCs are primitive cells typically derived from the fluid surrounding the fetus within the amniotic sac.[91] Induced pluripotent SCs (iPSCs) are differentiated cells that have been reprogrammed to a state analogous to embryonic stem cells.[92]

Cutting-edge 3D bioprinting techniques leverage therapies based on mesenchymal and pluripotent SCs, thereby effecting a paradigm shift in the domains of regenerative medicine, tissue engineering, and organ transplantation. The formulation of bioinks is of paramount importance, as they must provide a matrix conductive to cell support, growth, proliferation, and differentiation.[93] These materials are typically derived from synthetic or natural polymers. Natural hydrogels, including starch, chitosan, gelatin, collagen, alginate, decellularized ECM, hyaluronic acid, and κ-carrageenan, along with their composites, have emerged as a subject of interest in scientific research due to their potential applications in the field of 3D printing by extrusion. These hydrogels possess rheological properties such as pseudoplasticity and shear thinning, which are advantageous in minimizing shear stresses that can lead to cell lysis and compromise process efficiency.[94] Human adipose tissue-derived SCs were used to evaluate the cell viability of composite bioinks based on methacrylated κ-carrageenan with hydroxyapatite.[95] The studies demonstrated that cell viability was increased by nearly twofold, thus indicating the potential for biomedical applications.[95]

The sophistication of 3D bioprinted neural tissue models has notably increased in the last decade. Combining fibrin-based bioink formulations with drug-releasing microspheres validates environments conducive to culturing neural cells derived from induced pluripotent human SCs. This combination also increases the mechanical strength required for bioinspiring the target neural tissue.[96,97] Regenerative medicine has transformed plastic surgery, and combining SCs with bioprinting provides new solutions to tissue reconstruction challenges.[98] Mesenchymal SCs have been used to print scaffolds for critical-sized mandibular defects in animal models. The mechanical support provided good structural integration over time, and the addition of osteoinductive growth factors accelerated cell differentiation.[99] Thus, the relationship between SCs and 3D bioprinting signifies substantial advancements in tissue engineering.

Over time, strategies have been developed to guide cell differentiation and support specific tissue regeneration. Induced pluripotent SCs, which are commonly reprogrammed from blood mononuclear cell cultures, umbilical cord cells, or fibroblasts, are among the most promising tools in regenerative medicine. These cells have the ability to differentiate into cells from all three germ layers. However, this vast differentiation capacity can lead to a high risk of developing teratomas. Therefore, safe, ideal, and highly efficient differentiation protocols are necessary to obtain the desired differentiated cell culture.[100] Using pigment epithelium-derived factor and its associated peptides (44-mer and 17-mer) has been shown to have neuroprotective effects when differentiating human induced pluripotent SCs into retinal ganglion cells.[101] The study found significant increases in the expression of the neuroaxonal markers Tau and NFH, the retinal progenitor markers Pax6, and the retinal ganglion cell markers Brn3b and Sncg. This enables the development of therapies for treating optic neuropathies that cause ganglion cell degeneration and irreversible vision loss.[101]

Oldershaw's research team developed the first well-defined protocol for differentiating human embryonic SCs into chondrocytes.[102] This protocol requires two matrix substrates (gelatin and fibronectin), seven growth factors (NT-4, BMP4, WNT3A, GDF-5, FGF-2, Follistatin, and Activin-A), and chemically supplemented media. This protocol facilitates future studies on cell replacement therapies and cartilage repair.[102] Cell differentiation for target tissue regeneration is favored by correctly selecting growth factors, a support matrix, and substrates for cell supplementation.

Bioinspiration or biomimicry is crucial for designing bioprinted environments that reproduce the structure and function of the target tissue. Cardiac tissue, for example, has no regenerative capacity; therefore, its 3D bioprinting may be a promising alternative to transplants for treating end-stage heart failure. However, reproducing the native structure requires developing advanced cardiac bioinks. The main obstacles to this development include replicating the cardiac microenvironment, achieving precise 3Dorganization, and accurately characterizing their properties.[103] A new bioink consisting of hyaluronic acid functionalized with gallic acid, type I collagen, and multilayer carbon nanotubes coated with hyaluronic acid has shown positive responses with cardiomyocytes derived from induced pluripotent human SCs.[104] This response enables the 3D printing of functional cardiac ventricles responsive to pharmacological treatment. It overcomes the challenge of post-bioprinting matrix contraction due to the interaction of encapsulated cells with the collagen matrix. This ensures fidelity to the 3D design.[104]

Bioprinted vascular grafts require extreme geometric fidelity to be applicable. The main challenge for clinical applications is precisely positioning endothelial and smooth muscle cells to optimize tissue performance.[105,106] Small-caliber vessels were bioprinted using SCs from adipose tissue. Differentiation into endothelial cells was performed using the vascular endothelial growth factor (VEGF)-165 PODS® (Polyhedrin Delivery System), and TGF-β1 PODS® was applied to obtain smooth muscle cells.[106] The results indicated successful blood vessel biofabrication with a double layer of endothelial and epithelial cells and smooth muscle cells. There was also improved biocompatibility, low platelet adhesion, and desirable angiogenic properties.[106] Thus, combining SCs with strategies that guide cell differentiation and growth, along with 3D bioprinting technology, is a promising approach for regenerative medicine, tissue engineering, and cell therapies.

6.4 CHALLENGES AND CLINICAL ADVANCES

The advances in the 3D printing field have increasingly enabled not only the development of shape and dimensioned patient-specific materials but also the development of biologically active constructs that can mimic native tissue environments.[107,108] Despite these notable advances, key challenges concerning the overall biocompatibility, immune response, and the real clinical application of these materials remain to be overcome.

6.4.1 Key Obstacles: Vascularization, Immune Response, Functional Integration

Besides the challenges involved in reaching the required characteristics of a bioink, such as the stability of the final construct combined with a controlled degradation rate, the biocompatibility, and the ability to support cell proliferation, one of the key obstacles is the functional integration of the constructs with the local tissue. In this sense, to support the long-term survival of bioprinted constructs, it is essential to establish a connected vascular network with the host's native blood vessels.[107] Vascularization is a crucial element for providing not only nutrients and oxygen transport, but also the disposal of cell waste products, ensuring the maintenance of cell viability and tissue functionality.[109] Due to the lack of oxygen and nutrients, cells can die if they are distant from a blood vessel (more than 100–200 μm).[110] *In vivo*, the process can occur through two pathways: by angiogenesis, in which proangiogenic factors induce formation of new vessels from a vessel that already exists; or by vasculogenesis, where mesodermal cells differentiate into angioblasts and into endothelial cells during the embryonic phase.[111] In this sense, *in vitro* researchers have been looking for different ways to improve the vascularization process in the bioprinted materials, for example, using raw materials that can mimic ECM, adding proangiogenic factors in the bioink, such as VEGFs and basic fibroblast growth factors, to induce microvessels formation.[109] Researchers produced, through 3D bioprinting technique, a VEGF-controlled-releasing lobule-like hepatorganoid, based on gelatin methacryloyl (GelMA) loaded with VEGF and infused with human umbilical vein endothelial cells.[112] The authors observed a significant improvement in the hepatocytes' viability and functionality following orthotopic implantation, with a long viability and abundant angiogenesis in liver post the implantation.

Another key obstacle involved in 3D-printed biomaterials for regenerative medicine is related to the immune response from the host's tissue in contact with the construct. While the inflammatory response is a crucial process for wound healing and tissue repair, an uncontrolled process can lead to the formation of a fibrous capsule around the implant, isolating the material from the adjacent tissue in a process called as the foreign body response.[113] Generally, this process involves the adsorption of proteins onto the surface of the biomaterial, which creates an attractive environment for neutrophils, monocytes and macrophages, and mast cells.[113] Under unhealthy or inflammatory conditions, neutrophils can be produced in abundance and can phagocytose the material along with its surrounding microenvironment; monocytes differentiate into macrophages upon extravasation into the injured tissue; and mast cells can be activated, leading to the recruitment of neutrophils and macrophages. In this sense, the type of raw material used to produce the constructs, and the functionalization or modification over the biomaterial are crucial aspects to avoid inflammatory response.[113–115] Researchers developed a 3D-printed silicone implants of gelatin-based, a biocompatible and biodegradable natural polymer, loaded with a cytokine cocktail composed of interleukin-10 and prostaglandin-E2 as coating.[114] They showed that the immunomodulatory material presented a controlled release of the cocktail components (for at least 14 days), with a reduced inflammatory response and high survival rate when applied *in vivo*.

In addition to the importance to produce a construct that can improve the vascularization and reduce the inflammatory response in the host tissue, the biomaterial–tissue integration is also a key parameter for the regenerative medicine field. In this context, it's also expected from the biomaterial to have good mechanical and structural compatibility with the target tissue, a functional surface and an internal architecture that can support the regeneration process.[116,117] Regarding the structural features, in general, porous materials (with larger pore sizes, around 5–100 μm) show better integration with lower levels of fibrous encapsulation than nonporous constructs.[117,118] Shi et al.[119] developed an organic–inorganic nanoink system based on gelatin methacryloyl (GelMA), containing bone morphogenic protein-2 (BMP-2) and ultrasmall calcium phosphate oligomer for craniofacial bone repair grafts. *In vitro*, the biomaterial presented promising osteogenic and angiogenic potential, with an effective new bone formation induced by its hierarchical structure.

6.4.2 Promising Clinical Trials and Leading Biotech-Hospital Initiatives

Despite the various challenges involved in the development of 3D-printed constructs for regenerative medicine, in the *in vitro* and even *in vivo* tests inside the laboratory have been achieved success in general. However, the progress toward the clinical phase still represents a major barrier, involving ethical concerns and scale-up limitations.[120] Even with these limitations, some materials have been tested, as demonstrated in a report by Ivanovski et al.,[121] which showed an effective clinical application of a 3D-printed personalized PCL resorbable scaffold for staged alveolar bone augmentation. The case reported the improvement in the bone gain, with new bone presence and successful graft integration across the defected zone. The trial is registered with the Australian New Zealand Clinical Trials Registry, ACTRN12622000118707p.

Moreover, some studies currently in clinical trials are being developed in association with hospitals and companies that support research in the medical 3D printing field. A relevant example involves a personalized tracheobronchial splint composed of PCL that was developed by the University of Michigan in collaboration with Materialise, a company of 3D printing services and software. The device designed to help the treatment of severe tracheobronchomalacia in infants has already been tested in over 40 patients under Food and Drug Administration (FDA) compassionate use programs, and a pivotal clinical trial has recently been initiated to systematically assess safety and efficacy. The trial is registered under ClinicalTrials.gov ID NCT06406452. Another example of a clinically applied biomaterial is 3DMatrix™, an implant made of polydioxanone and developed by the PrintBio company. According to the company, the material was designed to provide temporary support and degrade completely within six months, possessing a directional porous structure with a great adaptation to soft tissues. In 2024, this device received the FDA 510(k) clearance (number K232602) and has been implemented in reconstructive procedures.

6.5 PERSPECTIVES

Over the past two decades, 3D bioprinting has emerged as a promising tool within regenerative medicine, offering new possibilities for personalized therapies, complex tissue reconstruction, and *in situ* tissue regeneration. As the field matures, a shift from experimental innovation to clinical translation is underway, raising important discussions around how this technology will be implemented in real-world healthcare systems. Central to these discussions are three interconnected themes: the balance between personalized and standardized therapeutic solutions, the integration of bioprinting with surgical and hospital-based technologies, and the anticipated trajectory of clinical adoption in the coming decade.

6.5.1 Personalized, Autologous Constructs vs. Standardized Off-the-Shelf Solutions

One of the most compelling promises of 3D bioprinting is the ability to produce fully personalized constructions that are anatomically and biologically tailored to individual patients. These patient-specific, autologous tissues are often produced using the patient's own cells, potentially reducing immune rejection and enhancing integration. Such approaches are particularly attractive in cases of congenital defects, trauma, and reconstructive surgeries where both structural and functional precision are critical.[122] However, personalization presents logistical challenges. Producing customized constructs is labor-intensive, often requiring extensive imaging, processing of patient-derived cells, and time-consuming manufacturing steps. These factors limit scalability and may not be practical in emergencies or high-volume clinical settings. For instance, in cases of large-scale trauma or organ failure, there may be insufficient time to culture autologous cells and prepare personalized grafts.[122]

In contrast, off-the-shelf, standardized constructions offer speed and efficiency. These ready-made biomaterials and scaffolds can be manufactured in bulk, stored, and made readily available for surgical use. While these products may not match the biological specificity of autologous constructs, they still provide substantial therapeutic values especially when designed to be bioactive, biodegradable, and modifiable.[123] Synthetic biomaterials can be preloaded with growth factors, seeded with allogeneic or SCs, and engineered to degrade at controlled rates to match tissue regeneration timelines.[122]

In future clinical workflows, it is likely that both approaches will coexist. Personalized bioprinting may become the gold standard for complex, high-risk procedures or for patients with specific medical needs, while off-the-shelf constructs may serve routine applications or bridge therapy. The development of hybrid strategies, such as semipersonalized constructs that combine standardized scaffolds with patient-specific cell populations, may help resolve this tension and offer a practical compromise between customization and scalability.

6.5.2 Integration with Surgical Robotics and Point-of-Care Bioprinting

Another frontier in bioprinting is its potential integration with surgical robotics and point-of-care systems. These technologies aim to bring bioprinting directly into the clinical environment, allowing real-time fabrication of tissue constructs during surgical procedures. This shift would significantly shorten the time between design and implantation, reduce dependence on external manufacturing facilities, and improve the responsiveness of treatment.[124] For example, robotic-assisted bioprinters could be used in operating rooms to deposit bioinks directly onto a patient's wound or defect site with high precision. Such approaches are already being explored in skin regeneration, where *in situ* bioprinting systems apply layers of bioink containing cells and hydrogel matrices onto burn wounds. The technology allows for the reconstruction of skin with patient-specific geometry and cell content, all within the same surgical session.[13]

The concept of "point-of-care bioprinting" also aligns well with hospital workflows and precision medicine initiatives. Embedding compact bioprinters in clinical laboratories or surgical suites could enable hospitals to fabricate constructs on demand, from diagnostic tissue models to patient-matched implants. This decentralization of bioprinting could reduce production costs, speed up therapeutic timelines, and enhance accessibility, especially in resource-limited settings or remote healthcare systems.[13]

However, several technical and regulatory hurdles remain. Point-of-care systems require reliable sterilization, quality control, and user-friendly interfaces suitable for clinical personnel who may not have specialized training in biofabrication.

Integration with existing surgical platforms and electronic health record systems will also be important. Moreover, *in situ* printing raises unique challenges in terms of biocompatibility, patient safety, and consistency, which regulators will need to address through new guidance and risk assessment frameworks.

Despite these obstacles, the potential of combining robotic surgery, real-time imaging, and on-site bioprinting is immense. It could allow for automated graft placement, intelligent adaptation to surgical conditions, and even intraoperative feedback mechanisms to adjust the bioprinting process in real time based on tissue response.

6.5.3 Outlook for Clinical Adoption in the Next Decade

While the laboratory success of 3D bioprinting is now well established, the question of when and how it will become standard in clinical practice remains open. Over the next ten years, several factors will shape the pace of clinical adoption.

First, regulatory frameworks are gradually adapting to biofabricated products. Agencies such as the FDA (United States), EMA (Europe), and PMDA (Japan) have started to evaluate 3D-printed implants and regenerative therapies, including customized airway splints and resorbable bone scaffolds. Some of these applications have already received limited approvals under compassionate use programs, and formal clinical trials are increasingly being registered. As more precedent is established, regulatory uncertainty should diminish, providing clearer pathways for developers.[125]

Second, clinical evidence will play a pivotal role. Current research is moving from proof-of-concept studies toward rigorous, multicenter clinical trials that assess long-term outcomes, safety, and cost-effectiveness. Trials involving tracheal implants, vascular grafts, and soft tissue repair have shown early promise, but widespread clinical use will depend on robust data demonstrating that 3D-printed constructs outperform traditional alternatives.[125]

Third, economic feasibility will determine how widely bioprinting is adopted. Currently, the cost of bioprinters, bioinks, and laboratory infrastructure remains high, limiting access to well-funded research institutions and specialty hospitals. However, ongoing innovation is reducing these costs, and the emergence of modular, compact, and automated systems may democratize access. Reimbursement policies, insurance coverage, and health economics analyses will also be critical in incentivizing hospital systems to adopt the technology.[125]

Fourth, interdisciplinary collaboration will be essential. Clinical adoption of bioprinting depends on effective partnerships among material scientists, engineers, biologists, clinicians, and industry stakeholders. Medical professionals will need to be trained not only in the surgical application of printed materials but also in understanding their biological behavior and limitations. Curriculum changes in medical education, alongside certification programs for bioprinting technologies, may help bridge the current skills gap.[125]

Finally, public perception and ethical considerations must not be overlooked. As bioprinting moves closer to organ fabrication and therapeutic cloning, debates surrounding the use of SCs, animal models, and genetic manipulation are likely to intensify. Transparent communication with patients and the public will be essential to build trust and address misconceptions about what bioprinting can and cannot do.

6.5.4 4D Bioprinting Technology

Figure 6.9 illustrates the concept of 4D bioprinting, an evolution of 3D printing that incorporates the dimension of time, enabling printed constructs to change their shape, properties, or function after fabrication. This is made possible using smart biomaterials, stimuli-responsive materials capable of reacting to environmental triggers such as temperature, pH, moisture, light, or magnetic fields. Once printed, these materials can undergo controlled morphogenesis or functional transformation, resulting in dynamic and adaptive structures. Such capabilities open promising opportunities in basic research, for modeling complex biological processes; in regenerative medicine, with implants able to adapt to the host environment; and in pharmacology, with drug delivery systems that respond to specific physiological stimuli.[126]

6.6 CONCLUSION

Bioprinting has emerged as a transformative technology at the interface of biofabrication, tissue engineering, and regenerative medicine, enabling the precise spatial organization of cells, biomaterials, and bioactive molecules to create functional, patient-specific constructs. Advances in bioink formulation, printing strategies, and post-fabrication maturation have broadened its applicability, from *in vitro* tissue models to implantable constructs for clinical use. Despite significant progress, challenges remain in replicating the full complexity of native tissues, ensuring vascularization and long-term functionality, and addressing regulatory and manufacturing constraints. Continued interdisciplinary efforts integrating materials science, biology,

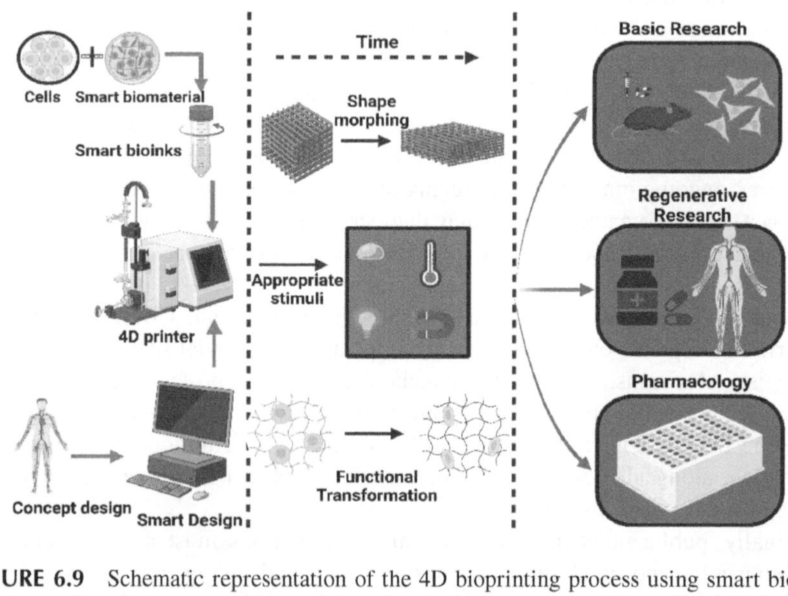

FIGURE 6.9 Schematic representation of the 4D bioprinting process using smart biomaterials capable of shape morphing and functional transformation, with applications in basic research, regenerative medicine, and pharmacology. (From Prakash et al.[126] Copyright 2024, Elsevier.)

engineering, and computational design are essential to overcome these limitations. Looking ahead, bioprinting holds immense potential to revolutionize personalized medicine, offering solutions for organ shortage, drug screening, and disease modeling, and paving the way for truly functional, lab-grown tissues and organs.

REFERENCES

1. D'Souza R, Her Y, Hussain N, Karri J, Schatman M, Calodney A, et al. Evidence-based clinical practice guidelines on regenerative medicine treatment for chronic pain: a consensus report from a multispecialty working group. *J Pain Res.* 2024;17:2951–3001. doi:10.2147/JPR.S480559
2. Kim J. Advanced strategies in 3D bioprinting for vascular tissue engineering and disease modelling using smart bioinks. *Virtual Phys Prototyp.* 2024;19:e2395470. doi:10.1080/TFOCOLL.2024.0.ISSUE-3D-BIOPRINTING
3. Lovett M, Lee K, Edwards A, Kaplan DL. Vascularization strategies for tissue engineering. *Tissue Eng Part B Rev.* 2009;15(3):353–370. doi:10.1089/ten.teb.2009.0085
4. Ukon Y, Hosoya S, Morita K, Yokozeki Y, Kataoka T, Kitahara T, et al. Identification of unapproved orthopedic regenerative medicine: usefulness of the act on safety of regenerative medicine. *Stem Cell Rep.* 2024;19(5):597–603. doi:10.1016/j.stemcr.2024.04.001
5. Berthiaume F, Maguire TJ, Yarmush ML. Tissue engineering and regenerative medicine: history, progress, and challenges. *Annu Rev Chem Biomol Eng.* 2011;2(1):403–430. doi:10.1146/annurev-chembioeng-061010-114257
6. Yang S, Sun Y, Yan C. Recent advances in the use of extracellular vesicles from adipose-derived stem cells for regenerative medical therapeutics. *J Nanobiotechnol.* 2024;22(1):316. doi:10.1186/S12951-024-02603-4
7. Boyce S, Lalley AL. Tissue engineering of skin and regenerative medicine for wound care. *Burns Trauma.* 2018;6:4. doi:10.1186/S41038-017-0103-Y/5680409
8. Mahdavi SS, Abdekhodaie MJ, Mashayekhan S, Baradaran-Rafii A, Djalilian AR. Bioengineering approaches for corneal regenerative medicine. *Tissue Eng Regen Med.* 2020;17(5):567–593. doi:10.1007/S13770-020-00262-8
9. Mastrogiacomo M, Muraglia A, Komlev V, Peyrin F, Rustichelli F, Crovace A, et al. Tissue engineering of bone: search for a better scaffold. *Orthod Craniofac Res.* 2005;8(4):277–284. doi:10.1111/j.1601-6343.2005.00350.x
10. Lee SJ, Jeong W, Atala A. 3D bioprinting for engineered tissue constructs and patient-specific models: current progress and prospects in clinical applications. *Adv Mater.* 2024;36(49). doi:10.1002/adma.202408032
11. Li H, Zhang Z, Liu J, Wang H. Antioxidant scaffolds for enhanced bone regeneration: recent advances and challenges. *Biomed Eng Online.* 2025;24(1). doi:10.1186/s12938-025-01370-z
12. Alam MI, Kashyap S, Balaji PG, Yadav AK, Flora SJS. 3D-printed medical implants: recent trends and challenges. *Biomed Mater Devices.* 2025;3(2):750–770. doi:10.1007/s44174-024-00221-0
13. Mirshafiei M, Rashedi H, Yazdian F, Rahdar A, Baino F. Advancements in tissue and organ 3D bioprinting: current techniques, applications, and future perspectives. *Mater Des.* 2024;240:112853. doi:10.1016/j.matdes.2024.112853
14. Wang J, Wang Y, Wang R, Wang Q, Wen M, Wang J, et al. A review on 3D printing processes in pharmaceutical engineering and tissue engineering: applications, trends and challenges. *Adv Mater Technol.* 2025;10(2). doi:10.1002/admt.202400620
15. Matai I, Kaur G, Seyedsalehi A, McClinton A, Laurencin CT. Progress in 3D bioprinting technology for tissue/organ regenerative engineering. *Biomaterials.* 2020;226:119536. doi:10.1016/J.BIOMATERIALS.2019.119536

16. Singh S, Kumar M, Kumar D, Kumar S, Chopra S, Bhatia A. Therapeutic precision: unveiling the potential of 3D printing in drug delivery, tissue engineering, and regenerative medicine. *3D Print Addit Manuf.* 2024. doi:10.1089/3dp.2023.0364
17. Bhardwaj H, Jangde R. Biomedical application of 3D printing. In: *3D Printing and Microfluidics in Dermatology*, eds. M Pradhan, K. Yadav. Taylor & Francis;2024:56–80. doi:10.1201/9781032690926-3
18. Dumic-Cule I, Peric M, Kucko L, Grgurevic L, Pecina M, Vukicevic S. Bone morphogenetic proteins in fracture repair. *Int Orthop.* 2018;42(11):2619–2626. doi:10.1007/s00264-018-4153-y
19. Jeraj AR, Zameer Z. AI-enhanced bioactive 3D-printed scaffolds for tissue regeneration: innovations in healing and functional additives. *J Comp Biomed Inform.* 2025;8(2). doi:10.56979/802/2025
20. Mota C, Camarero-Espinosa S, Baker MB, Wieringa P, Moroni L. Bioprinting: from tissue and organ development to *in vitro* models. *Chem Rev.* 2020;120(19):10547–10607. doi:10.1021/acs.chemrev.9b00789
21. Liu J, Song Q, Yin W, Li C, An N, Le Y, et al. Bioactive scaffolds for tissue engineering: a review of decellularized extracellular matrix applications and innovations. *Exploration.* 2025;5(1). doi:10.1002/EXP.20230078
22. Zhu X, Li H, Huang L, Zhang M, Fan W, Cui L. 3D printing promotes the development of drugs. *Biomed Pharmacother.* 2020;131:110644. doi:10.1016/J.BIOPHA.2020.110644
23. Parhi R, Jena GK. An updated review on application of 3D printing in fabricating pharmaceutical dosage forms. *Drug Deliv Transl Res.* 2022;12(10):2428–2462. doi:10.1007/s13346-021-01074-6
24. Zhu Y, Guo S, Ravichandran D, Ramanathan A, Sobczak MT, Sacco AF, et al. 3D-printed polymeric biomaterials for health applications. *Adv Healthc Mater.* 2025;14(1). doi:10.1002/adhm.202402571
25. Wu H, Diao J, Li X, Yue D, He G, Jiang X, et al. Hydrogel-based 3D printing technology: from interfacial engineering to precision medicine. *Adv Colloid Interface Sci.* 2025;341:103481. doi:10.1016/j.cis.2025.103481
26. Dong T, Ding R, Zhou R, Shen C, Sheridan W, Paez D, et al. A portable nucleic acid testing platform with photosensitization, a three-dimensionally printed multipiece chip, and digital color sensing. *Anal Chem.* 2024;96(17):6628–6633. doi:10.1021/acs.analchem.3c05897
27. Dong T, Ding R, Zhou R, Shen C, Sheridan W, Paez D, et al. A portable nucleic acid testing platform with photosensitization, a three-dimensionally printed multipiece chip, and digital color sensing. *Anal Chem.* 2024;96(17):6628–6633. doi:10.1021/acs.analchem.3c05897
28. Hoveidaei AH, Sadat-Shojai M, Mosalamiaghili S, Salarikia SR, Roghani-shahraki H, Ghaderpanah R, et al. Nano-hydroxyapatite structures for bone regenerative medicine: cell-material interaction. *Bone.* 2024;179:116956. doi:10.1016/j.bone.2023.116956
29. Albanna M, Binder KW, Murphy S V., Kim J, Qasem SA, Zhao W, et al. In situ bioprinting of autologous skin cells accelerates wound healing of extensive excisional full-thickness wounds. *Sci Rep.* 2019;9(1):1–15. doi:10.1038/S41598-018-38366-W
30. Christy PN, Basha SK, Kumari VS, Bashir AKH, Maaza M, Kaviyarasu K, et al. Biopolymeric nanocomposite scaffolds for bone tissue engineering applications – a review. *J Drug Deliv Sci Technol.* 2020;55:101452. doi:10.1016/J.JDDST.2019.101452
31. Liang J, Liu P, Yang X, Liu L, Zhang Y, Wang Q, et al. Biomaterial-based scaffolds in promotion of cartilage regeneration: recent advances and emerging applications. *J Orthop Translat.* 2023;41:54–62. doi:10.1016/J.JOT.2023.08.006
32. Unal A, Arora N. 3D printing in regenerative medicine. In: *Regenerated Organs*, ed. CP Sharma. Elsevier; 2021:305–330. doi:10.1016/B978-0-12-821085-7.00015-4

33. Murphy S V., Atala A. 3D bioprinting of tissues and organs. *Nat Biotechnol.* 2014;32(8):773–785. doi:10.1038/NBT.2958
34. Ma X, Liu J, Zhu W, Tang M, Lawrence N, Yu C, et al. 3D bioprinting of functional tissue models for personalized drug screening and in vitro disease modeling. *Adv Drug Deliv Rev.* 2018;132:235–251. doi:10.1016/J.ADDR.2018.06.011
35. Daly AC, Cunniffe GM, Sathy BN, Jeon O, Alsberg E, Kelly DJ. 3D bioprinting of developmentally inspired templates for whole bone organ engineering. *Adv Healthc Mater.* 2016;5(18):2353–2362. doi:10.1002/ADHM.201600182
36. Chimene D, Lennox KK, Kaunas RR, Gaharwar AK. Advanced bioinks for 3D printing: a materials science perspective. *Ann Biomed Eng.* 2016;44(6):2090–2102. doi:10.1007/S10439-016-1638-Y/METRICS
37. Nakagawa S, Okada R, Kushioka J, Kodama J, Tsukazaki H, Bal Z, et al. Effects of rhBMP-2-loaded hydroxyapatite granules/beta-tricalcium phosphate hydrogel (HA/β-TCP/hydrogel) composite on a rat model of caudal intervertebral fusion. *Sci Rep.* 2022;12(1):1–9. doi:10.1038/S41598-022-12082-Y
38. Lei B, Gao X, Zhang R, Yi X, Zhou Q. In situ magnesium phosphate/polycaprolactone 3D-printed scaffold induce bone regeneration in rabbit maxillofacial bone defect model. *Mater Des.* 2022;215:110477. doi:10.1016/J.MATDES.2022.110477
39. Tateiwa D, Nakagawa S, Tsukazaki H, Okada R, Kodama J, Kushioka J, et al. A novel BMP-2–loaded hydroxyapatite/beta-tricalcium phosphate microsphere/hydrogel composite for bone regeneration. *Sci Rep.* 2021;11(1):1–13. doi:10.1038/S41598-021-96484-4
40. Yang YP, Labus KM, Gadomski BC, Bruyas A, Easley J, Nelson B, et al. Osteoinductive 3D printed scaffold healed 5 cm segmental bone defects in the ovine metatarsus. *Sci Rep.* 2021;11(1):1–12. doi:10.1038/S41598-021-86210-5
41. Lu J, Gao Y, Cao C, Wang H, Ruan Y, Qin K, et al. 3D bioprinted scaffolds for osteochondral regeneration: advancements and applications. *Mater Today Bio.* 2025;32:101834. doi:10.1016/J.MTBIO.2025.101834
42. Phatchayawat PP, Khamkeaw A, Yodmuang S, Phisalaphong M. 3D bacterial cellulose-chitosan-alginate-gelatin hydrogel scaffold for cartilage tissue engineering. *Biochem Eng J.* 2022;184:108476. doi:10.1016/J.BEJ.2022.108476
43. Savsani C, Aitchison K, Allen AH, Adams NB, Adams EA, Savsani K, et al. The use of gelatin methacrylate (GelMA) in cartilage tissue engineering: a comprehensive review. *Bioengineering.* 2025;12(7):700. doi:10.3390/BIOENGINEERING12070700
44. Wang W, Zhang B, Li M, Li J, Zhang C, Han Y, et al. 3D printing of PLA/n-HA composite scaffolds with customized mechanical properties and biological functions for bone tissue engineering. *Compos B Eng.* 2021;224:109192. doi:10.1016/J.COMPOSITESB.2021.109192
45. Yan Y, Chen H, Zhang H, Guo C, Yang K, Chen K, et al. Vascularized 3D printed scaffolds for promoting bone regeneration. *Biomaterials.* 2019;190-191:97–110. doi:10.1016/J.BIOMATERIALS.2018.10.033
46. Ma K, Zhao T, Yang L, Wang P, Jin J, Teng H, et al. Application of robotic-assisted in situ 3D printing in cartilage regeneration with HAMA hydrogel: an in vivo study. *J Adv Res.* 2020;23:123–132. doi:10.1016/J.JARE.2020.01.010
47. Shi W, Sun M, Hu X, Ren B, Cheng J, Li C, et al. Structurally and functionally optimized silk-fibroin–gelatin scaffold using 3D printing to repair cartilage injury in vitro and in vivo. *Adv Mater.* 2017;29(29):1701089. doi:10.1002/ADMA.201701089
48. Li S, Xu Y, Zheng L, Fan C, Luo F, Zou Y, et al. High self-supporting chitosan-based hydrogel ink for in situ 3D printed diabetic wound dressing. *Adv Funct Mater.* 2025;35(5):2414625. doi:10.1002/ADFM.202414625

49. Cao Y, Cheng P, Sang S, Xiang C, An Y, Wei X, et al. 3D printed PCL/GelMA biphasic scaffold boosts cartilage regeneration using co-culture of mesenchymal stem cells and chondrocytes: in vivo study. *Mater Des.* 2021;210:110065. doi:10.1016/J.MATDES.2021.110065
50. Zhong Y, Cao X, Huang M, Lei Y, Liu AL. Biomimetic bone cartilage scaffolds based on trilayer methacrylated hydroxyapatite/GelMA composites for full-thickness osteochondral regeneration. *Int J Biol Macromol.* 2025;298:139860. doi:10.1016/J.IJBIOMAC.2025.139860
51. Lee V, Singh G, Trasatti JP, Bjornsson C, Xu X, Tran TN, et al. Design and fabrication of human skin by three-dimensional bioprinting. *Tissue Eng Part C Methods.* 2014;20(6):473–484. doi:10.1089/TEN.TEC.2013.0335
52. Zhou X, Luo Y, Gao Y, Ma J, Lin C, Zhou X, et al. Development and application of a mechanical arm-based in situ 3D bioprinting method for the repair of skin wounds. *Discover Applied Sciences.* 2024;6(8):1–16. doi:10.1007/S42452-024-06043-5
53. Fu H, Zhang D, Zeng J, Fu Q, Chen Z, Sun X, et al. Application of 3D-printed tissue-engineered skin substitute using innovative biomaterial loaded with human adipose-derived stem cells in wound healing. *Int J Bioprint.* 2023;9(2):674. doi:10.18063/IJB.V9I2.674
54. Isomi M, Sadahiro T, Ieda M. Progress and challenge of cardiac regeneration to treat heart failure. *J Cardiol.* 2019;73(2):97–101. doi:10.1016/j.jjcc.2018.10.002
55. Pashneh-Tala S, MacNeil S, Claeyssens F. The tissue-engineered vascular graft – past, present, and future. *Tissue Eng Part B Rev.* 2016;22(1):68–100. doi:10.1089/TEN.TEB.2015.0100,
56. Noor N, Shapira A, Edri R, Gal I, Wertheim L, Dvir T. 3D printing of personalized thick and perfusable cardiac patches and hearts. *Adv Sci.* 2019;6(11):1900344. doi:10.1002/ADVS.201900344
57. Chen EP, Toksoy Z, Davis BA, Geibel JP. 3D bioprinting of vascularized tissues for in vitro and in vivo applications. *Front Bioeng Biotechnol.* 2021;9:664188. doi:10.3389/FBIOE.2021.664188
58. Zhang YS, Arneri A, Bersini S, Shin SR, Zhu K, Goli-Malekabadi Z, et al. Bioprinting 3D microfibrous scaffolds for engineering endothelialized myocardium and heart-on-a-chip. *Biomaterials.* 2016;110:45–59. doi:10.1016/J.BIOMATERIALS.2016.09.003
59. Maiullari F, Costantini M, Milan M, Pace V, Chirivì M, Maiullari S, et al. A multicellular 3D bioprinting approach for vascularized heart tissue engineering based on HUVECs and iPSC-derived cardiomyocytes. *Sci Rep.* 2018;8(1):1–15. doi:10.1038/S41598-018-31848-X
60. Ajdary R, Ezazi NZ, Correia A, Kemell M, Huan S, Ruskoaho HJ, et al. Multifunctional 3D-printed patches for long-term drug release therapies after myocardial infarction. *Adv Funct Mater.* 2020;30(34):2003440. doi:10.1002/ADFM.202003440
61. Mei T, Cao H, Zhang L, Cao Y, Ma T, Sun Z, et al. 3D printed conductive hydrogel patch incorporated with MSC@GO for efficient myocardial infarction repair. *ACS Biomater Sci Eng.* 2024;10(4):2451–2462. doi:10.1021/ACSBIOMATERIALS.3C01837
62. Galván NTN, Paulsen SJ, Kinstlinger IS, Marini JC, Didelija IC, Yoeli D, et al. Blood flow within bioengineered 3d printed vascular constructs using the porcine model. *Front Cardiovasc Med.* 2021;8:629313. doi:10.3389/FCVM.2021.629313/BIBTEX
63. Jian H, Li X, Dong Q, Tian S, Bai S. In vitro construction of liver organoids with biomimetic lobule structure by a multicellular 3D bioprinting strategy. *Cell Prolif.* 2023;56(5):e13465. doi:10.1111/CPR.13465
64. Singh S, Kumar M, Kumar D, Kumar S, Chopra S, Bhatia A. Therapeutic precision: unveiling the potential of 3D printing in drug delivery, tissue engineering, and regenerative medicine. *3D Print Addit Manuf.* 2024. doi:10.1089/3dp.2023.0364

65. Jang J, Park HJ, Kim SW, Kim H, Park JY, Na SJ, et al. 3D printed complex tissue construct using stem cell-laden decellularized extracellular matrix bioinks for cardiac repair. *Biomaterials.* 2017;112:264–274. doi:10.1016/j.biomaterials.2016.10.026
66. Choi J, Lee EJ, Jang WB, Kwon SM. Development of biocompatible 3D-printed artificial blood vessels through multidimensional approaches. *J Funct Biomater.* 2023;14(10):497. doi:10.3390/JFB14100497
67. Schöneberg J, De Lorenzi F, Theek B, Blaeser A, Rommel D, Kuehne AJC, et al. Engineering biofunctional in vitro vessel models using a multilayer bioprinting technique. *Sci Rep.* 2018;8(1):1–13. doi:10.1038/S41598-018-28715-0
68. Kjar A, McFarland B, Mecham K, Harward N, Huang Y. Engineering of tissue constructs using coaxial bioprinting. *Bioact Mater.* 2021;6(2):460–471. doi:10.1016/J.BIOACTMAT.2020.08.020
69. Millik SC, Dostie AM, Karis DG, Smith PT, McKenna M, Chan N, et al. 3D printed coaxial nozzles for the extrusion of hydrogel tubes toward modeling vascular endothelium. *Biofabrication.* 2019;11(4):045009. doi:10.1088/1758-5090/AB2B4D
70. Lee H, Han W, Kim H, Ha DH, Jang J, Kim BS, et al. Development of liver decellularized extracellular matrix bioink for three-dimensional cell printing-based liver tissue engineering. *Biomacromolecules.* 2017;18(4):1229–1237. doi:10.1021/ACS.BIOMAC.6B01908
71. Mirdamadi ES, Kalhori D, Zakeri N, Azarpira N, Solati-Hashjin M. Liver tissue engineering as an emerging alternative for liver disease treatment. *Tissue Eng Part B Rev.* 2020;26(2):145–163. doi:10.1089/TEN.TEB.2019.0233
72. Gough A, Soto-Gutierrez A, Vernetti L, Ebrahimkhani MR, Stern AM, Taylor DL. Human biomimetic liver microphysiology systems in drug development and precision medicine. *Nat Rev Gastroenterol Hepatol.* 2020;18(4):252–268. doi:10.1038/s41575-020-00386-1
73. Bouwmeester MC, Bernal PN, Oosterhoff LA, van Wolferen ME, Lehmann V, Vermaas M, et al. Bioprinting of human liver-derived epithelial organoids for toxicity studies. *Macromol Biosci.* 2021;21(12):2100327. doi:10.1002/MABI.202100327
74. Homan KA, Kolesky DB, Skylar-Scott MA, Herrmann J, Obuobi H, Moisan A, et al. Bioprinting of 3D convoluted renal proximal tubules on perfusable chips. *Sci Rep.* 2016;6(1):1–13. doi:10.1038/SREP34845
75. Garreta E, Prado P, Tarantino C, Oria R, Fanlo L, Martí E, et al. Fine tuning the extracellular environment accelerates the derivation of kidney organoids from human pluripotent stem cells. *Nat Mater.* 2019;18(4):397–405. doi:10.1038/s41563-019-0287-6
76. Huang Y, Wu W, Liu H, Chen Y, Li B, Gou Z, et al. 3D printing of functional nerve guide conduits. *Burns Trauma.* 2021;9:tkab011. doi:10.1093/BURNST/TKAB011
77. Amalakanti S, Mulpuri RP, Avula VCR. Recent advances in biomaterial design for nerve guidance conduits: a narrative review. *Adv Technol Neurosci.* 2024;1(1):32–42. doi:10.4103/ATN.ATN-D-23-00005
78. Rodríguez-Sánchez DN, Pinto GBA, Cartarozzi LP, de Oliveira ALR, Bovolato ALC, de Carvalho M, et al. 3D-printed nerve guidance conduits multi-functionalized with canine multipotent mesenchymal stromal cells promote neuroregeneration after sciatic nerve injury in rats. *Stem Cell Res Ther.* 2021;12(1):1–20. doi:10.1186/S13287-021-02315-8/METRICS
79. Sadiq IZ, Abubakar FS, Katsayal BS, Ibrahim B, Adamu A, Usman MA, et al. Stem cells in regenerative medicine: unlocking therapeutic potential through stem cell therapy, 3D bioprinting, gene editing, and drug discovery. *Biomed Eng Adv.* 2025;9:100172. doi:10.1016/j.bea.2025.100172
80. Hussen BM, Taheri M, Yashooa RKh, Abdullah GH, Abdullah SR, Kheder RK, et al. Revolutionizing medicine: recent developments and future prospects in stem-cell therapy. *Int J Surg.* 2024;110(12):8002–8024. doi:10.1097/JS9.0000000000002109

81. Zhao J, Meng H, Liao S, Su Y, Guo L, Wang A, et al. Therapeutic effect of human umbilical cord mesenchymal stem cells in early traumatic osteonecrosis of the femoral head. *J Orthop Translat*. 2022;37:126–142. doi:10.1016/j.jot.2022.09.008
82. Suchanecka M, Grzelak J, Farzaneh M, Azizidoost S, Dari MAG, Józkowiak M, et al. Adipose derived stem cells – sources, differentiation capacity and a new target for reconstructive and regenerative medicine. *Biomed Pharmacother*. 2025;186:118036. doi:10.1016/j.biopha.2025.118036
83. Eskandar K. Regenerative medicine in plastic surgery: the role of stem cells and bioprinting. *Regen Repair Rehab*. 2025;1(2):51–59. doi:10.1016/j.rerere.2025.02.003
84. Du P, Wu J. Hallmarks of totipotent and pluripotent stem cell states. *Cell Stem Cell*. 2024;31(3):312–333. doi:10.1016/j.stem.2024.01.009
85. Gonzalez-Vilchis RA, Piedra-Ramirez A, Patiño-Morales CC, Sanchez-Gomez C, Beltran-Vargas NE. Sources, characteristics, and therapeutic applications of mesenchymal cells in tissue engineering. *Tissue Eng Regen Med*. 2022;19(2):325–361. doi:10.1007/s13770-021-00417-1
86. Lee JY, Hong SH. Hematopoietic stem cells and their roles in tissue regeneration. *Int J Stem Cells*. 2020;13(1):1–12. doi:10.15283/ijsc19127
87. Moyo MTG, Adali T, Tulay P. Exploring gellan gum-based hydrogels for regenerating human embryonic stem cells in age-related macular degeneration therapy: a literature review. *Regen Ther*. 2024;26:235–250. doi:10.1016/j.reth.2024.05.018
88. Gonzalez-Vilchis RA, Piedra-Ramirez A, Patiño-Morales CC, Sanchez-Gomez C, Beltran-Vargas NE. Sources, characteristics, and therapeutic applications of mesenchymal cells in tissue engineering. *Tissue Eng Regen Med*. 2022;19(2):325–361. doi:10.1007/s13770-021-00417-1
89. Sagar R, David AL. Fetal therapies – (stem cell transplantation; enzyme replacement therapy; in utero genetic therapies). *Best Pract Res Clin Obstet Gynaecol*. 2024;97:102542. doi:10.1016/j.bpobgyn.2024.102542
90. Sun Y, Zhao H, Yang S, Wang G, Zhu L, Sun C, et al. Urine-derived stem cells: promising advancements and applications in regenerative medicine and beyond. *Heliyon*. 2024;10(6):e27306. doi:10.1016/j.heliyon.2024.e27306
91. Shi J, Yao H, Chong H, Hu X, Yang J, Dai X, et al. Tissue-engineered collagen matrix loaded with rat adipose-derived stem cells/human amniotic mesenchymal stem cells for rotator cuff tendon-bone repair. *Int J Biol Macromol*. 2024;282:137144. doi:10.1016/j.ijbiomac.2024.137144
92. Zhen X, Park SJ, Choe SH, Lee DS, Lee JH. Generation of induced pluripotent stem cells (cmESF-iPS-C5) derived from cynomolgus monkey ear skin fibroblasts (cmESF). *Stem Cell Res*. 2022;65:102977. doi:10.1016/j.scr.2022.102977
93. Maturavongsadit P, Narayanan LK, Chansoria P, Shirwaiker R, Benhabbour SR. Cell-laden nanocellulose/chitosan-based bioinks for 3D bioprinting and enhanced osteogenic cell differentiation. *ACS Appl Bio Mater*. 2021;4(3):2342–2353. doi:10.1021/acsabm.0c01108
94. Michel R, Auzély-Velty R. Hydrogel-colloid composite bioinks for targeted tissue-printing. *Biomacromolecules*. 2020;21(8):2949–2965. doi:10.1021/acs.biomac.0c00305
95. Kansız S, Vurat MT, Parmaksiz M, Elçin AE, Elçin YM. Methacrylated-κ-carrageenan/hydroxyapatite composite bioinks for extrusion-based bioprinting: physicochemical, rheological, mechanical, and in vitro biological investigations. *Int J Biol Macromol*. 2025;316:144745. doi:10.1016/j.ijbiomac.2025.144745
96. Sharma R, Smits IPM, De La Vega L, Lee C, Willerth SM. 3D bioprinting pluripotent stem cell derived neural tissues using a novel fibrin bioink containing drug releasing microspheres. *Front Bioeng Biotechnol*. 2020;8. doi:10.3389/fbioe.2020.00057

97. Sharma R, Kirsch R, Valente KP, Perez MR, Willerth SM. Physical and mechanical characterization of fibrin-based bioprinted constructs containing drug-releasing microspheres for neural tissue engineering applications. *Processes*. 2021;9(7):1205. doi:10.3390/pr9071205
98. Eskandar K. Regenerative medicine in plastic surgery: the role of stem cells and bioprinting. *Regen Repair Rehab*. 2025;1(2):51–59. doi:10.1016/j.rerere.2025.02.003
99. Liang W, Zhou C, Liu X, Xie Q, Xia L, Liu L, et al. Current status of nano-embedded growth factors and stem cells delivery to bone for targeted repair and regeneration. *J Orthop Translat*. 2025;50:257–273. doi:10.1016/j.jot.2024.12.006
100. Lach MS, Rosochowicz MA, Richter M, Jagiełło I, Suchorska WM, Trzeciak T. The induced pluripotent stem cells in articular cartilage regeneration and disease modelling: are we ready for their clinical use? *Cells*. 2022;11(3):529. doi:10.3390/cells11030529
101. Lin CW, Yang SC, Klochkov V, Chen TC, Huang WK, Chen WL. The effects of pigment epithelium-derived factor and associated peptides on the differentiation of retinal ganglion cells from human-induced pluripotent stem cells. *Exp Eye Res*. 2025;257:110440. doi:10.1016/j.exer.2025.110440
102. Oldershaw RA, Baxter MA, Lowe ET, Bates N, Grady LM, Soncin F, et al. Directed differentiation of human embryonic stem cells toward chondrocytes. *Nat Biotechnol*. 2010;28(11):1187–1194. doi:10.1038/nbt.1683
103. Akter MZ, Tufail F, Ahmad A, Oh YW, Kim JM, Kim S, et al. Harnessing native blueprints for designing bioinks to bioprint functional cardiac tissue. *iScience*. 2025;28(3):111882. doi:10.1016/j.isci.2025.111882
104. Roshanbinfar K, Evans AD, Samanta S, Kolesnik-Gray M, Fiedler M, Krstic V, et al. Enhancing biofabrication: shrink-resistant collagen-hyaluronan composite hydrogel for tissue engineering and 3D bioprinting applications. *Biomaterials*. 2025;318:123174. doi:10.1016/j.biomaterials.2025.123174
105. Augustine R, Dan P, Hasan A, Khalaf IM, Prasad P, Ghosal K, et al. Stem cell-based approaches in cardiac tissue engineering: controlling the microenvironment for autologous cells. *Biomed Pharmacother*. 2021;138:111425. doi:10.1016/j.biopha.2021.111425
106. Priya S, Boyd AS, Torres-Bautista A, Sawadkar P, Mosahebi A, Narayan Rath S, et al. Accelerating vascular graft development: adipose-derived stem cells and PODS® (polyhedrin delivery system with tissue-specific growth factors) – enhanced 3D bioprinting for functional blood vessels. *Chem Eng J*. 2024;494:152934. doi:10.1016/j.cej.2024.152934
107. Sousa AC, Alvites R, Lopes B, Sousa P, Moreira A, Coelho A, et al. Three-dimensional printing/bioprinting and cellular therapies for regenerative medicine: current advances. *J Funct Biomater*. 2025;16(1):28. doi:10.3390/jfb16010028
108. Ma Y, Deng B, He R, Huang P. Advancements of 3D bioprinting in regenerative medicine: exploring cell sources for organ fabrication. *Heliyon*. 2024;10(3). doi:10.1016/j.heliyon.2024.e24593
109. Dell AC, Maresca J, Davis BA, Isaji T, Dardik A, Geibel JP. Development and deployment of a functional 3D-bioprinted blood vessel. *Sci Rep*. 2025;15(1). doi:10.1038/s41598-025-93276-y
110. Yeo M, Sarkar A, Singh YP, Derman ID, Datta P, Ozbolat IT. Synergistic coupling between 3D bioprinting and vascularization strategies. *Biofabrication*. 2024;1(12003). doi:10.1088/1758-5090/ad0b3f
111. Carmeliet P, Jain RK. Molecular mechanisms and clinical applications of angiogenesis. *Nature*. 2011;473(7347):298–307. doi:10.1038/nature10144
112. Yan J, Ye Z, Lu Y, Yuan Y, Wang X, Yan T, et al. 3D bioprinting lobule-like hepatorganoids with induced vascularization for orthotopic implantation. *Mater Today Bio*. 2025;31. doi:10.1016/j.mtbio.2025.101515

113. Whitaker R, Hernaez-Estrada B, Hernandez RM, Santos-Vizcaino E, Spiller KL. Immunomodulatory biomaterials for tissue repair. *Chem Rev.* 2021;121(18):11305–11335. doi:10.1021/acs.chemrev.0c00895
114. Barthes J, Lagarrigue P, Riabov V, Lutzweiler G, Kirsch J, Muller C, et al. Biofunctionalization of 3D-printed silicone implants with immunomodulatory hydrogels for controlling the innate immune response: an in vivo model of tracheal defect repair. *Biomaterials.* 2021;268. doi:10.1016/j.biomaterials.2020.120549
115. Wang T, Yu Z, Lin S, Chen Z, Jin H, Liang L, et al. 3D-printed Mg-incorporated PCL-based scaffolds improves rotator cuff tendon-bone healing through regulating macrophage polarization. *Front Bioeng Biotechnol.* 2024;12. doi:10.3389/fbioe.2024.1407512
116. Kim YS, Shin YS. Surface functionalization of 3D-printed bio-inspired scaffolds for biomedical applications: a review. *Biomimetics.* 2024;9(11). doi:10.3390/biomimetics9110703
117. Huang D, Li Z, Li G, Zhou F, Wang G, Ren X, et al. Biomimetic structural design in 3D-printed scaffolds for bone tissue engineering. *Mater Today Bio.* 2025;32. doi:10.1016/j.mtbio.2025.101664
118. Madden LR, Mortisen DJ, Sussman EM, Dupras SK, Fugate JA, Cuy JL, et al. Proangiogenic scaffolds as functional templates for cardiac tissue engineering. *Proc Natl Acad Sci USA.* 2010;107(34):15211–15216. doi:10.1073/pnas.1006442107
119. Shi Y, Shi J, Sun Y, Liu Q, Zhang C, Shao C, et al. A hierarchical 3D graft printed with nanoink for functional craniofacial bone restoration. *Adv Funct Mater.* 2023;33(40). doi:10.1002/adfm.202301099
120. Briones Y, Pascua B, Tiangco N, Crisostomo I, Casiguran S, Remenyi R. Assessing the landscape of clinical and observational trials involving bioprinting: a scoping review. *3D Print Med.* 2025;11(1). doi:10.1186/s41205-025-00253-2
121. Ivanovski S, Staples R, Arora H, Vaquette C, Alayan J. Alveolar bone regeneration using a 3D-printed patient-specific resorbable scaffold for dental implant placement: a case report. *Clin Oral Implants Res.* 2024;35(12):1655–1668. doi:10.1111/clr.14340
122. Goswami DR, Saxena DD, Kumari DP. Precision in practice: the evolution of patient-specific implants in modern surgery. *Int J Environ Sci.* 2025;11(12s):425–430. doi:10.64252/0mcby283
123. Chen FM, Liu X. Advancing biomaterials of human origin for tissue engineering. *Prog Polym Sci.* 2016;53:86–168. doi:10.1016/j.progpolymsci.2015.02.004
124. Liu S, Chen Y, Wang Z, Liu M, Zhao Y, Tan Y, et al. The cutting-edge progress in bioprinting for biomedicine: principles, applications, and future perspectives. *MedComm.* 2024;5(10). doi:10.1002/mco2.753
125. Khan SB, Irfan S, Zhang Z, Yuan W. Redefining medical applications with safe and sustainable 3D printing. *ACS Appl Bio Mater.* 2025. doi:10.1021/acsabm.4c01923
126. Prakash A, Malviya R, Sridhar SB, Shareef J. 4D printing in dynamic and adaptive bone implants: progress in bone tissue engineering. *Bioprinting.* 2024;44:e00373. doi:10.1016/j.bprint.2024.e00373

7 Engineering Scaled-Up Tissues via 3D Bioprinting

Gabriela S. Kronemberger,
Francesca D. Spagnuolo,
Aliaa S. Karam, and Kaoutar Chattahy

7.1 3D BIOPRINTING OUTLOOK

Three-dimensional (3D) bioprinting, a rapidly evolving branch of additive manufacturing, offers great potential in the field of regenerative medicine and tissue engineering (TE). Bioprinting allows the precise deposition of living cells in predefined spatial arrangements, closely mimicking the complex architecture of native tissues. This capability not only enhances the reproducibility and scalability of engineered constructs but also provides extended control over the graft structure and therefore the engineered tissue architecture [1,2].

One of the key advantages of bioprinting is its ability to generate anatomically accurate and user-defined designs (Figure 7.1a), tailored to the patient contributing significantly to the evolution of personalized medicine. This customization minimizes the risk of immune rejection and improves integration within host tissues. Moreover, the use of computer-aided design coupled with advanced medical imaging technologies enables rapid prototyping of complex geometries, facilitating the reconstruction of tissues. Preclinical and early-stage clinical studies have demonstrated the feasibility of bioprinted skin [3], cartilage [4], bone [5], and vascularized tissue grafts [6,7]. For example, 3D bioprinted skin grafts are being developed for burn patients [8,9], offering improved wound healing outcomes. Moreover, several studies have demonstrated the feasibility of creating anatomically shaped musculoskeletal tissue grafts (Figure 7.1b)—such as chondrogenic grafts—using various bioinks (alginate, gelatin methacryloyl or GelMA) [10,11] and clinically relevant cell sources (bone marrow mesenchymal/stromal stem cells, MSCs). However, these advances are still at the preclinical stage. A key limitation in those approaches that can impact the clinical translation after implantation is the poor mechanical properties of the soft hydrogel-based bioinks which are required to provide cell viability and extracellular matrix (ECM) deposition. Recent approaches have focused on reinforcing soft bioinks with supportive polymeric scaffolds, where researchers demonstrated how the integration of polycaprolactone (PCL) scaffolds with inkjet bioprinting can result into a tissue that not only supports tissue differentiation but also exhibits improved mechanical properties and zonal architecture [12].

Furthermore, recent studies are investigating the potential of 3D bioprinting to mimic and regenerate even more complex tissue or organ structures such as blood

DOI: 10.1201/9781032638164-7

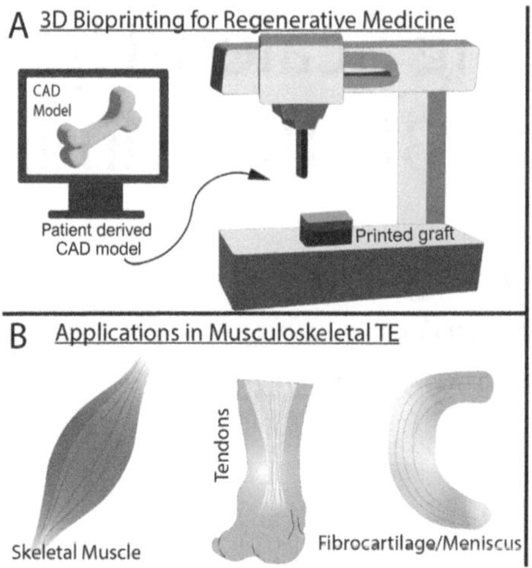

FIGURE 7.1 Overview of 3D bioprinting for regenerative medicine and tissue engineering. (a) Schematic of the bioprinting process using CAD-guided deposition of bioinks (e.g., GelMA, alginate) to fabricate customized tissue constructs. (b) Clinical and preclinical applications in musculoskeletal tissue engineering include skeletal muscle, tendons, cartilage, and bone, with increasing focus on replicating ECM composition and structure. (c) Future directions for bioprinting in regenerative medicine include whole organ bioprinting, *in situ* bioprinting during surgery, and use of bioprinted tissues for high-throughput drug screening.

vessels and the heart [13–15]. Although full organ replacement by 3D bioprinting strategies remains a long-term goal, the ability to bioprint functional tissue units represents a significant step toward addressing organ shortages and improving patient outcomes. Another significant benefit of 3D bioprinting is the potential to streamline drug discovery and toxicology screening (Figure 7.1c). By bioprinting human-relevant, 3D tissue models, researchers can evaluate drug responses in a physiologically relevant context *in vitro*, reducing reliance on animal testing and accelerating the translational pipeline. Looking ahead, 3D bioprinting holds immense promise for reshaping the landscape of personalized medicine. The convergence of stem cell biology, biomaterials science, and advanced manufacturing is expected to enable the creation of fully functional, patient-specific organs. Additionally, the optimization of bioinks and the development of new bioprinting platforms to support scaled-up tissue biofabrication are also accelerating the preclinical translation of bioprinted tissues. Of note, the integration with emerging technologies such as artificial intelligence, robotics (Figure 7.1c), and real-time imaging will likely further enhance the precision and efficiency of bioprinting processes. In addition, future bioprinting platforms may support *in situ* tissue regeneration—directly bioprinting tissues within the body during surgery [16,17]—opening new avenues for minimally invasive therapies. As regulatory frameworks and ethical guidelines evolve, the path toward clinical translation will become clearer, paving the way for broader adoption of bioprinting in the healthcare system.

7.2 CELL-ONLY BIOPRINTING TO ENGINEER SCALED-UP TISSUES

As previously discussed, 3D bioprinting is an emerging approach that is increasingly recognized as one of the most promising technologies for large-scale tissue biofabrication in the coming years. Originating from additive manufacturing, 3D bioprinting enables the precise layer-by-layer arrangement of cells, biomaterials, and soluble factors [18]. This technique allows for the hierarchical organization of tissues that closely replicates their native in vivo architecture, facilitating the reproduction of both morphological and functional properties. Moreover, the bioprinted constructs can be further matured either *in vitro* or in vivo to acquire the desired biomechanical functionality [19]. There are three primary 3D bioprinting techniques currently in use: (1) inkjet-based, (2) extrusion-based, and (3) laser-assisted bioprinting [20] (Figure 7.2).

Inkjet bioprinting offers precise control over the spatial patterning and cell density within each droplet, allowing for accurate regulation of the volume, size, and number of printed samples. A notable advantage of this technique is the ability to control the number of cells per droplet, which enhances cell seeding efficiency—particularly beneficial when working with scaffolds [21]. Laser-assisted bioprinting is based on the principle of laser-induced forward transfer, which allows for highly accurate deposition of cells, growth factors, and biomaterial droplets at MHz-scale frequency. This technique is capable of achieving high-resolution outputs [22]. Nonetheless, a major drawback is the potential for reduced cell viability due to laser exposure [23].

Extrusion bioprinting is one of the most used bioprinting technologies due to its ease of use and wide biomaterial compatibility [24,25]. For pneumatic printheads, compressed air is used to generate a user-defined pressure to extrude the bioink. While in piston- or rotation-driven printheads, the bioink is extruded by mechanical force generated by the movement of the piston or screw. Such mechanical extrusion methods have been shown to have a higher printing accuracy but lower cell viability when compared to pneumatic extrusion [24,26]. In extrusion bioprinting, the building material or bioink can be cell only, cellular, or acellular (Figure 7.5) [24,27,28]. A cell-only bioink will experience high shear stresses and potential nutrient diffusion issues [27]. Cellular bioinks consist of cells with one or more biomaterials, usually hydrogels, and/or other bioactive components. The addition of a biomaterial reduces the stresses experienced by cells during the printing process, maintaining a high cell viability [29]. Acellular bioinks are composed of one or a combination of different biomaterials [27,28].

Key rheological factors that affect the printability of a bioink include its shear-thinning properties, viscosity, and yield stress [30]. Shear-thinning bioinks have great printability with extrusion-based bioprinters. While under shear, a shear-thinning material would become less viscous. This would allow a bioink to easily deform and flow through a nozzle when pressure is applied. Once extruded there is no longer applied stress, and the bioink would regain its initial viscosity maintaining its shape [29]. This is highly advantageous because it allows for the biofabrication of high-resolution constructs while using low printing pressures. Thus, various additives have been added to bioinks to enhance their shear-thinning behavior [30,31]. Such polymers include gellan gum and poloxamer such as pluronic [31,32]. In addition

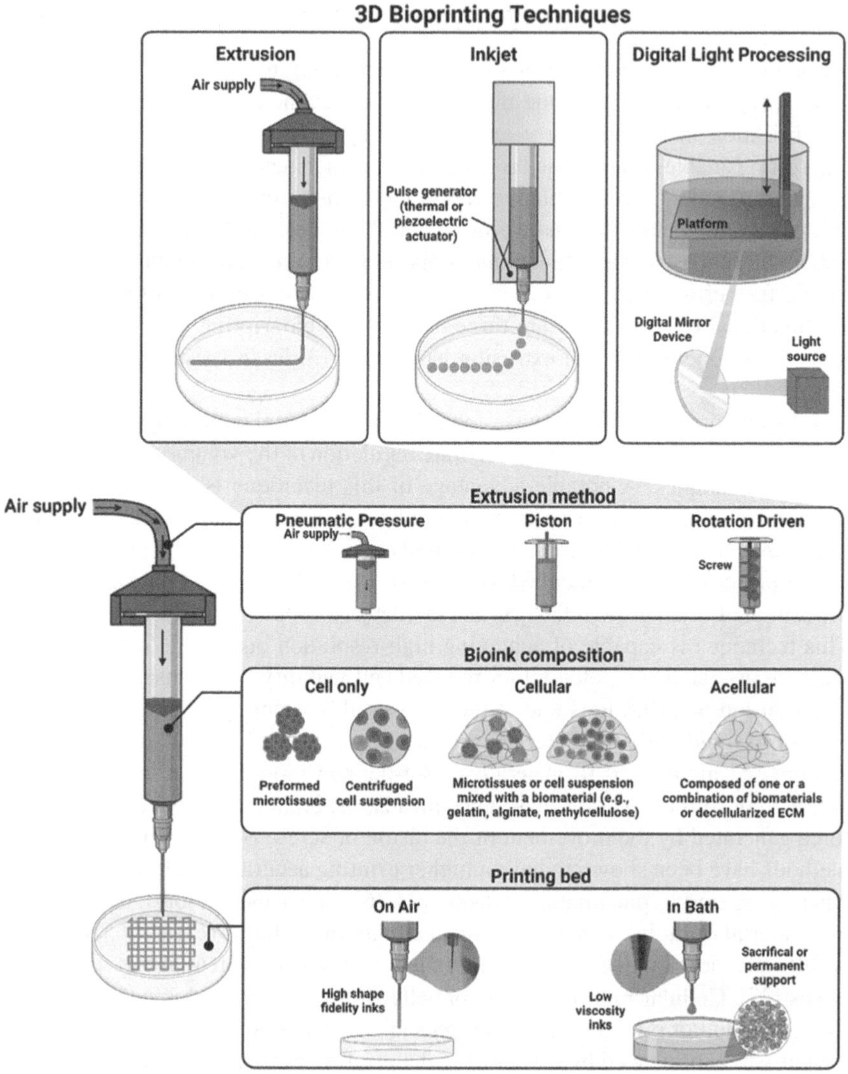

FIGURE 7.2 Diagrammatic representation of extrusion, inkjet, and digital light processing bioprinting. In extrusion bioprinting, the extrusion methods are either pneumatic or mechanically driven. Bioinks used in extrusion bioprinting can be cell-free composed of only biomaterials, cell-only containing cells, or cellular containing both cells and biomaterials. Depending on the viscosity of a bioink it may require a support bath to improve print fidelity. (Created with BioRender.com.)

to the printability of a bioink, it is important to ensure that it can support cellular growth, proliferation, and differentiation. Depending on the viscosity of a bioink it may require a support bath during bioprinting. High viscosity bioinks will generally have a good shape fidelity in air. However, these viscous inks need high extrusion pressures which will affect cell viability and would be limited by a maximum number of layers before a construct would collapse. Emerging support baths have paved the way for extrusion bioprinting of low-viscosity bioinks and the bioprinting of gravity-defying shapes and structures [33,34].

However, the potential toxicity and immunogenicity associated with classic biomaterial-based scaffolds have spurred the development of scaffold-free approaches in 3D bioprinting. One of these approaches is cell-only bioprinting [35]. In this technique, no exogenous supporting hydrogel or biomaterial is used; instead, the bioinks consist exclusively of living cells, either as single-cell suspensions, spheroids, organoids, or preformed microtissues that can self-assemble into functional tissue architectures post-printing. This approach offers a more physiologically relevant microenvironment that closely mimics native tissue neoformation, enabling enhanced cell–cell and cell–ECM interactions. Interestingly, it eliminates concerns related to scaffold degradation and the potential immunogenicity of biomaterials. However, cell-only bioprinting presents several challenges, the foremost being the requirement for extremely high cell numbers to obtain a workable volume. During bioprinting of a cell-only bioink, clogging issues may arise as cells begin to adhere to one another and form aggregates. To alleviate this, an enzyme such as hyaluronidase can be added to the cells before bioprinting [35]. Additionally, due to the absence of porous biomaterials that typically facilitate diffusion, these dense constructs often suffer from limited nutrient and oxygen transport, especially in larger constructs. To address these limitations and support the maturation of complex, thicker tissues, the development of perfusion bioreactors or other dynamic culture systems is often necessary. These systems enable continuous media flow, improving nutrient delivery and waste removal, thereby enhancing cell viability and function during long-term culture and tissue development. As the field advances, integrating vascularization strategies and optimizing bioreactor conditions will be critical for translating cell-only bioprinting into scalable, clinically relevant TE platforms [13,36].

7.3 CELLULAR SPHEROIDS, MICROTISSUES, AND ORGANOIDS IN THE CONTEXT OF BOTTOM-UP TISSUE ENGINEERING

Spheroids are cellular aggregates formed by a process called *self-assembly*. In this biophysical process, cell-to-cell and cell-to-ECM interactions prevail to allow the compaction and final aggregation of cells into spheroids. It is a process that happens during embryogenesis, and this is one of the main reasons why microtissues are more similar to our 3D microenvironment when compared to classical monolayer cell culture [37]. After spheroids are fully compact, they can be differentiated to fabricate a desired tissue with induction growth factors cocktails. After spheroids are induced and can secrete a tissue-specific ECM, they can be called microtissues [38] (Figure 7.3). Therefore, many studies are exploring the potential of microtissues in the TE field to mimic the native tissue microenvironment. The main advantages of using microtissues for TE strategies are: (1) they produce their own ECM, (2) they have high cell density in one unit, (3) they can secrete tissue-specific soluble mediators, (4) they can be produced on a large scale by automated systems, and (5) they can fuse with one another to generate more complex tissue structures [39].

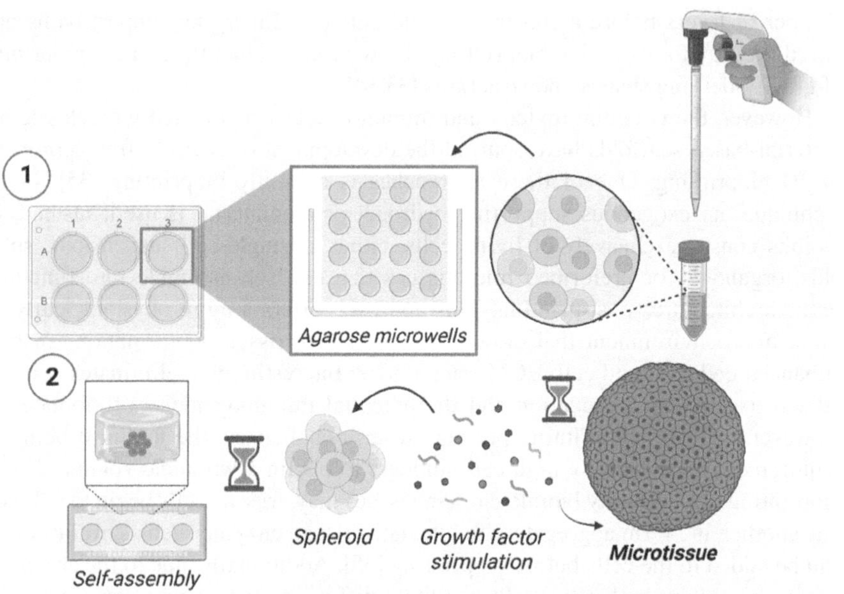

FIGURE 7.3 Fabrication of spheroids via self-assembly. (1) One common technique for spheroids via self-assembly involves the use of agarose microwells. These microwells are created using a positive mold. Once the cell suspension is added to the microwells, (2) the self-assembly process begins. Over approximately 12 hours of incubation, cells aggregate and form spheroids. Following stimulation with appropriate growth factors to mimic the target tissue environment, these spheroids develop into microtissues, complete with relevant extracellular matrix components. (Created with BioRender.com.)

As microtissues can be produced on large scale, they are being largely explored in regenerative medicine for high-throughput drug screening tests, which are highly interesting because they have the potential to reduce the need for animal testing in the long term. In this application, microtissues can be fabricated using the patient's own cells to develop a personalized treatment [40]. Furthermore, as microtissues show an intrinsic fusion capacity, they can be used as biological building blocks for 3D bioprinting approaches [41]. 3D bioprinting will be explored next in detail, but it is currently the technique with the highest potential to biofabricate functional tissues *in vitro*, which can address in the future one of the biggest challenges in regenerative medicine that is organ transplantation. Microtissues can be fabricated using different 3D cell culture strategies, such as: pellet culture, magnetic and acoustic fields, hanging droplets, non-adherent surfaces, and microfluidics. Each technique has its own advantages and disadvantages. However, the literature describes non-adherent surfaces as the one with more advantages nowadays [37]. The main reason is because microtissues are homogeneous in size and shape, which is crucial for high-throughput drug testing and bioprinting and is a technique that can be scaled up to address the challenges of the applications mentioned. Microtissues can also be produced by using microfluidics in organ-on-a-chip devices. However, one disadvantage is that it is difficult to keep the size and shape homogeneity of the microtissues. Microtissues were already successfully applied in TE strategies to biofabricate cartilage and bone. For cartilage TE, the application of microtissues is interesting because of the hypoxia core that is naturally formed inside these units. In addition, microtissues were already implanted to evaluate the formation of those tissues in animal models [42]. The implantation of microtissues in defect sites is interesting as it is a scaffold-free approach, which reduces the biocompatibility concern of the use of hydrogel and polymeric biomaterials. Furthermore, the microtissues can be produced from autologous cells which reduces even more immunological risks.

Organoids are 3D cellular structures derived from pluripotent stem cells, progenitor, or mesenchymal cells that recapitulate the phenotype and functions of the target tissue *in vitro*. Often, microtissues and organoids are still described as synonyms in the literature. However, organoids are multicellular structures that show intra- or inter-organ self-organization. The use of organoids has been largely explored in the last years to develop especially heart, brain, liver, intestines, and pancreas models [43,44]. Interestingly, if organoids are used in regenerative medicine, it is possible to mimic the native organ environment to later engineer complex disease models and perform drug screening tests. Different disease models have been investigated in organoids and the application of organ-on-a-chip models has become a key tool to integrate them and create systems similar to the human body [45]. One example is the development of an organ-on-a-chip to accommodate liver, intestine, and pancreas organoids in different channels to investigate the action of a desired drug. In that way, organoids can be produced with the patients' own cells, and it potentially reduces the need for animal testing which is crucial for the 3Rs (replacement, reduction and refinement). Organoids are also currently being produced on a large scale because of this interest in high-throughput drug testing, especially from the pharmacological industry. Furthermore, studies are being developed to 3D bioprint organoids to hierarchically biofabricate layer by layer even more complex tissue models that can also be used for high-throughput drug screening [46]. Differently from microtissues, organoids usually do not show homogeneity in size and shape, but they can be all consistently produced using a standard number of cells from the beginning of the *in vitro* culture. One of the main techniques to produce organoids was developed by Lancaster for brain organoids, and it is easily adapted to any cell culture room and relies on the use of Matrigel and constant agitation for the formation of the organoids [47]. Through this method, the brain organoids could be maintained for a long term in culture and showed complex levels of neural tissue organization. Besides, tumor organoids are being explored to replicate the intricate and complex microenvironment of tumors. In this approach, patient tumor cells are isolated by biopsy to generate biobanks that are used to fabricate the organoids. Once the organoids are fabricated, they can be applied for drug testing. Therefore, the fabrication of microtissues and organoids for regenerative medicine has the potential to address crucial clinical translation challenges of the current strategies such as the use of polymeric scaffolds for tissue regeneration or monolayer classical methods. The innovation of those scaffold-free approaches can be interesting not only for 3D bioprinting as the applications will be discussed further but also for high-throughput drug testing and personalized medicine.

7.4.1 Bioprinting Methods Using Microtissues as Biological Building Blocks

Spheroids and microtissues have been increasingly utilized in bioprinting approaches, primarily due to their inherent tissue fusion properties, with the number of studies in this area growing substantially in recent years [48,49]. To overcome technical challenges associated with using spheroids as components of bioinks, novel biofabrication methods have been developed, including assisted bioprinting techniques, the Kenzan method, extrusion-based bioprinting in supporting baths, and hybrid approaches combining existing methodologies.

The "Kenzan" method enables the automated positioning of spheroids into 3D arrangements by placing them onto microneedles spaced sufficiently to allow spheroid fusion. The deformation forces exerted on the spheroids during assembly do not negatively impact cell viability, ECM production, or fusion processes [50]. Using layers of spheroids arranged via the Kenzan method, tubular structures and heterogeneous tissues have been successfully fabricated by selecting appropriate spheroid types and spatial configurations. For instance, this technique has facilitated the formation of microvascular fragments through the fusion of induced pluripotent stem cell-derived spheroids and endothelial cells [50].

Another approach that has gained significant attention recently is assisted bioprinting through precise positioning, which allows for the automated placement of individual spheroids within a supportive hydrogel according to a predefined structure. Following placement, the spheroids fuse to form more complex tissue constructs. In a study by Daly and Kelly [51], assisted bioprinting of induced pluripotent stem cell spheroids was employed to engineer microscale cardiac tissue. This technique also holds potential for fabricating microvascular and perfusable structures.

Conventional bioprinting techniques are often constrained by their inability to maintain complex geometries and structural fidelity, particularly when working with soft or scaffold-free constructs. Embedded 3D bioprinting has emerged as a promising solution to these limitations. In this approach, the bioink is extruded within a secondary hydrogel that acts as a temporary, biocompatible support material during and/or after the printing process [52]. This method has shown significant potential for fabricating and scaling up "soft" tissue constructs, particularly when using cellular aggregates or spheroids, without the need for permanent synthetic scaffolds. One of the most widely known embedded bioprinting strategies is the Freeform Reversible Embedding of Suspended Hydrogels (FRESH™) technique [53]. FRESH utilizes a thermoreversible support bath composed of gelatin microparticles, which enables the deposition of soft bioinks at both millimeter and centimeter scales. After printing, the gelatin bath can be liquefied at physiological temperatures (37°C), while the printed construct retains its form through the natural fusion and self-assembly of its biological constituents [54]. Another notable embedded printing approach is Suspended Layer Additive Manufacturing (SLAM), which employs a 0.5% agarose solution as the support matrix for low-viscosity bioinks. Unlike FRESH, the agarose used in SLAM is not thermoreversible. However, it provides greater optical transparency and improved reproducibility [55]. Following the introduction of these methods, a wide range of support baths with tunable physical and biological properties have been developed to better match specific bioink formulations and cell types.

While embedded bioprinting offers clear advantages for soft tissue fabrication, the application of these methods to microtissue-based printing presents unique challenges. In particular, when using thermoreversible support baths like gelatin, the bath degrades after printing, potentially leading to dispersion of the microtissues in the culture medium before sufficient fusion occurs. This affects structural integrity and prevents the formation of robust tissue grafts. To address this, researchers have explored more permanent support baths. For example, a xanthan gum (XG)-based bath has been employed to maintain low shear stress conditions while supporting printed spheroids [56]. Although this approach facilitated excellent microtissue fusion, the resulting constructs exhibited significant shrinkage over time and poor shape fidelity—limitations that pose challenges for clinical translation. To overcome this, Spagnuolo et al. developed a bioprinting platform utilizing a previously developed modified XG support bath functionalized with methacrylate groups [6], allowing it to be permanently stabilized through photocrosslinking [57]. This approach prevented post-fusion tissue shrinkage and preserved construct geometry. Furthermore, by tuning the stiffness of the support bath, the researchers were able to direct the phenotype of MSC-derived microtissues, enabling the engineering of diverse musculoskeletal tissues with zone-specific characteristics.

Microtissue-based bioprinting represents a significant advancement in TE, offering several key advantages over traditional single-cell bioprinting approaches. By leveraging the inherent cellular organization and ECM content of microtissues, this strategy enables enhanced cell viability, improved biological function, and more robust tissue formation post-printing. The use of predifferentiated or zonally conditioned microtissues allows for the engineering of complex, heterogeneous tissues that more closely mimic native structure and function. Moreover, microtissue fusion following printing facilitates scaffold-free tissue maturation, reducing the need for synthetic biomaterials and minimizing the risk of long-term foreign body response. When combined with tailored support baths that promote structural integrity and controlled fusion, microtissue printing holds immense promise for scalable, clinically relevant fabrication of musculoskeletal and other soft tissues.

7.5 BIOFABRICATION STRATEGIES TO ENGINEER SCALED-UP MUSCULOSKELETAL TISSUES USING CELL- AND MICROTISSUES-DERIVED BIOINKS

7.5.1 Cartilage

The poor self-healing potential of articular cartilage (AC) and the increasing prevalence of osteoarthritis (OA) have motivated the need for cartilage TE [58]. It is a challenging goal to engineer functional AC grafts because of the complex structure and zonal organization of the native tissue. Classically, TE grafts for AC repair were fabricated by seeding cells onto 3D scaffolds. For example, almost 50 years ago the first AC graft was designed and paved the way for cartilage TE [59]. The engineered graft was composed of rabbit chondrocytes seeded onto a decalcified bone scaffold and was implanted into rabbit knee joints [59]. Ever since, different cell types and numerous biomaterials have been explored for cartilage TE.

Early attempts in the field of cartilage TE-fabricated hydrogels and polymeric scaffolds that were seeded with cells and/or other bioactive factors to stimulate the production of cartilage ECM components by the seeded cells and/or the patient's own cells in vivo [60–63]. However, these hydrogels and scaffolds were both uniform in structure and composition, and recognizing that the function of AC is dependent on its complex structural organization, heterogeneous bilayered scaffolds and hydrogels emerged as a promising approach [64–71]. These bilayered scaffolds were somewhat successful in recapitulating some aspects of the zonal composition or anisotropic properties of native AC, but were unsuccessful in mimicking the intricate architecture of the tissue including the arcade-like collagen network which is critical for its load-bearing properties. This was demonstrated through computational modeling which indicated that achieving the characteristic arcade-like collagen organization of AC is the most important parameter in determining the functional success of an engineered graft for cartilage repair [72].

During organogenesis, the external forces sensed by cells play a crucial role in their differentiation, development, and morphogenesis [73–75]. Similarly, stem cells *in vitro* can still sense their surrounding microenvironment and respond to mechanical, physical, and geometrical cues [76]. Leveraging this, another strategy involves using bioreactors to mechanically condition and/or perfuse an engineered graft with the aim of creating a more biomimetic environment that will enhance chondrogenesis. Such dynamic culture conditions were observed to increase both sulfated glycosaminoglycan (sGAG) and collagen production of chondrocytes seeded on agarose hydrogels or polymeric scaffolds but fail to control the microscale spatial organization of this secreted matrix [77–79]. This motivates the need for novel TE strategies that can direct neotissue collagen organization into a biomimetic arcade-like architecture. Emerging 3D bioprinting techniques could potentially be used to address limitations of classical TE strategies by providing spatially and temporally defined biochemical and biophysical cues to self-organizing cells to engineer structurally anisotropic and mechanically functional AC grafts (Figure 7.4). These cues or boundaries would serve as guiding structures for neotissue growth and cell alignment. 3D bioprinting would also enable a reproducible scale-up production of large grafts with the freedom of having patient-specific geometries.

Many different bioinks have been developed for cartilage engineering. For example, methacrylated gelatin has been widely used. It is usually crosslinked with UV light post-bioprinting while still maintaining a high cell viability [80]. GelMA contains the RGD cell attachment ligand, and has tunable mechanical properties based on the concentration, degree of crosslinking, and methacryloyl used [81,82]. It is seen to support the chondrogenic differentiation of MSCs and chondrocytes which can be further enhanced by the addition of native cartilage ECM components such as hyaluronic acid (HA) and chondroitin sulfate [83,84]. However, a main disadvantage of GelMA is that it is seen to induce a more fibrocartilage-like phenotype rather than stable hyaline cartilage [85]. Alginate has also been popular in cartilage bioinks because it has a fast and easy gelation method, shear-thinning properties, and a tunable degradation rate [11]. Multiple studies have shown that MSCs and chondrocytes

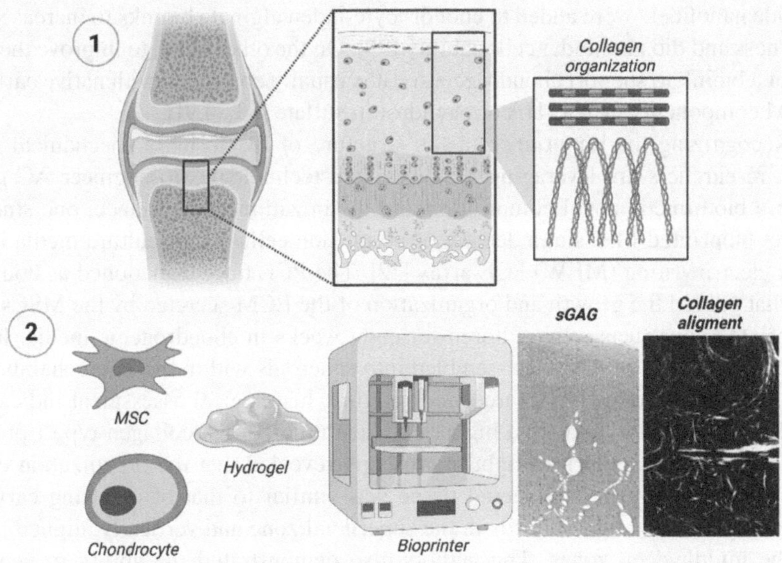

FIGURE 7.4 Structure of articular cartilage and 3D bioprinting as a strategy in tissue engineering (TE) for neocartilage grafts. (1) Articular cartilage exhibits a distinct hierarchical structure, characterized by an arcade-like organization of collagen fibers that is closely tied to its biomechanical function. (2) Traditional TE approaches typically utilize cells (primarily mesenchymal stem cells [MSCs] and/or chondrocytes), hydrogels, and polymeric scaffolds to create cartilage grafts; however, these often lack native tissue organization. The emergence of 3D bioprinting has enabled the fabrication of larger, more complex cartilage constructs using the same bioink components, while also imparting anisotropic properties and improved phenotypic fidelity. sGAG: sulfated glycosaminoglycans. (Created with BioRender.com.)

exhibit a high viability and hyaline-like phenotype when bioprinted using alginate-based bioinks [85,86–88]. To improve the cell adhesion properties of alginate, it can be modified with RGD ligands [89]. It can also be sulfated which would allow it to bind transforming growth factors and improve chondrogenesis by providing a local delivery of growth factors to encapsulated cells [90]. Similarly, the addition of HA and chondroitin sulfate to alginate-based bioinks improves chondrogenesis [91]. Decellularized cartilage ECM has also been evaluated for cartilage bioprinting. These bioinks support robust chondrogenesis as they are chondro inductive, providing encapsulated cells with a more biomimetic microenvironment [92–97].

Different additives are added to bioinks for cartilage TE to improve their mechanical properties or to further support a more robust chondrogenesis. To improve the mechanical stability of ECM-based bioinks they can be methacrylated to allow for crosslinking post-bioprinting or combined with another material including norbornene-modified polyvinyl alcohol, sericin methacrylate, or combined with a PCL scaffold [92–96]. The shear-thinning properties and hence the extrusion of a bioink can be improved with the addition of nanofibers. This was demonstrated with silk fibroin nanofibers which improved the rheological properties of HA-based bioinks allowing for a high shape fidelity in air without impacting cell viability [98]. Likewise, polylactide nanofibers were added to chondrocyte-laden alginate bioinks to increase their stiffness and did not hinder cell viability [99]. On the other hand, to improve the ability of a bioink to support chondrogenesis, it is usually combined with native cartilage ECM components such as HA or chondroitin sulfate [83,84,91].

Recognizing the importance of the structure of AC to its biomechanical function, researchers are leveraging 3D bioprinted technologies to engineer AC grafts with a biomimetic zonal composition and organization. For instance, one study of inkjet-bioprinted MSCs at a density of 30 million cells/mL of culture media into a melt electrowriting (MEW) PCL array [12]. The PCL fibers functioned as boundaries that guided the growth and organization of the ECM secreted by the MSCs. The bioprinted constructs were cultured for eight weeks in chondrogenic media. It was observed that the MSCs self-assembled into spheroids within the microchambers of the PCL array. Following a three-week culture, histological assessment indicated a hyaline-like phenotype with a higher collagen type II than collagen type I production. Importantly, polarized light microscopy revealed that the organization of the collagen fibrils in the engineered tissue was similar to that of maturing cartilage with horizontally aligned fibrils in the superficial zone and vertically aligned fibrils in the middle/deep zones. The authors also demonstrated the ability to generate scaled-up versions of the bioprinted graft. However, the mechanical properties of the engineered tissue following the eight-week *in vitro* maturation were still lower than native AC. Another study aimed to recapitulate the cell density gradient in native AC [100]. The bioink used was biomimetic being composed of collagen type II and chondrocytes. The bioprinting constructs were cultured for three weeks in chondrogenic media. Histological evaluation indicated a cell density gradient post-bioprinting. The mechanical properties of the construct were not evaluated, and there was poor sGAG deposition. It is also important to note that even though a cell density gradient is present in native AC, it is not the most critical parameter in determining graft functionality.

7.5.2 Bone

Bone is a specialized type of connective tissue that is highly vascularized and innervated, forming, together with cartilage, the skeletal system. Among the various functions of bone tissue in the body, three stand out: (1) providing mechanical support and serving as an attachment site for muscles to enable locomotion; (2) protecting vital organs and the bone marrow, which is housed within long and flat bones; and (3) acting as a reservoir for calcium and phosphate, essential for maintaining homeostasis [101]. Bone is a dynamic tissue capable of self-repair to noncritical lesions [102]. Bone defects resulting from extensive tumor removals, trauma-induced fractures, biochemical imbalances, infections, or genetic skeletal disorders are major contributors to disability and diminished quality of life worldwide. Effectively treating these defects to restore normal bone structure and function remains a substantial clinical challenge, particularly in cases where natural bone healing is impaired. Over time, numerous surgical methods have been developed to support bone regeneration, including the application of synthetic bone substitutes and bone grafts, in which the autologous grafts remain the clinical gold standard for repairing critical-sized or nonhealing bone defects. However, they are associated with significant risks including complications from general anesthesia, infections, secondary fractures, pain, and donor-site morbidity. Consequently, there is a pressing need for effective bone substitutes that can support native bone remodeling, and TE approaches have been continuously developed over the years to overcome this challenge [103]. Most of the studies in classical TE focused on the fabrication of biomimetic scaffolds to be implanted in preclinical critical and noncritical bone defects to evaluate the regeneration capacity. Therefore, a high number of animal studies were performed in the last decades in bone TE to test the bone regenerative capacity of these constructs [104,105].

With the advent of 3D bioprinting, bottom-up TE has emerged as a highly promising approach for scaling up bone biofabrication. This is largely due to its ability to precisely position multicellular components in a controlled, layer-by-layer manner using osteoinductive hydrogels and polymers, which can ultimately undergo functional maturation within bioreactor systems (Figure 7.5). Bioprinted bone grafts offer a compelling alternative to traditional allografts, with the potential to reduce immune rejection and chronic inflammation. While conventional approaches, such as seeding cells onto prefabricated 3D-printed scaffolds, have been explored for bone TE, they often suffer from limitations like uneven cell distribution. In contrast, 3D bioprinting allows for precise and uniform multicellular placement, supports the fabrication of complex, anatomically relevant geometries, and provides greater control over structural parameters, such as porosity, which is crucial for replicating the native bone microenvironment [106]. In this context, the following section highlights recent

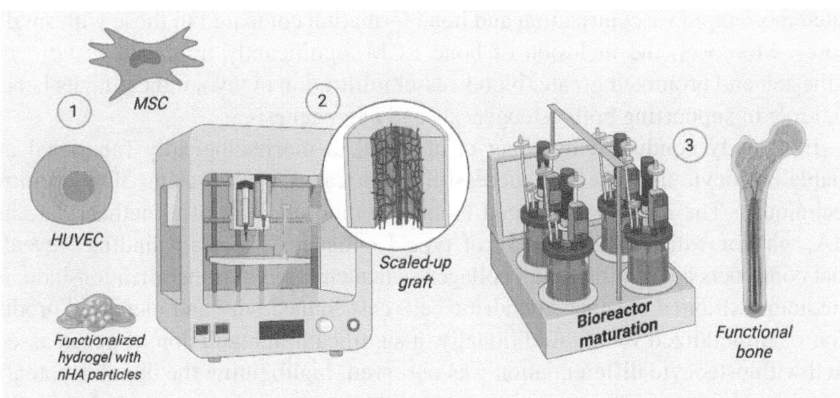

FIGURE 7.5 Biofabrication of functional bone grafts via 3D bioprinting. (1) Mesenchymal stem cells (MSCs) and human umbilical vein endothelial cells (HUVECs) can be combined with osteoinductive materials, such as nanohydroxyapatite (nHA)-based hydrogels, to formulate bioinks for engineering vascularized bone grafts. (2) Using extrusion-based 3D bioprinting, these bioinks can be deposited in a controlled, layer-by-layer manner to fabricate scaled-up constructs with defined architecture. (3) The printed grafts can then be cultured in bioreactor systems to promote their final maturation and functional integration. (Created with BioRender.com.)

advancements in bone tissue biofabrication achieved through the application of 3D bioprinting technologies over the past several years.

In a study by Daly et al. [85], the authors proposed a 3D bioprinting strategy that leveraged bioinks with enhanced mechanical properties, inspired by the developmental biology of bone formation. The engineered construct was based on a gelatin methacrylate bioink formulation containing bone marrow-derived MSCs that were predifferentiated along the chondrogenic lineage. This cellular component was combined with a PCL scaffold, both with and without incorporated vascular channels. The main findings demonstrated that, once implanted in vivo, the bioprinted constructs successfully supported endochondral ossification. Significant bone tissue formation and the development of vascularized regions were observed at the subcutaneous implantation site.

Another study conducted by Byambaa et al. [107] reported the fabrication of a complex construct targeting both bone tissue and its vascular component using extrusion-based bioprinting. The authors employed GelMA-based hydrogels functionalized with soluble endothelial factors, nanoparticles, and MSCs. At the core of the construct, a low-concentration GelMA bioink containing endothelial cells was used as a sacrificial material. The results demonstrated that the sacrificial bioink degraded at physiological temperature, leading to the formation of a perfusable channel. Furthermore, the endothelial cells adhered to the surrounding biomaterial and self-organized into a vascular-like structure.

In a study by Freeman et al. [108], 3D bioprinting was used to fabricate PCL scaffolds incorporated with bone-derived ECM, aiming to enhance mechanical performance and promote improved cell adhesion on the scaffold surface. Following in vivo implantation, the authors observed that scaffolds with larger pore sizes facilitated more rapid vascularization and bone formation compared to those with smaller pores. Moreover, the inclusion of bone ECM significantly improved *in vitro* cell adhesion and promoted greater blood vessel infiltration in vivo, indicating its beneficial role in supporting both osteogenesis and angiogenesis.

In a study conducted by Yang et al. [109], a morphologically functional and viable osteocyte network was successfully fabricated *in vitro* using 3D bioprinting techniques. The authors developed bioinks composed of gelatin methacrylate and HA, with or without the addition of type I collagen. The main findings revealed that constructs containing type I collagen, when cultured in mineralization-inducing medium, exhibited enhanced dendritic cell–cell connectivity and increased production of mineralized ECM. Additionally, a significant upregulation of genes associated with osteocyte differentiation was observed, highlighting the bioink's potential for promoting osteocytogenesis in engineered bone tissue.

Pitacco et al. [110] 3D bioprinted cartilage templates were employed as an endochondral ossification strategy for the treatment of large bone defects in a rat model. Human MSCs were encapsulated within fibrin-based bioinks and bioprinted into PCL scaffolds fabricated using the fused deposition modeling technique. The key findings demonstrated that the hypertrophic bioprinted constructs effectively supported vascularization and bone formation in vivo. These results highlight the potential of 3D bioprinting as a scalable and clinically relevant approach for engineering bone grafts.

Kim et al. [111] developed a novel biofabrication platform to enable the scalable production of tissue constructs through the precise, simultaneous deposition of spheroids into a gel-based substrate. The platform's efficiency was evaluated in the context of bone TE *in situ* using a rat calvarial defect model. Constructs derived from the spheroids remained viable and significantly enhanced bone volume formation. Notably, mature bone tissue was observed in the group receiving high-density bioprinted constructs. One year later, Duan et al. [112] also utilized 3D cellular structures as biological building blocks. In their study, the team engineered bone organoids by combining MSCs, human umbilical vein endothelial cells, and osteogenic microparticles. These organoids exhibited strong osteogenic potential and were incorporated into prevascularized hydrogel constructs, which were then 3D bioprinted at high cell density. Post-printing results demonstrated rapid formation of vascularized bone tissue, ultimately leading to successful regeneration of cranial bone defects. This approach shows significant promise for scaling up bone graft production in regenerative medicine.

In conclusion, various strategies have been developed to biofabricate bone grafts using 3D bioprinting technologies in a versatile manner, enabling the integration of diverse biomaterials and cell types to more accurately replicate the hierarchical structure of native bone tissue. Despite these advancements, the translation of such models to preclinical applications remains limited by the need to scale up constructs to clinically relevant sizes. To overcome these challenges, several approaches can be employed, including: (1) the implementation of bioreactors, (2) the controlled delivery of growth factors, and (3) the automation of cell culture procedures.

7.5.3 Meniscus

The meniscus, a crescent-shaped fibrocartilaginous structure located between the femur and tibia, plays a crucial role in knee joint function by transmitting and distributing loads across the tibial plateau. It is composed of two wedge-shaped discs: the medial and lateral menisci, which act as shock absorbers and stabilizers of the joint [113,114]. The meniscus originates during fetal development through mesenchymal condensation between the eighth and tenth weeks of gestation and is initially highly cellular and vascular. However, postnatal maturation results in a significant reduction in cellularity, increased collagen organization, and regression of blood vessels to the outer 10%–30% of the tissue, leaving the inner region avascular with a limited capacity for repair [113]. This inner avascular region is predominantly composed of chondrocyte-like cells that secrete an ECM rich in sGAG and type II collagen, with fibers aligned radially to resist compressive forces. In contrast, the outer region consists mainly of fibroblast-like cells and a mix of type I and II collagen fibers aligned circumferentially, adapted to handle tensile and shear stresses, and facilitates tissue repair through its higher blood supply [115] (Figure 7.6).

Meniscal injuries, especially in the avascular zone, remain a significant clinical challenge due to poor intrinsic healing potential [116,117]. Current surgical treatments, including meniscectomy and meniscal allografting, are common but often fail to fully restore function and long-term outcomes, particularly in the case of large meniscal defects [118,119]. This is largely due to the complex and

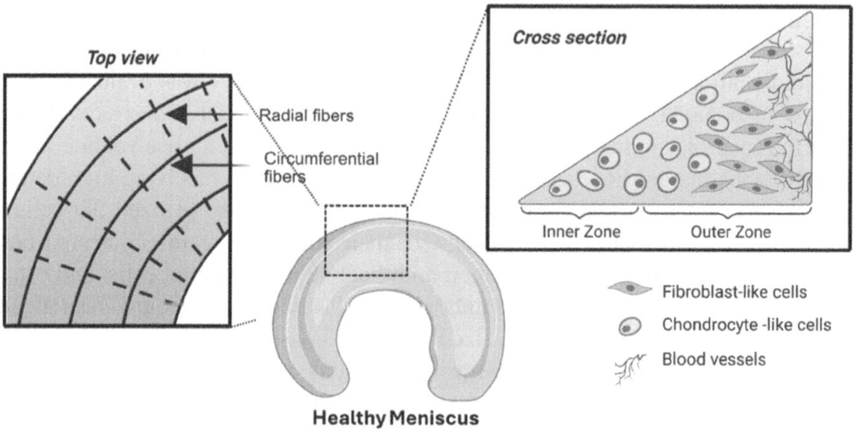

FIGURE 7.6 Structural and cellular organization of the native meniscus: regional variations in collagen fiber alignment, cell phenotype, and vascularization. (Created with BioRender.com.)

heterogeneous structure of the native meniscus, which exhibits distinct zonal variations in cellular phenotype, ECM composition, vascularity, and collagen fiber orientation. The inner zone is composed mainly of chondrocyte-like cells producing type II collagen and sGAGs, with radially oriented collagen fibers that withstand compressive forces. In contrast, the outer zone contains fibroblast-like cells, is richer in type I collagen arranged circumferentially to bear tensile loads, and is better vascularized, making it more capable of healing [120]. In addition to its structural and compositional complexity, the meniscus harbors a population of clonogenic and multipotent meniscal progenitor cells (MPCs), which have been shown to migrate to injury sites and participate in endogenous repair. Damage to the meniscus disrupts this sophisticated architecture, impairs joint biomechanics, and increases the risk of developing osteoarthritis [121,122]. These challenges underscore the importance of engineering meniscal grafts that replicate the native tissue's zonal complexity and structural integrity. However, regenerating the meniscus at a clinically relevant size scale remains difficult due to its avascular nature, limited healing, and the demanding mechanical environment of the knee joint [113,119]. Engineering a successful graft requires mimicking not only the meniscus's shape and geometry, but also the zonal variations in ECM composition, collagen fiber orientation, and cell phenotype [123]. A critical barrier to this goal is the limited diffusion of nutrients and oxygen into the inner regions of larger constructs, often resulting in cell death and insufficient ECM formation [124]. Moreover, the mechanical demands of the joint environment require engineered tissues to have anisotropic and viscoelastic properties that can withstand compressive, tensile, and shear forces [125]. Failure to recreate these regional features can lead to reduced mechanical integrity and poor integration postimplantation [126].

In this context, 3D bioprinting technologies offer the spatial control necessary to design scaled-up anatomically accurate and regionally defined meniscal constructs [11]. Extrusion-based bioprinting, in particular, enables the use of multiple printheads to deposit distinct cell populations and biomaterials with high precision, while advanced techniques such as embedded printing in support baths can enhance structural resolution and mechanical reinforcement without compromising cell viability [127,128]. A critical component of successful bioprinting is the selection of appropriate bioinks and cell sources. Bioinks must meet rheological requirements for printability, such as shear-thinning behavior to enable smooth extrusion, sufficient yield stress to maintain the shape of printed structures, and rapid gelation or crosslinking (e.g., via temperature, UV, or ionic mechanisms) to stabilize constructs post-printing, all while supporting cell viability, differentiation, and long-term tissue development [128–130]. Natural hydrogels like gelatin methacryloyl (GelMA), collagen and decellularized ECM provide bioactivity and cell-instructive cues, while synthetic polymers such as polyethylene glycol or polyurethane add mechanical robustness. Many strategies involve blending natural and synthetic materials to balance print fidelity and biological functionality. Bioinks can also be functionalized with growth factors or peptides to direct zone-specific tissue formation, mimicking the meniscus's native gradients in mechanical and biochemical cues [129,130]. In line with bioink development, researchers at the University of South Korea [129] created a 3D-printed bioink using a decellularized meniscus ECM, which supported stem cell growth and differentiation. Sathish et al. [131] optimized a tricomposite bioink using gelatin, carboxymethylcellulose, and alginate for both direct and indirect 3D printing of meniscal scaffolds, demonstrating enhanced cellular proliferation and collagen deposition. Collectively, these studies underscore how tailored bioink formulations can recapitulate key aspects of the native meniscal microenvironment while improving the structural and functional performance of engineered constructs.

Various cell types have been explored for meniscus bioprinting. MSCs, derived from bone marrow, adipose tissue, or synovium, are widely used due to their multipotency and ease of expansion. Adipose-derived stem cells are particularly attractive because they are easily harvested with minimal invasiveness. However, MSCs are prone to hypertrophic differentiation and matrix calcification, which can limit their long-term functionality in fibrocartilaginous tissues. Strategies such as co-culturing MSCs with meniscal cells or culturing them within decellularized meniscus ECM have been employed to promote their fibrochondrogenic potential and suppress hypertrophy [11]. MPCs, isolated from the inner and outer zones of the meniscus, retain region-specific phenotypes and are well adapted to the native microenvironment. Because of their native specialization and immuno compatibility, MPCs are considered ideal for autologous applications and for recapitulating zonal heterogeneity. Combining inner and outer MPCs in engineered constructs enables the fabrication of meniscal grafts with region-specific biochemical and biomechanical properties, improving their capacity to restore normal joint function.

An emerging strategy in meniscus engineering is the use of preformed cellular microtissues as biological building blocks for 3D bioprinting. These spheroidal aggregates offer high cell density, enhanced cell–cell interaction, and the capacity to self-organize and fuse into cohesive scaled-up tissues post-bioprinting. The potential of microtissue-based approaches for meniscus repair has been demonstrated in vivo, where transplantation of synovial MSC aggregates led to superior meniscal regeneration compared to single-cell suspensions in rat models [132]. The effectiveness of this approach was further demonstrated in aged primates, where autologous synovial MSC aggregates promoted functional meniscus repair and delayed cartilage degeneration [133]. Microtissue-based 3D bioprinting more closely mirrors natural developmental processes and offers a bottom-up approach to creating modular, scalable, and reproducible constructs [134]. Building on this concept, our recent study focused on bio-assembling region-specific MPC-derived microtissues to closely mimic the meniscus's native zonal heterogeneity. These constructs demonstrated promising integration, underscoring the potential of microtissue-based strategies for meniscal regeneration [135].

7.5.4 Tendon and Ligament

Tendons and ligaments are characterized by their hierarchical, collagen-rich ECM, high tensile strength, and fibroblast-dominant cellular composition [136–138] (Figure 7.7). They exhibit gradient mechanical properties and region-specific matrix organization, particularly at the tendon-to-bone or ligament-to-bone insertion sites, which transition from soft tissue to mineralized interface [139]. These structural and functional complexities pose a significant challenge for traditional scaffold-based approaches.

Tendon and ligament injuries are common musculoskeletal disorders with limited regenerative capacity and suboptimal outcomes following surgical repair. Traditional grafting techniques, including autografts and allografts [140], are often associated with donor-site morbidity, immunogenicity, and mechanical mismatch. As a result, there is a growing interest in TE approaches, particularly 3D bioprinting, to fabricate scaled-up, functional, biomimetic tendon and ligament constructs [141–143].

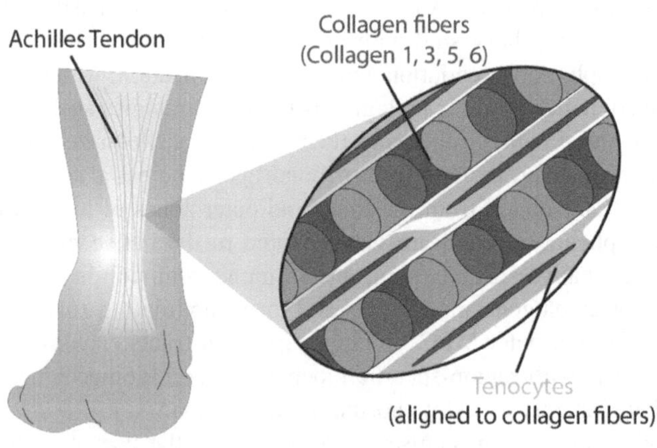

FIGURE 7.7 Hierarchical structure of tendon tissue. Tendons are composed of highly aligned collagen fibers (primarily types 1, 3, 5, and 6) that provide tensile strength and mechanical integrity. These fibers are aligned alongside elongated tenocytes, which are responsible for maintaining and renewing the extracellular matrix composition. The zoomed-in view highlights the organized, parallel arrangement of collagen bundles and resident tenocytes, which is primarily responsible for the tissue's high tensile strength.

Preclinical studies in small and large animal models have demonstrated the feasibility of bioprinted tendon and ligament constructs [129,144,145]. These grafts have shown encouraging results in terms of biomechanical integrity, host integration, and histological resemblance to native tissue. However, extrusion-based bioprinting, while widely used due to its versatility and cell-friendly conditions, often lacks the resolution needed to reproduce the fine microarchitecture characteristic of these load-bearing tissues. To address this challenge, the Zenobi-Wong research group in ETH (Zurich, Switzerland) developed a novel light-based 3D bioprinting method known as Filamented Light (FLight) bioprinting [146]. This approach builds on the principles of digital light processing (DLP) but uniquely leverages optical modulation instability and self-focusing of light within a photocrosslinkable hydrogel to generate aligned filament-like structures *in situ*. By dynamically manipulating the intensity and pattern of the light, the FLight technique enables the rapid formation of parallel microchannels or fibers that guide cell alignment and matrix organization. This method is particularly well suited for musculoskeletal TE, where directional cues are essential for cellular orientation and mechanical function. In proof-of-concept studies, the FLight bioprinting platform was used to fabricate mini-tendon and mini-muscle constructs with native-like alignment [147], showing promise for both fundamental biological studies and potential therapeutic applications. By overcoming the resolution and anisotropy limitations of extrusion-based systems, light-based printing techniques such as FLight bioprinting represent a critical advancement in the fabrication of structurally and functionally relevant tendon and ligament grafts. However, a key limitation of this approach lies in the size of the constructs that can be engineered. This is due to the depth-dependent nature of light-crosslinkable resins, where the ability of light to penetrate and effectively crosslink material diminishes as tissue thickness increases.

Using extrusion-based or DLP bioprinting, researchers have been able to fabricate aligned fiber architectures that guide cell orientation and ECM deposition. Such approaches are essential for replicating the native load-bearing capacity and directional strength of tendon and ligament tissues. The choice of bioink is critical for the bioprinting process and ultimately successful tendon and ligament regeneration once in vivo. Hydrogels such as GelMA, collagen, and fibrin offer cell compatibility and tunable mechanical properties but often require reinforcement to match the tensile properties of native tissue. To address this, hybrid printing strategies have been developed, combining soft hydrogels with stiffer polymers like PCL to create mechanically robust, cell-supportive constructs. Advanced strategies have also explored the use of a decellularized ECM derived from tendon or ligament tissue as a bioink component. These materials retain native biochemical cues and have shown promise in guiding tissue-specific differentiation and ECM remodeling.

While no bioprinted tendon or ligament constructs have yet reached clinical trials, the progress in scaffold design, bioink development, and bioreactor conditioning brings this application closer to engineering scaled-up grafts and therefore to clinical translation. Future directions include integrating vascularization strategies, refining mechanical stimulation protocols, and developing scalable, GMP-compliant manufacturing processes, advancements that will also support the generation of tissues at clinically relevant sizes for human applications in future clinical trials.

7.5.5 Skeletal Muscle

Skeletal muscle injuries resulting from trauma or tumor ablation often require reconstructive procedures to restore normal tissue function. In most cases, these injuries lead to significant functional impairment, severe physical deformities, and a profound impact on quality of life. The current gold standard for treatment involves the use of autologous muscle pedicle flaps harvested from regions adjacent to the injury. However, limited availability of donor muscle tissue and the risk of donor-site morbidity make this approach highly challenging. Recent advances in cell therapies, such as the injection of cultured cells, have demonstrated some potential for functional tissue augmentation. Nevertheless, this strategy faces major limitations due to low cell engraftment and poor survival of the injected cells. As a result, TE has emerged as a promising alternative for the fabrication of implantable muscle constructs capable of restoring the biological and functional integrity of the damaged area. Recently, research has been focused on mimicking the microstructure of the native skeletal muscle tissue, where the myofibers (resident skeletal muscle cells) are highly oriented toward one direction. This organization of the myofibers is vital for the muscle to contract and function physiologically. Therefore, controlling the organization of the engineered myofibers is crucial to engineer a biomechanically functionable graft.

3D bioprinting has emerged as a promising strategy for engineering functional skeletal muscle tissues, which require precise cellular organization, contractile capability, and vascular integration to function properly. In a recent study by Stang et al. [148], the researchers utilized FRESH printing to engineer biomimetic 3D skeletal muscle architectures [148]. Type I collagen was printed within a FRESH support bath in various designs to replicate the native structural organization of muscle. Subsequently, myoblasts were seeded onto the scaffolds to guide myogenesis. The engineered constructs demonstrated aligned cells and fusion into myotubes—a critical process for the maturation of myoblasts into functional myofibers.

In another study, cells were directly bioprinted using a decellularized ECM derived from muscle tissue as a bioink. ECM-derived materials are frequently employed in bioprinting due to their ability to retain bioactive molecules and growth factors that promote cell differentiation and recapitulate skeletal muscle tissue function. They also provide an instructive microenvironment, offering biochemical and biophysical cues that modulate key cellular processes such as migration, differentiation, tissue growth, and development [149,150]. In this study, cells were bioprinted into defined patterns to generate 3D muscle constructs with tailored architectures. Collectively, these studies highlight the potential of 3D bioprinting and cell printing to fabricate customized, functional muscle substitutes, offering promising avenues for the treatment of skeletal muscle injuries.

7.6 CONCLUSION AND FUTURE DIRECTIONS

3D bioprinting represents a major advancement in the field of TE, offering precise spatial control, scalability, and the ability to recapitulate native tissue complexity. By leveraging both cell-only bioinks and microtissue-based building blocks such as spheroids and organoids, this technology allows for the fabrication of highly organized, functional tissue constructs. Recent developments in bottom-up biofabrication strategies have enhanced the fidelity and maturation potential of engineered grafts, particularly in musculoskeletal applications including cartilage, bone, meniscus, tendon, and skeletal muscle. However, despite significant progress, several challenges remain. These include improving vascularization of large constructs, standardizing bioink formulations, and ensuring reproducible outcomes across different bioprinting platforms. Additionally, translating bioprinted tissues from bench to bedside requires the integration of robust bioreactor systems, scalable manufacturing protocols, and compliance with regulatory standards. Looking forward, advances in stem cell biology, bioactive materials, and machine learning-driven design optimization are expected to further accelerate the clinical applicability of 3D bioprinting. As interdisciplinary collaboration continues to expand, the prospect of fabricating patient-specific, functional tissues for transplantation and disease modeling becomes increasingly realistic. Ultimately, 3D bioprinting holds the potential to transform regenerative medicine by enabling the fabrication of complex, personalized tissue constructs at clinically relevant scales.

REFERENCES

[1] Gu Z, Fu J, Lin H, He Y. Development of 3D bioprinting: From printing methods to biomedical applications. *Asian J Pharm Sci.* 2020 Sep;15(5):529–557. doi: 10.1016/j.ajps.2019.11.003.

[2] Tripathi S, Mandal SS, Bauri S, Maiti P. 3D bioprinting and its innovative approach for biomedical applications. *MedComm.* 2022 Dec 24;4(1):e194. doi: 10.1002/mco2.194.

[3] Weng T, et al. 3D bioprinting for skin tissue engineering: Current status and perspectives. *J Tissue Eng.* 2021 Jul 13;12:20417314211028574. doi: 10.1177/20417314211028574.

[4] Galarraga JH, Kwon MY, Burdick JA. 3D bioprinting via an in situ crosslinking technique towards engineering cartilage tissue. *Sci Rep.* 2019 Dec 27;9(1):19987. doi: 10.1038/s41598-019-56117-3.

[5] Shen M, et al. 3D bioprinting of in situ vascularized tissue engineered bone for repairing large segmental bone defects. *Mater Today Bio.* 2022 Aug 8;16:100382. doi: 10.1016/j.mtbio.2022.100382.

[6] Patrício SG, et al. Freeform 3D printing using a continuous viscoelastic supporting matrix. *Biofabrication.* 2020 May 15;12(3):035017. doi: 10.1088/1758-5090/ab8bc3.

[7] Chen EP, Toksoy Z, Davis BA, Geibel JP. 3D bioprinting of vascularized tissues for in vitro and in vivo applications. *Front Bioeng Biotechnol.* 2021 May 13;9:664188. doi: 10.3389/fbioe.2021.664188.

[8] He P, et al. Bioprinting of skin constructs for wound healing. *Burns Trauma.* 2018 Jan 23;6:5. doi: 10.1186/s41038-017-0104-x.

[9] Varkey M, et al. Skin bioprinting: The future of burn wound reconstruction? Burns Trauma. 2019 Feb 12;7:4. doi: 10.1186/s41038-019-0142-7.

[10] Freeman FE, Kelly DJ. Tuning alginate bioink stiffness and composition for controlled growth factor delivery and to spatially direct msc fate within bioprinted tissues. *Sci Rep.* 2017 Dec 6;7(1):17042. doi: 10.1038/s41598-017-17286-1.

[11] Barceló X, Eichholz KF, Garcia O, Kelly DJ. Tuning the degradation rate of alginate-based bioinks for bioprinting functional cartilage tissue. *Biomedicines.* 2022 Jul 7;10(7):1621. doi: 10.3390/biomedicines10071621.

[12] Dufour A, et al. Integrating melt electrowriting and inkjet bioprinting for engineering structurally organized articular cartilage. *Biomaterials* 2022;283:121405. doi: 10.1016/j.biomaterials.2022.121405.

[13] Skylar-Scott MA, et al. Biomanufacturing of organ-specific tissues with high cellular density and embedded vascular channels. *Sci Adv.* 2019 Sep 6;5(9): eaaw2459. doi: 10.1126/sciadv.aaw2459.

[14] Ahrens JH, et al. Programming cellular alignment in engineered cardiac tissue via bioprinting anisotropic organ building blocks. *Adv Mater.* 2022 Jul;34(26): e2200217. doi: 10.1002/adma.202200217.

[15] Hwang DG, et al. Bioprinting-assisted tissue assembly for structural and functional modulation of engineered heart tissue mimicking left ventricular myocardial fiber orientation. *Adv Mater.* 2024 Aug;36(34): e2400364. doi: 10.1002/adma.202400364.

[16] Xie M, et al. In situ 3D bioprinting with bioconcrete bioink. *Nat Commun.* 2022 Jun 23;13(1):3597. doi: 10.1038/s41467-022-30997-y.

[17] Pagan E, et al. A handheld bioprinter for multi-material printing of complex constructs. *Biofabrication.* 2023 May 2;15(3). doi: 10.1088/1758-5090/acc42c.

[18] Mandrycky C, Wang Z, Kim K, Kim DH. 3D bioprinting for engineering complex tissues. *Biotechnol Adv.* 2016 Jul–Aug;34(4):422–434. doi: 10.1016/j.biotechadv.2015.12.011.

[19] Datta P, et al. Essential steps in bioprinting: From pre- to post-bioprinting. *Biotechnol Adv.* 2018 Sep–Oct;36(5):1481–1504. doi: 10.1016/j.biotechadv.2018.06.003.

[20] Huang Y, et al. 3D bioprinting and the current applications in tissue engineering. *Biotechnol J.* 2017 Aug;12(8). doi: 10.1002/biot.201600734.

[21] Zhang X, Zhang Y. Tissue engineering applications of three-dimensional bioprinting. *Cell Biochem Biophys.* 2015 Jul;72(3):777–782. doi: 10.1007/s12013-015-0531-x.

[22] Devillard R, et al. Cell patterning by laser-assisted bioprinting. *Methods Cell Biol.* 2014; 119:159–174. doi: 10.1016/B978-0-12-416742-1.00009-3.

[23] Hall GN, et al. Laser-assisted bioprinting of targeted cartilaginous spheroids for high density bottom-up tissue engineering. *Biofabrication.* 2024 Aug 22;16(4). doi: 10.1088/1758-5090/ad6e1a.

[24] Zhang YS, et al. 3D extrusion bioprinting. *Nat Rev Methods Primers.* 2021;1:75. doi: 10.1038/s43586-021-00073-8.

[25] Ozbolat IT, Hospodiuk M. Current advances and future perspectives in extrusion-based bioprinting. *Biomaterials.* 2016;76:321–343.

[26] Ning L, et al. Process-induced cell damage: pneumatic versus screw-driven bioprinting. *Biofabrication* 2020;12(2):025011. doi: 10.1088/1758-5090/ab5f53.

[27] Gungor-Ozkerim PS, et al. Bioinks for 3D bioprinting: An overview. *Biomater Sci.* 2018;6(5):915–946. doi: 10.1039/c7bm00765e.

[28] Ashammakhi N, et al. Bioinks and bioprinting technologies to make heterogeneous and biomimetic tissue constructs. *Mater Today Bio.* 2019;1:100008. doi: 10.1016/j.mtbio.2019.100008.

[29] Garcia-Cruz MR, Postma A, Frith JE, Meagher L. Printability and bio-functionality of a shear thinning methacrylated xanthan-gelatin composite bioink. *Biofabrication.* 2021;13(3). doi: 10.1088/1758-5090/abec2d.

[30] Malda J, et al. 25th anniversary article: Engineering hydrogels for biofabrication. *Adv Mater.* 2013;25(36):5011–5028. doi: 10.1002/adma.201302042.

[31] McGivern S, et al. Translational application of 3D bioprinting for cartilage tissue engineering. *Bioengineering.* 2021;8(10):144. doi: 10.3390/bioengineering8100144.

[32] Chopin-Doroteo M, Mandujano-Tinoco EA, Krötzsch E. Tailoring of the rheological properties of bioinks to improve bioprinting and bioassembly for tissue replacement. *Biochim Biophys Acta.* 2021;1865(2):129782. doi: 10.1016/j.bbagen.2020.129782.

[33] McCormack A, Highley CB, Leslie NR Melchels FPW. 3D printing in suspension baths: Keeping the promises of bioprinting afloat. *Trends Biotechnol.* 2020;38(6):584–593. doi: 10.1016/j.tibtech.2019.12.020.

[34] Zhou K, et al. Hydrogels for 3D embedded bioprinting: A focused review on bioinks and support baths. *J Mater Chem B.* 2022;10(12):1897–1907. doi: 10.1039/d1tb02554f.

[35] Bhattacharjee T, et al. Liquid-like solids support cells in 3D. *ACS Biomater Sci Eng.* 2016;2(10):1787–1795. doi: 10.1021/acsbiomaterials.6b00218.

[36] Kolesky DB, et al. 3D bioprinting of vascularized, heterogeneous cell-laden tissue constructs. *Adv Mater.* 2014;26(19):3124–3130.

[37] Achilli TM, Meyer J, Morgan JR. Advances in the formation, use and understanding of multi-cellular spheroids. *Expert Opin Biol Ther.* 2012, 12(10):1347–1360. doi: 10.1517/14712598.2012.707181.

[38] Kronemberger GS, et al. Growth factor stimulation regimes to support the development and fusion of cartilage microtissues. *Tissue Eng Part C Methods.* 2025 Jan;31(1):36–48. doi: 10.1089/ten.tec.2024.0309.

[39] Kronemberger GS, et al. Cartilage and bone tissue engineering using adipose stromal/stem cells spheroids as building blocks. *World J Stem Cells.* 2020 Feb 26;12(2):110–122. doi: 10.4252/wjsc.v12.i2.110.

[40] Gonzales-Aloy E, et al. From cells to organoids: The evolution of blood-brain barrier technology for modelling drug delivery in brain cancer. *Adv Drug Deliv Rev.* 2023;196:114777. doi: 10.1016/j.addr.2023.114777.

[41] Mironov V, et al. Organ printing: Tissue spheroids as building blocks. *Biomaterials.* 2009;30(12):2164–2174. doi: 10.1016/j.biomaterials.2008.12.084.

[42] Burdis R, Kelly DJ. Biofabrication and bioprinting using cellular aggregates, microtissues and organoids for the engineering of musculoskeletal tissues. *Acta Biomater.* 2021;126:1–14. doi: 10.1016/j.actbio.2021.03.016.

[43] Marti-Figueroa CR, Ashton RS. The case for applying tissue engineering methodologies to instruct human organoid morphogenesis. *Acta Biomater.* 2017;54:35–44. doi: 10.1016/j.actbio.2017.03.023.

[44] Ko J, et al. Revealing the clinical potential of high-resolution organoids. *Adv Drug Deliv Rev.* 2024;207:115202. doi: 10.1016/j.addr.2024.115202.

[45] Shinde A, et al. Recent advances of biosensor-integrated organ-on-a-chip technologies for diagnostics and therapeutics. *Anal Chem.* 2023;95(6):3121–3146. doi: 10.1021/acs.analchem.2c05036.

[46] Chliara MA, Elezoglou S, Zergioti I. Bioprinting on organ-on-chip: Development and applications. *Biosensors.* 2022;12(12):1135. doi: 10.3390/bios12121135.

[47] Lancaster MA, Knoblich JA. Generation of cerebral organoids from human pluripotent stem cells. *Nat Protoc.* 2014, 9(10):2329–2340. doi: 10.1038/nprot.2014.158.

[48] Kim SJ, et al. Engineering multi-cellular spheroids for tissue engineering and regenerative medicine. *Adv Healthc Mater.* 2020;9(23):e2000608. doi: 10.1002/adhm.202000608.

[49] Kronemberger GS, et al. The hypertrophic cartilage induction influences the building-block capacity of human adipose stem/stromal cell spheroids for biofabrication. *Artif Organs.* 2021 Oct;45(10):1208–1218. doi: 10.1111/aor.14000.

[50] Dalton PD, Woodfield TBF, Mironov V, Groll J. Advances in hybrid fabrication toward hierarchical tissue constructs. *Adv Sci.* 2020;7(11):1902953. doi: 10.1002/advs.201902953.

[51] Daly AC, Kelly DJ. Biofabrication of spatially organised tissues by directing the growth of cellular spheroids within 3D printed polymeric microchambers. *Biomaterials.* 2019 Mar;197:194–206. doi: 10.1016/j.biomaterials.2018.12.028.

[52] Brunel LG, Hull SM, Heilshorn SC. Engineered assistive materials for 3D bioprinting: support baths and sacrificial inks. *Biofabrication.* 2022 May 19;14(3): ac6bbe. doi: 10.1088/1758-5090/ac6bbe.

[53] Shiwarski DJ, et al. 3D bioprinting of collagen-based high-resolution internally perfusable scaffolds for engineering fully biologic tissue systems. *Sci Adv.* 2025 Apr 25;11(17):eadu5905. doi: 10.1126/sciadv.adu5905.

[54] Mirdamadi E, et al. FRESH 3D bioprinting a full-size model of the human heart. *ACS Biomater Sci Eng.* 2020 Nov 9;6(11):6453–6459. doi: 10.1021/acsbiomaterials.0c01133.

[55] Yang Y, et al. Bioprinting of an osteocyte network for biomimetic mineralization. *Biofabrication*. 2020;12:1–26.
[56] Trikalitis VD, et al. Embedded 3D printing of dilute particle suspensions into dense complex tissue fibers using shear thinning xanthan baths. *Biofabrication*. 2022 Dec 6;15(1). doi: 10.1088/1758-5090/aca124.
[57] Spagnuolo FD, Kronemberger GS, Kelly DJ. A 4D bioprinting platform to engineer anisotropic musculoskeletal tissues by spatially patterning microtissues into temporally adapting support baths. *BioRxiv*. doi: 10.1101/2025.05.01.651636.
[58] Allen KD, et al. Epidemiology of osteoarthritis. *Osteoarthritis Cartilage*. 2022;30(2):184–195. doi: 10.1016/j.joca.2021.04.020.
[59] Green WT, Jr. Articular cartilage repair. Behavior of rabbit chondrocytes during tissue culture and subsequent allografting. *Clin Orthopaed Relat Res*. 1977;(124): 237–250.
[60] Elisseeff J, et al. Transdermal photopolymerization of poly (ethylene oxide)-based injectable hydrogels for tissue-engineered cartilage. *Plast Reconstr Surg*. 1999;104(4):1014–1022. doi: 10.1097/00006534-199909040-00017.
[61] Elisseeff J, et al. Photoencapsulation of chondrocytes in poly (ethylene oxide)-based semi-interpenetrating networks. *J Biomed Mater Res*. 2000;51(2): 164–71. doi: 10.1002/(sici)1097-4636(200008)51:2<164:aid-jbm4>3.0.co;2–w.
[62] Kim WS, et al. Cartilage engineered in predetermined shapes employing cell transplantation on synthetic biodegradable polymers. *Plast Reconstr Surg*. 1994;94(2):233–237; discussion 238–240.
[63] Elisseeff J, et al. Controlled-release of IGF-I and TGF-beta1 in a photopolymerizing hydrogel for cartilage tissue engineering. *J Orthop Res*. 2001;19(6):1098–1104. doi: 10.1016/S0736-0266(01)00054-7.
[64] Owida HA, et al. Induction of zonal-specific cellular morphology and matrix synthesis for biomimetic cartilage regeneration using hybrid scaffolds. *J R Soc Interf*. 2018;15(143). doi: 10.1098/rsif.2018.0037.
[65] Nguyen LH, et al.. Unique biomaterial compositions direct bone marrow stem cells into specific chondrocytic phenotypes corresponding to the various zones of articular cartilage. *Biomaterials*. 2011;32(5):1327–1338. doi: 10.1016/j.biomaterials.2010.10.020.
[66] Nguyen LH, et al. Engineering articular cartilage with spatially-varying matrix composition and mechanical properties from a single stem cell population using a multilayered hydrogel. *Biomaterials*. 2011;32(29):6946–6952. doi: 10.1016/j.biomaterials.2011.06.032.
[67] Steele JA, et al. Combinatorial scaffold morphologies for zonal articular cartilage engineering. *Acta Biomater*. 2014;10(5):2065–2675. doi: 10.1016/j.actbio.2014.01.030.
[68] Klein TJ, et al. Tissue engineering of articular cartilage with biomimetic zones. *Tissue Eng Part B: Rev*. 2009;15(2):143–157. doi: 10.1089/ten.TEB.2008.0353.
[69] Ng KW, Ateshian GA, Hung CT. Zonal chondrocytes seeded in a layered agarose hydrogel create engineered cartilage with depth-dependent cellular and mechanical inhomogeneity. *Tissue Eng Part A*. 2009;15(9):2315–2324. doi: 10.1089/ten.tea.2008.0429.
[70] Moroni L, et al. Design of biphasic polymeric 3-dimensional fiber deposited scaffolds for cartilage tissue engineering applications. *Tissue Eng*. 2007;13(2):361–371. doi: 10.1089/ten.2006.0127.
[71] Semitela Â, et al. Boosting in vitro cartilage tissue engineering through the fabrication of polycaprolactone-gelatin 3D scaffolds with specific depth-dependent fiber alignments and mechanical stimulation. *J Mech Behav Biomed Mater*. 2021;117:104373. doi: 10.1016/j.jmbbm.2021.104373.
[72] Khoshgoftar M, et al. The effect of tissue-engineered cartilage biomechanical and biochemical properties on its post-implantation mechanical behavior. *Biomech Model Mechanobiol*. 2013;12(1):43–54. doi: 10.1007/s10237-012-0380-0.

[73] Mammoto T, Ingber DE. Mechanical control of tissue and organ development. *Development*. 2010;137(9):1407–1420. doi: 10.1242/dev.024166.
[74] Gjorevski N, Ranga A, Lutolf MP. Bioengineering approaches to guide stem cell-based organogenesis. *Development*. 2014;141(9):1794–1804. doi: 10.1242/dev.098418.
[75] Chanet S, Martin AC. Mechanical force sensing in tissues. *Prog Mol Biol Transl Sci*. 2014;126:317–352. doi: 10.1016/B978-0-12-394624-9.00013-0.
[76] Théry M. Micropatterning as a tool to decipher cell morphogenesis and functions. *J Cell Sci*. 2010;123(24): 4201–4213.
[77] Seidel JO, et al. Long-term culture of tissue engineered cartilage in a perfused chamber with mechanical stimulation. *Biorheology*. 2004;41(3–4):445–458.
[78] Vunjak-Novakovic G, et al. Bioreactor cultivation conditions modulate the composition and mechanical properties of tissue-engineered cartilage. *J Orthop Res*. 1999;17(1):130–138. doi: 10.1002/jor.1100170119.
[79] Mauck RL, et al. Functional tissue engineering of articular cartilage through dynamic loading of chondrocyte-seeded agarose gels. *J Biomech Eng*. 2000;122(3):252–260. doi: 10.1115/1.429656.
[80] Jahangir S, et al. Cell-laden 3D printed GelMA/HAp and THA hydrogel bioinks: Development of osteochondral tissue-like bioinks. *Materials*. 2023;16(22):7214. doi: 10.3390/ma16227214.
[81] Chen YC, et al. Functional human vascular network generated in photocrosslinkable gelatin methacrylate hydrogels. *Adv Funct Mater*. 2012;22:2027–2039. doi: 10.1002/adfm.201101662.
[82] Wei D, et al. A biocompatible hydrogel with improved stiffness and hydrophilicity for modular tissue engineering assembly. *J Mater Chem B*. 2015;3:275363. doi: 10.1039/c5tb00129c.
[83] Schuurman W, et al. Gelatin-methacrylamide hydrogels as potential biomaterials for fabrication of tissue-engineered cartilage constructs. *Macromol Biosci*. 2013;13(5):551–561. doi: 10.1002/mabi.201200471.
[84] Levett PA, et al. A biomimetic extracellular matrix for cartilage tissue engineering centered on photocurable gelatin, hyaluronic acid and chondroitin sulfate. *Acta Biomater*. 2014;10(1):214–223. doi: 10.1016/j.actbio.2013.10.005.
[85] Daly AC, et al. A comparison of different bioinks for 3D bioprinting of fibrocartilage and hyaline cartilage. *Biofabrication*. 2016;8(4):045002. doi: 10.1088/1758-5090/8/4/045002.
[86] Lafuente-Merchan M, et al. Chondroitin and dermatan sulfate bioinks for 3D bioprinting and cartilage regeneration. *Macromol Biosci*. 2022;22(3):e2100435. doi: 10.1002/mabi.202100435.
[87] Markstedt K, et al. 3D bioprinting human chondrocytes with nanocellulose-alginate bioink for cartilage tissue engineering applications. *Biomacromolecules*. 2015;16(5):1489–96. doi: 10.1021/acs.biomac.5b00188.
[88] Catros S, et al. Layer-by-layer tissue microfabrication supports cell proliferation in vitro and in vivo. *Tissue Eng Part C Methods*. 2012;18(1):62–70. doi: 10.1089/ten.TEC.2011.0382.
[89] Rowley JA, et al. Alginate hydrogels as synthetic extracellular matrix materials. *Biomaterials*. 1999;20(1):45–53. doi: 10.1016/s0142-9612(98)00107-0.
[90] Öztürk E, et al. Sulfated hydrogel matrices direct mitogenicity and maintenance of chondrocyte phenotype through activation of FGF signaling. *Adv Funct Mater*. 2016;26(21):3649–3662. doi: 10.1002/adfm.201600092.
[91] Costantini M, et al. 3D bioprinting of BM-MSCs-loaded ECM biomimetic hydrogels for in vitro neocartilage formation. *Biofabrication*. 2016;8(3):035002. doi: 10.1088/1758-5090/8/3/035002.

[92] Visscher DO, et al. A photo-crosslinkable cartilage-derived extracellular matrix bioink for auricular cartilage tissue engineering. *Acta Biomater.* 2021;121:193–203. doi: 10.1016/j.actbio.2020.11.029.
[93] Meng X, et al. A sturgeon cartilage extracellular matrix-derived bioactive bioink for tissue engineering applications. *Int J Bioprint.* 2023;9(5):768. doi: 10.18063/ijb.768.
[94] Setayeshmehr M, et al. Bioprinting via a dual-gel bioink based on poly(vinyl alcohol) and solubilized extracellular matrix towards cartilage engineering. *Int J Mol Sci.* 2021;22(8):3901. doi: 10.3390/ijms22083901.
[95] Rathan S, et al. Fiber reinforced cartilage ECM functionalized bioinks for functional cartilage tissue engineering. *Adv Healthc Mater.* 2019;8(7):e1801501. doi: 10.1002/adhm.201801501.
[96] Jia L, et al. Bioprinting and regeneration of auricular cartilage using a bioactive bioink based on microporous photocrosslinkable acellular cartilage matrix. *Bioact Mater.* 2022;16:66–81. doi: 10.1016/j.bioactmat.2022.02.032.
[97] Jung CS, et al. Development of printable natural cartilage matrix bioink for 3D printing of irregular tissue shape. *Tissue Eng Regen Med.* 2017;15(2):155–162. doi: 10.1007/s13770-017-0104-8.
[98] Sakai S, et al. Silk fibroin nanofibers: A promising ink additive for extrusion three-dimensional bioprinting. *Mater Today Bio.* 2020;8:100078. doi: 10.1016/j.mtbio.2020.100078.
[99] Kosik-Kozioł A, et al. PLA short sub-micron fiber reinforcement of 3D bioprinted alginate constructs for cartilage regeneration. *Biofabrication.* 2017;9(4):044105. doi: 10.1088/1758-5090/aa90d7.
[100] Ren X,et al. Engineering zonal cartilage through bioprinting collagen type II hydrogel constructs with biomimetic chondrocyte density gradient. *BMC Musculoskelet Disord.* 2016;17:301. doi: 10.1186/s12891-016-1130-8.
[101] Baron R. Anatomy and ultrastructure of bone – Histogenesis, growth and remodeling. In *Endotext,* edited by LJ De Groot, G Chrousos, K Dungan, et al. MDText.com, Inc. 2008.
[102] Mansoorifar A, Gordon R, Bergan R, Bertassoni LE. Bone-on-a-chip: Microfluidic technologies and microphysiologic models of bone tissue. *Adv Funct Mater.* 2021;31(6):2006796. doi: 10.1002/adfm.202006796.
[103] De Pace R, Molinari S, Mazzoni E, Perale G. Bone regeneration: A review of current treatment strategies. *J Clin Med.* 2025;14(6):1838. doi: 10.3390/jcm14061838.
[104] Dec P, Modrzejewski A, Pawlik A. Existing and novel biomaterials for bone tissue engineering. *Int J Mol Sci.* 2022;24(1):529. doi: 10.3390/ijms24010529.
[105] Yuan X, et al. Recent advances in 3D printing of smart scaffolds for bone tissue engineering and regeneration. *Adv Mater.* 2024;36(34):e2403641. doi: 10.1002/adma.202403641.
[106] Maresca JA, et al. Three-dimensional bioprinting applications for bone tissue engineering. *Cells.* 2023;12(9):1230. doi: 10.3390/cells12091230.
[107] Byambaa B, et al. Bioprinted osteogenic and vasculogenic patterns for engineering 3D bone tissue. *Adv Healthc Mater.* 2017;6:1–15.
[108] Freeman S, et al. A bioink blend for rotary 3D bioprinting tissue engineered small-diameter vascular constructs. *Acta Biomater.* 2019;95:152–164.
[109] Yang Y, et al. Bioprinting of an osteocyte network for biomimetic mineralization. *Biofabrication.* 2020;12:1–26.
[110] Pitacco P, Sadowska JM, O'Brien FJ, Kelly DJ. 3D bioprinting of cartilaginous templates for large bone defect healing. *Acta Biomater.* 2023;156:61–74. doi: 10.1016/j.actbio.2022.07.037.
[111] Kim MH, et al. High-throughput bioprinting of spheroids for scalable tissue fabrication. *Nat Commun.* 2024;15(1):10083. doi: 10.1038/s41467-024-54504-7.

[112] Duan J, et al. 3D bioprinting of prevascularized bone organoids for rapid in situ cranial bone reconstruction. *Adv Healthc Mater.* 2025;14(16):e2501376. doi: 10.1002/adhm.202501376.
[113] Fox AJ, Bedi A, Rodeo SA. The basic science of human knee menisci: Structure, composition, and function. *Sports Health.* 2012 Jul;4(4):340–351. doi: 10.1177/1941738111429419.
[114] Du MZ, et al. Meniscus heterogeneity and 3D-printed strategies for engineering anisotropic meniscus. *Int J Bioprint.* 2023 Feb 27;9(3):693. doi: 10.18063/ijb.693.
[115] Patel H, et al. Illustrative review of knee meniscal tear patterns, repair and replacement options, and imaging evaluation. *Clin Imaging.* 2021 Jan;69:4–16. doi: 10.1016/j.clinimag.2020.06.045.
[116] Englund M. The role of the meniscus in osteoarthritis genesis. *Rheum Dis Clin North Am.* 2008 Aug;34(3):573–579. doi: 10.1016/j.rdc.2008.05.009.
[117] López-Franco M, et al. Meniscal degeneration in human knee osteoarthritis: In situ hybridization and immunohistochemistry study. *Arch Orthop Trauma Surg.* 2016 Feb;136(2):175–183. doi: 10.1007/s00402-015-2378-4.
[118] Sukopp M, et al. Influence of menisci on tibiofemoral contact mechanics in human knees: A systematic review. *Front Bioeng Biotechnol.* 2021 Dec 3;9:765596. doi: 10.3389/fbioe.2021.765596.
[119] Makris EA, Hadidi P, Athanasiou KA. The knee meniscus: Structure-function, pathophysiology, current repair techniques, and prospects for regeneration. *Biomaterials.* 2011 Oct;32(30):7411–7431. doi: 10.1016/j.biomaterials.2011.06.037.
[120] Furumatsu T, et al. Inner meniscus cells main_tain higher chondrogenic phenotype compared with outer meniscus cells. *Connect Tissue Res.* 2011;52(6):459–465. doi:10.3109/03008207.2011.562061.
[121] Seol D, et al. Characteristics of meniscus progenitor cells migrated from injured meniscus. *J Orthop Res.* 2017 Sep;35(9):1966–1972. doi: 10.1002/jor.23472.
[122] Wang J, Roberts S, Li W, Wright K. Phenotypic characterization of regional human meniscus progenitor cells. *Front Bioeng Biotechnol.* 2022;10:1003966. doi: 10.3389/fbioe.2022.1003966.
[123] Bilgen B, Jayasuriya CT, Owens BD. Current concepts in meniscus tissue engineering and repair. *Adv Healthc Mater.* 2018 Jun;7(11):e1701407. doi: 10.1002/adhm.201701407. Epub 2018 Mar 15.
[124] Place ES, Evans ND, Stevens MM. Complexity in biomaterials for tissue engineering. *Nat Mater.* 2009 Jun;8(6):457–470. doi: 10.1038/nmat2441.
[125] Ionescu LC, Lee GC, Huang KL, Mauck RL. Growth factor supplementation improves native and engineered meniscus repair in vitro. *Acta Biomater.* 2012 Oct;8(10):3687–3694. doi: 10.1016/j.actbio.2012.06.005.
[126] Huey DJ, Hu JC, Athanasiou KA. Unlike bone, cartilage regeneration remains elusive. *Science.* 2012 Nov 16;338(6109):917–921. doi: 10.1126/science.1222454.
[127] Critchley SE, Kelly DJ. Bioinks for bioprinting functional meniscus and articular cartilage. *J 3D Print Med.* 2017;1(4):269–290. doi: 10.2217/3dp-2017-0012.
[128] Lu J, et al. The design and characterization of a strong bio-ink for meniscus regeneration. *Int J Bioprint.* 2022 Aug 8;8(4):600. doi: 10.18063/ijb.v8i4.600.
[129] Chae S, et al. 3D cell-printing of tendon-bone interface using tissue-derived extracellular matrix bioinks for chronic rotator cuff repair. *Biofabrication.* 2021 Apr 2;13(3). doi: 10.1088/1758-5090/abd159.
[130] Heydarigoojani M, Farokhi M, Simorgh S. Bioinks for engineering gradient-based osteochondral and meniscal tissue substitutes: A review. *Biofabrication.* 2025 Feb 13;17(2). doi: 10.1088/1758-5090/adb0f4.
[131] Sathish PB, et al. Tricomposite gelatin-carboxymethylcellulose-alginate bioink for direct and indirect 3D printing of human knee meniscal scaffold. *Int J Biol Macromol.* 2022 Jan 15;195:179–189. doi: 10.1016/j.ijbiomac.2021.11.184.

[132] Hiroki K, et al. Transplantation of aggregates of synovial mesenchymal stem cells regenerates meniscus more effectively in a rat massive meniscal defect. *Biochem Biophys Res Commun*. 2013. doi: 10.1016/j.bbrc.2013.05.026.

[133] Shimpei K, et al. Transplantation of autologous synovial mesenchymal stem cells promotes meniscus regeneration in aged primates. *J Orthop Res*. 2017 Jun;35(6):1274–1282. doi: 10.1002/jor.23211.

[134] Luis E, et al. 3D direct printing of silicone meniscus implant using a novel heat-cured extrusion-based printer. *Polymers*. 2020 May 1;12(5):1031. doi: 10.3390/polym12051031.

[135] Kronemberger GS, et al. Bioassembly of region-specific fibrocartilage microtissues to engineer zonally defined meniscal grafts. *BioRxiv*. 2025. doi: doi: 10.1101/2025.04.25.650568.

[136] Provenzano PP, Vanderby R Jr. Collagen fibril morphology and organization: Implications for force transmission in ligament and tendon. *Matrix Biol*. 2006 Mar;25(2):71–84. doi: 10.1016/j.matbio.2005.09.005.

[137] Franchi M, et al. Collagen structure of tendon relates to function. *Sci World J*. 2007 Mar 30;7:404–420. doi: 10.1100/tsw.2007.92.

[138] Van Gulick L, Saby C, Morjani H, Beljebbar A. Age-related changes in molecular organization of type I collagen in tendon as probed by polarized SHG and Raman microspectroscopy. *Sci Rep*. 2019 May 13;9(1):7280. doi: 10.1038/s41598-019-43636-2.

[139] Benjamin M, et al. Where tendons and ligaments meet bone: Attachment sites ("enthuses") in relation to exercise and/or mechanical load. *J Anat*. 2006 Apr;208(4):471–490. doi: 10.1111/j.1469-7580.2006.00540.x.

[140] Lim WL, et al. Current progress in tendon and ligament tissue engineering. *Tissue Eng Regen Med*. 2019 Jun 26;16(6):549–571. doi: 10.1007/s13770-019-00196-w.

[141] Merceron TK, et al. A 3D bioprinted complex structure for engineering the muscle-tendon unit. *Biofabrication*. 2015 Jun 17;7(3):035003. doi: 10.1088/1758-5090/7/3/035003.

[142] Laternser S, et al. A novel microplate 3D bioprinting platform for the engineering of muscle and tendon tissues. *SLAS Technol*. 2018 Dec;23(6):599–613. doi: 10.1177/2472630318776594.

[143] Al-Hakim Khalak F, et al. Decellularized extracellular matrix-based bioinks for tendon regeneration in three-dimensional bioprinting. *Int J Mol Sci*. 2022 Oct 26;23(21):12930. doi: 10.3390/ijms232112930.

[144] Zhang AY, et al. Tissue engineered intrasynovial tendons: in vivo graft survival and tensile strength. *Eur J Plast Surg*. 2010;33:283–289. doi: 10.1007/s00238-010-0398-4.

[145] Lee KI, et al. In vitro and in vivo performance of tissue-engineered tendons for anterior cruciate ligament reconstruction. *Am J Sports Med*. 2018 Jun;46(7):1641–1649. doi: 10.1177/0363546518759729.

[146] Liu H, et al. Filamented light (FLight) biofabrication of highly aligned tissue-engineered constructs. *Adv Mater*. 2022 Nov;34(45):e2204301. doi: 10.1002/adma.202204301.

[147] Liu H, et al. Filamented light (FLight) biofabrication of mini-tendon models show tunable matrix confinement and nuclear morphology. *Biofabrication*. 2025 Apr 28;17(3). doi: 10.1088/1758-5090/adce35.

[148] Stang M, et al. Engineering 3D skeletal muscle tissue with complex multipennate myofiber architectures. *BioRxiv*. 2025. doi: doi: 10.1101/2025.01.06.631119.

[149] Frantz C, Stewart KM, Weaver VM. The extracellular matrix at a glance. *J Cell Sci*. 2010 Dec 15;123(Pt 24):4195–4200. doi: 10.1242/jcs.023820.

[150] Zhang Y, et al. Tissue-specific extracellular matrix coatings for the promotion of cell proliferation and maintenance of cell phenotype. *Biomaterials*. 2009 Aug;30 (23–24):4021–4028. doi: 10.1016/j.biomaterials.2009.04.005.

8 Bioprinting on Organ-on-Chip Technology

Aliakbar Ebrahimi, Hamed Ghorbanpoor, Shadab Dabagh, Somayeh Asadi Haris, Ergün Alperay Tarım, Ayça Bal Öztürk, and Huseyin Avci

8.1 INTRODUCTION

Conventional two-dimensional (2D) and three-dimensional (3D) cultures with alternative *in vitro* methodologies fail to replicate the dynamic 3D microenvironment of *in vivo* tissues and human physiology [1]. Microfabricated multichannel 3D cell-culture systems and organ-on-chip (OoC) platforms are flexible instruments that can reduce the need for animal models by bridging the gap between the necessary *in vivo* investigations and standardized two-dimensional culture tests [2]. OoC technologies facilitate disease metabolism research, therapeutic screening, and discovery applications by simulating complex tissues *in vitro* for the study of human physiology [3,4]. Additionally, by getting beyond the main limitations of both *in vitro* and *in vivo* models, OoC devices increase the accuracy of preclinical testing [5]. To create *ex vivo* models, suitable cell populations that replicate physiological behaviors in tissue microenvironments must be included [3,6,7]. By combining 3D cell-culture models with microfluidics, this method enables more accurate simulation of pathological *in vivo* settings and careful control of system properties [5].

Traditional manufacturing methods, including photopatterning [8], soft lithography [9], injection molding and micromolding [10], are typically employed to construct OoC platforms. Soft lithography employs an elastomeric stamp to create molds with nanoscale-to-microscale features, into which polydimethylsiloxane (PDMS) is poured and sealed with glass. Photo-lithography utilizes a photoresist-coated silicon wafer, which is patterned using UV light and etching to fabricate molds for PDMS channels [11]. Nevertheless, these strategies are inadequate as they necessitate multistep lithographic procedures, masks, and specific tools, rendering manufacturing costly and time-consuming. Moreover, these technologies are solely adept in fabricating the microfluidic chip itself, whereas the additional components (i.e., microtissues, stimulus loading elements, and result-readout sensors) demand further processing [12]. Recent progress in microfabrication methods, cell biology, microfluidics, and 3D bioprinting has made it possible to quickly

DOI: 10.1201/9781032638164-8

make OoC systems and biomimetic tissue microarchitectures [13]. These can be used as a basis for preclinical studies with better predictive accuracy [3,14].

On the other hand, 3D bioprinting is a cutting-edge and promising method that is better than traditional manufacturing methods because it allows for unlimited design options, complex shapes, and less waste [1]. Moreover, it provides an effective technique for generating complex *in vitro* 3D structures, facilitating the precise deposition, localization, and assembly of cells along with their supporting scaffolds in user-specified topologies and dimensions [15]. In addition, 3D bioprinting enables the simultaneous printing of several materials and cell types with excellent spatial resolution and repeatability. This makes it easier to obtain a biomimetic environment with diverse 3D complex structures that closely mimic genuine tissues [16–18]. An OoC platform can also be used with certain 3D-printed sensors to track the screening of biological, chemical, and physical indicators in real time [7]. Microfluidic technology combined with 3D bioprinting has the potential to transform bioengineering by accuratcly simulating human physiology for improved drug testing, personalized medicine, and novel treatments [17].

In this chapter, the current progress of organs-on-chips platforms formed with 3D bioprinting technologies is discussed. First, fabrication technologies and methodologies are introduced with their strengths and weaknesses. Automation, sensor integration, and high-throughput production strategies are also presented as emerging approaches shaping the advancement of bioprinted OoC platforms. Then, recent advancements in the applications of 3D bioprinted OoC platforms are categorized on the basis of drug screening, toxicology, disease modeling (i.e., tumor microenvironment (TME) replication), and personalized medicine. In the final section, the current challenges in using bioprinting to fabricate OoC systems and some directions for future research are highlighted, along with a summary of key insights.

8.2 FABRICATION TECHNOLOGIES AND METHODOLOGIES

OoC-based microfluidic systems have continued to be of great importance in drug development, toxicity testing, and disease modeling through their ability to simulate the microenvironment of cells in their natural physiological conditions [19]. These systems, combined with bioprinting, permit the cell-specific spatial localization, formation of 3D tissues, and construction of functional tissue architectures. This section presents an overview of fabrication methods, encompassing, but not limited to, bioprinting techniques, microfluidic chip design and materials, and bioink formulations. The overall process of 3D printing can be described as follows: (1) computer-aided design, (2) convert to stereolithography file format (STL) format, and (3) layer-by-layer printing through the selected printing technology to produce microfluidic chips.

In OoC-based microfluidic systems, vat photopolymerization (VP), material extrusion (ME), and material jetting (MJ) techniques are of particular importance. VP is a 3D printing method of high precision, which is modeled on the regulated solidification of photosensitive polymers. UV or visible light causes polymerization. There are three subtypes of VP: stereolithography, in which a laser beam is used to polymerize the parts, point by point (Figure 8.1a); digital light processing, which

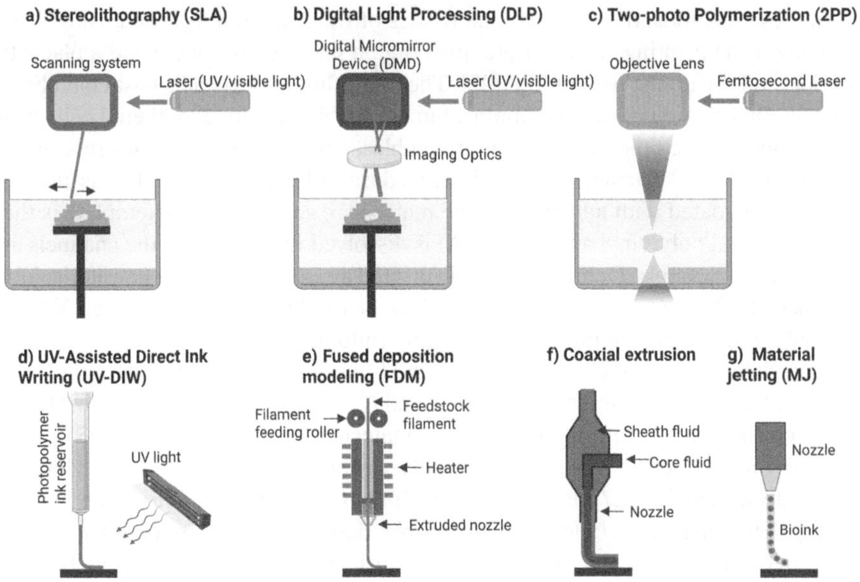

FIGURE 8.1 Illustration of 3D printing approaches that can be used for the fabrication of OoC systems: (a) SLA, (b) DLP, (c) 2PP, (d) UV-DIW, (e) FDM, (f) coaxial extrusion, and (e) MJ. (From BioRender.)

polymerizes the parts using a layer at a time, based on a digital micromirror device (Figure 8.1b); and two-photon polymerization, which uses femtosecond lasers to polymerize parts at a nanoscale (Figure 8.1c). Whereas VP is accurate, it has a limitation, like material variety [20].

The workings of ME methods are premised on the issue of polymer or bioink layered through a nozzle. There are UV-assisted direct ink writing, in which photocurable inks are extruded and which is simultaneously cured (Figure 8.1d); fused deposition modeling, where thermoplastic filaments are melted and deposited (Figure 8.1e); and coaxial extrusion, whereby a coaxial nozzle simultaneously deposits an outer layer of bioink and an inner layer of sacrificial material, enabling the fabrication of complex embedded microchannels (Figure 8.1f). ME allows the use of diverse polymers and hydrogels, making it highly versatile, although its resolution is lower than that of VP [21].

MJ relies on inkjet-based deposition of liquid droplets onto a substrate, followed by curing via photopolymerization or cooling (Figure 8.1g). Depending on droplet formation mechanisms, MJ can be thermal, piezoelectric, or electrostatic. Its advantages include high surface quality and multi-material capability, but limitations involve slower processing and restricted material compatibility [20].

In summary, VP provides superior resolution and accuracy but limited material diversity; ME offers wide material compatibility at lower resolution; and MJ provides multi-material capacity with high-quality surfaces, although at the expense of speed. The selection of a printing method should therefore be guided by the specific requirements of the intended biomedical application [7].

In these methods, the channels and tissues of the chip are fabricated using direct or indirect 3D printing. To illustrate this point, a previous study created a placental barrier model with the help of 2PP [22]. The microfluidic chip had a basal membrane printed. On one side of this membrane, human umbilical vein endothelial cells were seeded, and on the other side, human trophoblast cells were seeded, thus resembling the maternal–fetal barrier. Under this procedure, a temporary template is initially printed and coated with a biocompatible material, e.g., PDMS. The template is then dissolved (e.g., poly(vinyl alcohol) (PVA) is dissolved in water), and the channels are empty. As an example, Dahlberg et al. 3D printed an example of PVA (a water-soluble polymer). PDMS was then cast over it [23]. Once the PDMS hardened, the PVA was washed out in water, leaving behind clear microfluidic channels.

Materials used in OoC fabrication can be broadly classified into two groups: (1) structural materials for microfluidic chips and (2) bioprinting materials (bioinks) for tissue construction. Commonly employed materials include resins, PDMS, hydrogels, polymethylmethacrylate (PMMA), polyethylene terephthalate, and acrylonitrile butadiene styrene [24–27]. Resins allow high-resolution channel fabrication but may pose cytotoxicity risks unless biocompatible derivatives like polyethylene glycol diacrylate [28]. PDMS remains a gold standard for cell culture due to its biocompatibility and transparency, although its hydrophobicity can hinder cell adhesion. PMMA, PET glycol, and other polymers offer optical transparency and mechanical strength, often combined with PDMS in hybrid systems [29,30].

On the contrary, bioinks are generally hydrogel-based, providing support for cell adhesion, proliferation, and differentiation. Examples of natural hydrogels include alginate, gelatin, collagen, and silk fibroin, whereas synthetic hydrogels are also designed to fulfill these requirements [31–36]. While alginate is easy to handle, it lacks intrinsic cell-adhesion motifs and is therefore often blended with other biomaterials. Collagen and gelatin enhance cell physiology, whereas decellularized extracellular matrix (dECM)-based inks mimic native environments for long-term culture. Among synthetic options, gelatin methacryloyl (GelMA) is widely used for its biocompatibility and print fidelity, while hyaluronic acid methacryloyl provides rapid crosslinking [37]. Nanocomposites can also be incorporated to enhance mechanical stability.

OoC fabrication integrates both structural polymers for microfluidic chips and bioink-based hydrogels for tissue remodeling. Through appropriate selection of bioprinting techniques, bioink formulations, and scaffold materials, OoC platforms hold the potential to transform drug discovery and disease modeling. By offering physiologically relevant responses, these systems present a promising alternative to conventional cell culture and animal testing, paving the way for more ethical, efficient, and predictive biomedical research.

8.3 MICROENVIRONMENT CONSTRUCTING AND BIOLOGICAL INTEGRATION

An accurate replication of native tissue microenvironments (Figure 8.2), including customized biophysical and biochemical cues and structured tissue architecture, is necessary for the integration of bioprinting with OoC technology.

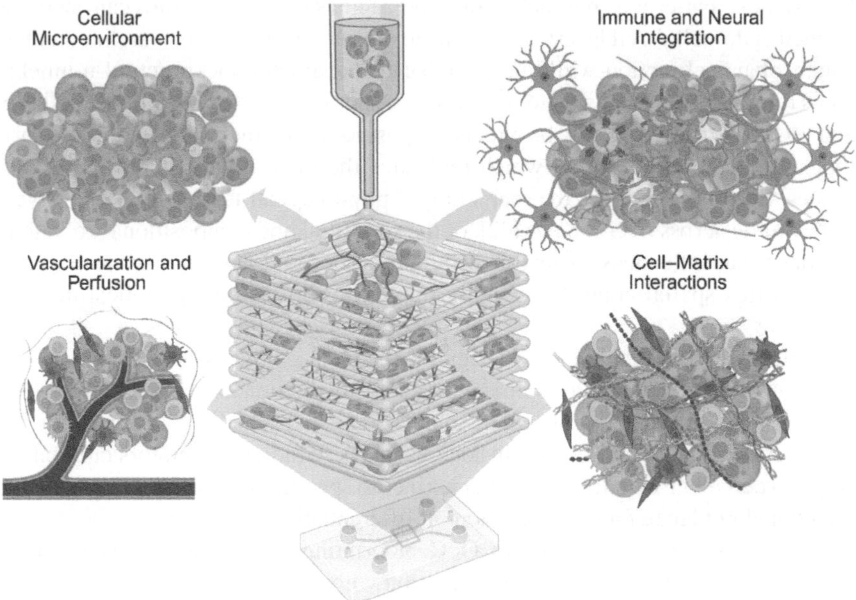

FIGURE 8.2 Schematic illustration of microenvironment formation for constructing functional bioprinted organ-on-chip models. cellular microenvironment, ensuring heterogeneous cell populations and signaling molecules are maintained; vascularization and perfusion, recreating functional blood vessel networks for nutrient and oxygen delivery; immune and neural integration, incorporating immune and neural cell types to mimic tissue-level responses; and cell–matrix interactions, emphasizing the dynamic interplay between cells and ECM components that regulate structural and functional outcomes. (From BioRender. Avci, H. (2025) https://BioRender.com/3irn7vm.)

This microenvironment is not just a passive scaffold; rather, it is an actively controlled, dynamic environment made up of extracellular matrix (ECM) components, mechanical forces, spatial organization, and biochemical signaling cues [38]. Producing predictive *in vitro* systems that enhance drug development, regenerative medicine, and disease modeling requires this level of complexity.

In bioprinted OoC models, biomaterials replicate ECM functions, with natural hydrogels such as GelMA, alginate, collagen, hyaluronic acid, fibrin, chitosan, Matrigel, agarose, silk fibroin, dECM, and synthetic polymers like polyethylene glycol favored for their biocompatibility, bioactivity, high water content, and tunable mechanics [39]. In addition to providing a structural framework, ECM is a dynamic regulator of cellular behavior that affects gene expression, migration, differentiation, and proliferation. Researchers can alter cell fate by fine-tuning stiffness, surface texture, and bioactive signaling. For example, harder matrices (10–40 kPa) more closely resemble the surroundings of muscle or cartilage, whereas soft matrices (0.1–1 kPa) encourage neuronal development [40]. In bioprinted OoC platforms, surface topography and patterning influence cell migration, alignment, and tissue organization, allowing for the replication of physiologically appropriate microarchitectures.

For example, patterned endothelial adhesive regions in vascular chips can encourage aligned endothelial cell layers that replicate the native vessel lumen architecture and enhance barrier function, while integrated surface characteristics in neural-mimicking chips direct axonal extension to form precise neural circuits [41]. Multiple cell types and ECM components can be precisely positioned in bioprinted OoC platforms thanks to spatial patterning, which replicates the intricate architecture of natural tissues. Because it enables the recreation of physiological features like the oxygenation profile across liver lobules [42], or the structural and compositional zonation of cartilage that influences its load-bearing properties and nutrient diffusion dynamics [43], this spatial control is equally important for accurately replicating native function.

Furthermore, it is possible to design biochemical gradients of oxygen, nutrients, and signaling molecules to mimic physiological circumstances and direct tissue development [44]. It can be shown as soluble components added by microfluidic perfusion or as immobilized ligands inside the matrix. Gradient generators built into the chip can deliver growth factors or chemokines to specific compartments, establishing directional guidance for cell migration or differentiation.

Building on these advances in OoC bioprinting, one critical consideration is how to achieve vascularization and perfusion within the constructs. Vascularization and perfusion strategies are approaches designed to recreate functional blood vessel networks and dynamic fluid flow inside microengineered tissue systems, so that cells receive adequate oxygen, nutrients, and waste removal over prolonged culture periods [45]. From the bioprinting perspective, strategies generally fall into direct bioprinting of vascular channels, biological induction of vascular networks, and microfluidic-integrated perfusions.

Coaxial extrusion, sacrificial bioink, and embedded printing techniques are defined as the direct bioprinting models for the vascular network in OoCs [46]. Coaxial extrusion uses a core–sheath nozzle to simultaneously print a sacrificial core and a cell-laden matrix shell, creating perfusable channels. A coaxially printed vessel network can be integrated into a microfluidic chip and perfused with growth factors and supplemented media to encourage capillary sprouting into surrounding tissue. Another approach, sacrificial bioink printing, involves depositing a temporary fugitive material (such as gelatin, Pluronic F-127, agarose, alginate, PVA, or carbohydrate glass) within a matrix. This material is later removed under mild conditions such as temperature or pH shifts, ionic changes, or enzymatic digestion, leaving behind a hollow, perfusable channel that can be lined with cells [47]. Thus, removing the sacrificial material within a microfluidic chip enables the formation of in-chip and pericellular nutrient-delivering matrices precisely tailored to the requirements of the target tissue. Embedded printing allows the creation of intricate vascular networks by depositing bioinks within a supportive, yield-stress medium (such as gelatin or agarose slurry, laponite, Carbopol, or xanthan gum), which stabilizes the structure during fabrication and enables accurate 3D positioning of complex vessel architecture while preventing structural collapse and enabling the fabrication of intricate, freeform geometries [48]. Once printing is complete, the support bath is gently removed, leaving behind stable, perfusable channels or tissues with high structural fidelity. Using this approach, even the chip itself can be fabricated as a matrix or allowing the matrix formed within the chip to be produced in a manner fully compatible with the target tissue.

Biological induction of vascular networks self-assembles into functional microvessels by incorporating biological cues and supportive microenvironments. Using the spatial precision of bioprinting, endothelial cells can be co-deposited with perivascular support cells such as fibroblasts, smooth muscle cells, or pericytes within ECM-mimicking hydrogels, enabling close cell–cell interactions that drive angiogenesis and vasculogenesis [49]. Pro-angiogenic factors such as vascular endothelial growth factor to stimulate endothelial proliferation and sprouting, basic fibroblast growth factor to enhance endothelial migration and matrix remodeling, and angiopoietin-1 to promote vessel stabilization and maturation are often incorporated directly into the bioink or encapsulated within controlled-release carriers such as microspheres, nanoparticles, or hydrogel microdomains, creating spatial and temporal concentration gradients that precisely direct capillary sprouting, lumen formation, branching, and long-term network stability [50]. In some designs, pre-vascularized spheroids or organoids are embedded in the printed tissue to accelerate inosculation with perfused microchannels in the chip [51]. When combined with dynamic flow in microfluidic circuits, these biologically driven processes yield stable, functional vascular networks that enhance nutrient and oxygen delivery, improve tissue viability, and provide physiologically relevant models for drug testing and disease research.

After being printed, the cells begin to interact with each other and their engineered matrix. They migrate, form cell-to-cell junctions, and remodel their surroundings. This self-assembly process is crucial for forming cohesive and functional tissue layers. Incorporating immune components into OoC platforms is another essential layer of physiological relevance, particularly when studying inflammatory diseases, immune surveillance, or responses to immunotherapy [52]. The integration of immune cells can be achieved through several approaches, each offering unique insights into immune-to-tissue interactions.

One strategy involves perfusing circulating immune cells through microvascular channels, allowing processes such as adhesion to endothelial surfaces, transendothelial migration, and cytokine secretion [53]. Alternatively, tissue-resident immune cells, including macrophages or dendritic cells, can be embedded directly within the parenchymal compartment to provide a localized perspective of immune activity in a tissue-specific context. Another approach is the timed introduction of immune cells at defined intervals, which is particularly useful for simulating transient inflammatory episodes. Common readouts in immune-integrated OoC models include cytokine profiling, live-cell imaging to track immune cell migration, and functional assays evaluating outcomes like pathogen clearance or tumor cell killing [54].

Neural integration is equally impactful, particularly for modeling organ–brain axis, neurovascular units, or neuromuscular junctions [55]. Bioprinting allows the co-deposition of neurons with glial support cells in ECM permissive to neurite outgrowth. Incorporating axon guidance cues, such as microgrooves or patterned adhesive ligands, supports the establishment of directional connectivity in the chip. When combined with vascular and immune components, neural elements enable the study of complex multi-system interactions, such as neuroinflammation or nerve-mediated vascular regulation [56].

Conversely, cells have active interactions with their surrounding matrix and constantly remodel their microenvironment by secreting enzymes, rearranging fibers, and altering stiffness [50]. Bioprinting now can support dynamic bioinks, materials whose properties change over time or in response to stimuli, allowing them to mimic these evolving conditions. Bioinks which polymerized due to enzymatic crosslinking to model fibrotic progression or photoresponsive materials whose ligand presentation can be altered with light to trigger differentiation cues [57]. Such programmable environments can simulate processes like wound healing, where ECM stiffness, porosity, degradability, deformability, and growth factor composition evolve rapidly [58]. Mechanotransduction refers to the process by which cells sense and respond to mechanical cues, which can be modeled on-chip using deformable membranes or cyclic stretch modules. For example, applying physiological strain to a bioprinted lung alveolar model promotes surfactant production and barrier function [59]. By designing systems that capture these dynamic feedback loops, the gap between simplified *in vitro* models and the adaptive nature of living tissues can be bridged.

8.4 AUTOMATION, SENSOR INTEGRATION, AND HIGH-THROUGHPUT PRODUCTION

The U.S. Food and Drug Administration (FDA) Modernization Act 2.0, enacted in 2022, eliminated the requirement for mandatory animal testing before clinical trials and has sparked interest in preclinical methods like using OoC systems [60]. This technology can recreate human-specific physiology and predict therapeutic effectiveness and toxicity. However, manufacturing, vascularization, and scalability constraints hinder widespread adoption [61]. Automated and standardized biofabrication is needed to maximize the OoC platform potential. The incorporation of automated bioprinting into microfluidic OoC technologies signifies a transformative change in this domain. In contrast to conventional manual seeding methods, which depend on pipetting and are prone to variability and contamination, bioprinters functioning under sterile conditions enable accurate, consistent, and scalable placement of the cells and the bioinks. This not only optimizes the production of vascularized tissue models but also facilitates high-throughput testing, overcoming significant translational obstacles for the pharmaceutical sector.

Bioprinting offers a promising road ahead, allowing for accurate spatial deposition of different cell types and bioinks directly within microfluidic chips [62,63]. This enables the regulated integration of parenchymal and vascular compartments, overcoming a long-standing barrier to physiological relevance. However, the intricacy of this biofabrication stage requires automation to assure repeatability, sterility, and throughput. Fully automated procedures, which include robotic chip handling, on-demand bioink deposition, and connection with perfusion-ready microfluidics, directly address manual assembly restrictions, contamination risk, and uneven results.

Fritschen et al. present a notable example of an automated platform that integrates on-demand bioprinting with robotic manipulation of microfluidic chips, enabling the fast, unattended construction of multi-organ chips in under 60 seconds (Figure 8.3a–c) [64]. Their design, featuring sealable post-printing microfluidic chips suitable for direct

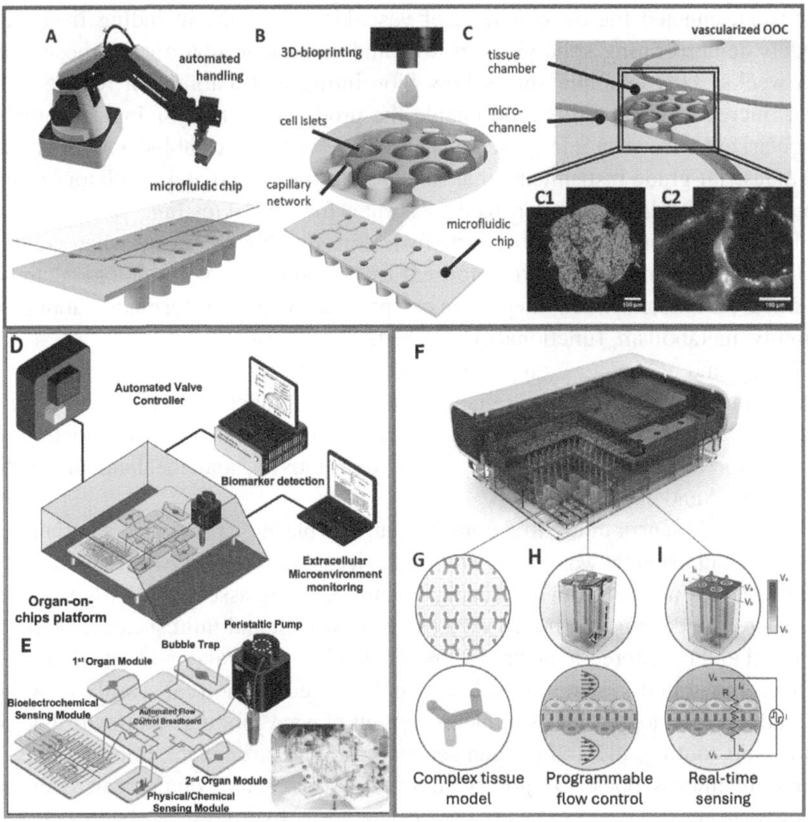

FIGURE 8.3 Automated fabrication of OoC models. (a) Robotic handling of custom microfluidic chips before and after 3D bioprinting. (b) Drop-on-demand bioprinting deposits parenchymal and vascular bioinks, forming cell islets within a capillary network. (c) The sealed perfusable chip supports long-term culture of vascularized tissues. (C1–C2) Bioprinted HepG2 islets proliferate, form spheroids, and establish stable microvascular networks over 14 days. (Figure is recreated under a Creative Commons Attribution (CC BY-NC 4.0) Wiley license [64].) Integrated automated multi-OoC and sensing platform. (d) Schematic of the complete multi-OoC system, housed in a custom benchtop incubator and integrated with an automated pneumatic valve controller, physical sensors, a potentiostat, and a central computer for system coordination. (e) Schematic of the modular microfluidic device with microbioreactors, reservoir, bubble trap, breadboard, and embedded physical/electrochemical biosensors. Inset shows a photograph of the integrated platform days. (Figure is recreated under a Creative Commons Attribution (CC BY-NC-ND 4.0) PNASlicense [65].) High-throughput organ-on-chip platform with integrated pumping and sensing. (f) Cutaway view of the high-throughput organ-on-chip platform, showing microfluidic channels of the MCP with integrated micropumps, TEER electrodes, and electronics of the MPSA. (g) The MCP hosts 96 independent tissue models, each with two channels divided by a permeable membrane. Channels connect to a 384-well-plate reservoir, allowing flexible co-culture of different cell types. (h) Independent micropumps drive fluid through each microchannel by transferring media between wells, generating pressure differentials for controlled flow. (i) Four micropump-associated electrodes enable four-point TEER measurements: one pair delivers current pulses, while the other senses potential to calculate tissue resistance. (Figure is recreated under a Creative Commons Attribution CC BY-NC 3.0 RSC license [68].)

perfusion, enabled the development of vascularized tissue, including liver cancer models demonstrating spheroidal growth and consistent albumin synthesis within two weeks. This example shows how bioprinting and automation reduce human error, increase repeatability, and enable the production of physiologically realistic vascularized tissues on a large scale. These developments establish OoCs as practical industrial-grade instruments that satisfy pharmaceutical and regulatory requirements for high-fidelity, standardized substitutes for animal testing.

The value of bioprinted OoC systems is considerably increased when combined with embedded sensors that allow for real-time monitoring of physiological and biochemical parameters. Such integration can provide dynamic information about tissue viability, metabolism, functionality, and response to stimuli.

Zhang and colleagues emphasize the essential requirement for sensors that can monitor environmental parameters, including temperature, pH, oxygen levels, and nutrient concentrations, alongside direct indicators of cellular function such as adhesion, detachment, mortality, metabolic activity, and mechanical reactions (Figure 8.3d and e) [65,66].

Established sensor modalities comprise surface plasmon resonance, photonic crystal fibers, and resonant waveguide grating devices. Platforms like heart-on-a-chip get significant advantages from measuring calcium levels to assess cardiomyocyte activity, whereas mechanical stimuli, such as cyclic stretch and fluid shear, must be both provided and monitored to accurately replicate physiological conditions [67].

Such integrated systems have been implemented in the real world. To monitor 3D cells morphology, one example design employs a modular platform that combines fluid routing, pH and oxygen sensors, immunobiosensors, microfluidics, and miniature microscopes. Long-term toxicity assessment of dual-organ liver–heart and liver–cancer–heart chips for periods of up to five days has been made possible by an in situ, automated equipment [65]. Commercial-scale, high-content OoC systems are the embodiment of these developments. Programmable perfusion pumps, trans-epithelial electrical resistance (TEER) sensors for evaluating barrier performance, and optical access for monitoring renal active transport and oxygen consumption are all included in one such 96-device-per-plate system. The system enables high-content screening and genomic studies, which allows for the simultaneous production and monitoring of several physiologically relevant tissues [68]. Moreover, advanced OoC research integrates high-resolution bioimaging techniques, including brightfield, fluorescence, multiphoton, and light-sheet modalities, with integrated sensors to provide multimodal, time-resolved investigations. This synergy allows the monitoring of cellular dynamics, metabolite release, pH levels, oxygen concentrations, and barrier integrity, which is particularly crucial in drug screening and toxicity assessment [69].

Lastly, electromechanical sensor technologies like electrical impedance spectroscopy, TEER–microelectrode array (MEA) platforms, and interdigitated electrodes make it possible to monitor both electrophysiology and contractile activity at the same time in cardiac OoC systems. These instruments make it easier to measure how drugs affect the body in real time. For example, they can show how calcium levels change or how muscles contract when drugs like verapamil or isoproterenol are present.

Scalability remains a critical challenge in translating bioprinted OoC platforms from research laboratories to high-throughput industrial applications. Bridging this gap necessitates systems capable of mass-producing uniform and functional microtissues, while ensuring compatibility with standard analytical workflows. One notable approach is the development of microfluidic culture plates in standard well-plate formats (e.g., 96-well) integrating automated pumps and sensor arrays. These platforms facilitate the culture and analysis of dozens of organ models in parallel, thus elevating throughput to industrially relevant scales [68] (Figure 8.3f–i).

Bioprinting itself accelerates cellular patterning and deposition. In standard pipetting seeding workflows, cells typically require six to eight hours to adhere and spread before flow can be applied within a microfluidic device. Bioprinting circumvents this delay by rapidly immobilizing cells, enabling immediate perfusion and culture initiation, and significantly reducing experiment turnaround time while maintaining reproducibility [70]. Emerging bioprinting technologies are enhancing speed and efficiency. The "HITS-Bio" system can manipulate multiple spheroids concurrently, achieving speeds up to ten times faster than conventional methods [71]. It supports in-surgery bioprinting into wounds. Advanced biosensing modalities and bioprinting are combined in high-throughput screening frameworks to enable massively multiplexed, high-speed detection and functional analysis. Finally, the integration of biofabrication principles with microfluidic automation points to the establishment of future systems capable of independently producing and maturing complex OoC structures—basically, a step toward "robot scientists" and self-driven tissue formation platforms.

In summary, bioengineering is evolving due to automation, sensor integration, and high-throughput manufacturing in OoC bioprinting. Automation increases reproducibility, decreases manual variability, and expedites the production of microfluidic tissue structures. Real-time monitoring of cellular activity and microenvironmental factors is made possible by sensor integration, which provides dynamic feedback for more responsive and accurate models. Scalability is added by high-throughput bioprinting for toxicological testing, industrial drug screening, and personalized therapy. These advances lay the groundwork for standardized, monitorable, and scalable bioprinted organoids, bringing OoC technology closer to biomedical use.

8.5 APPLICATIONS

8.5.1 Bioprinted OoC in Drug Screening and Toxicology

Bioprinted OoC systems are a significant advancement in drug screening and toxicology, offering a more physiological mimicry of human organ functions. These systems utilize microfluidics and bioprinting technologies to recreate the cellular environments of various organs, enabling more accurate assessments of drug efficacy and toxicity. The incorporation of vascularization in these systems enables vital waste removal and nutrient exchange, preserving cellular viability and functionality in long-term studies [72]. This design is essential for precise drug testing because these models outperform older systems in simulating the intricate reactions of the human body to pharmacological agents [73]. The production of bioprinted OoC modules can make an efficient automated fabrication which can improve the scalability and reproducibility of drug screening procedures. According to Thakare et al., this approach can significantly speed up the preclinical evaluation of drugs and lessen the need for animal testing by accelerating the development of numerous organ models, such as those for the liver and lung systems [11]. Lee et al. also point out that the creation of particular organ microenvironments is made possible by microfluidic technologies, which are essential for accurate metabolic and toxicological evaluations [74]. Additionally, as demonstrated by Wang et al., the incorporation of multi-OoC systems enables the simultaneous modeling of numerous organ interactions, which is very helpful in understanding systemic drug toxicity and responses [75]. These models are very useful for assessing how medications affect organ systems as a whole, as opposed to separately, which is a drawback of traditional models. According to research like that of Paek et al., artificial intelligence (AI)-enhanced image analysis adds a new level of data analysis capability that makes it easier to identify morphological and functional changes brought on by medications [76]. This integration improves early-stage drug discovery procedures in addition to supporting thorough data collection. OoC systems' clinically relevant prediction powers, which have been demonstrated to correspond with human clinical outcomes, make them crucial tools in regulatory drug testing frameworks. Ye et al. highlight how these platforms have been used to find drug toxicity markers, demonstrating how they can expedite the drug approval process by providing a testing mode that is more relevant to humans [73]. Pharmacology, toxicology, and personalized medicine will all be greatly impacted by the rapidly developing field of bioprinted OoCs. These systems may result in safer and more efficient treatments by facilitating a more sophisticated understanding of drug interactions and organ responses. 3D bioprinting is a cutting-edge method of additive manufacturing that combines biomaterials, bioactive compounds, and living cells to create engineered structures for OoC and tissue engineering applications. Cells are cultured and harvested first, followed by the preparation of bioinks by combining them with appropriate matrices and confirming their biological and physicochemical characteristics, as shown in Figure 8.4a [4]. A 3D bioprinter is used to deposit the bioinks layer by layer after they have been characterized and packaged to create functional scaffolds inside hydrogels. A variety of biomimetic materials and forms, including direct cell with organoid patterns, vascularized tissues, biological barriers, and hybrid material–cell assemblies, can be produced using 3D bioprinting in conjunction with OoC fabrication (Figure 8.4b). These structures provide a viable platform for drug testing, disease modeling, and regenerative medicine by making it easier to form complex microarchitectures that closely mimic the functions of target human tissues or diseases [77].

8.5.2 Disease Modeling Using Bioprinted Organ Chips

The integration of bioprinting technology with OoC platforms has opened new avenues for disease modeling and preclinical research. By enabling the fabrication of physiologically relevant tissue architectures, bioprinted OoCs offer significant advantages

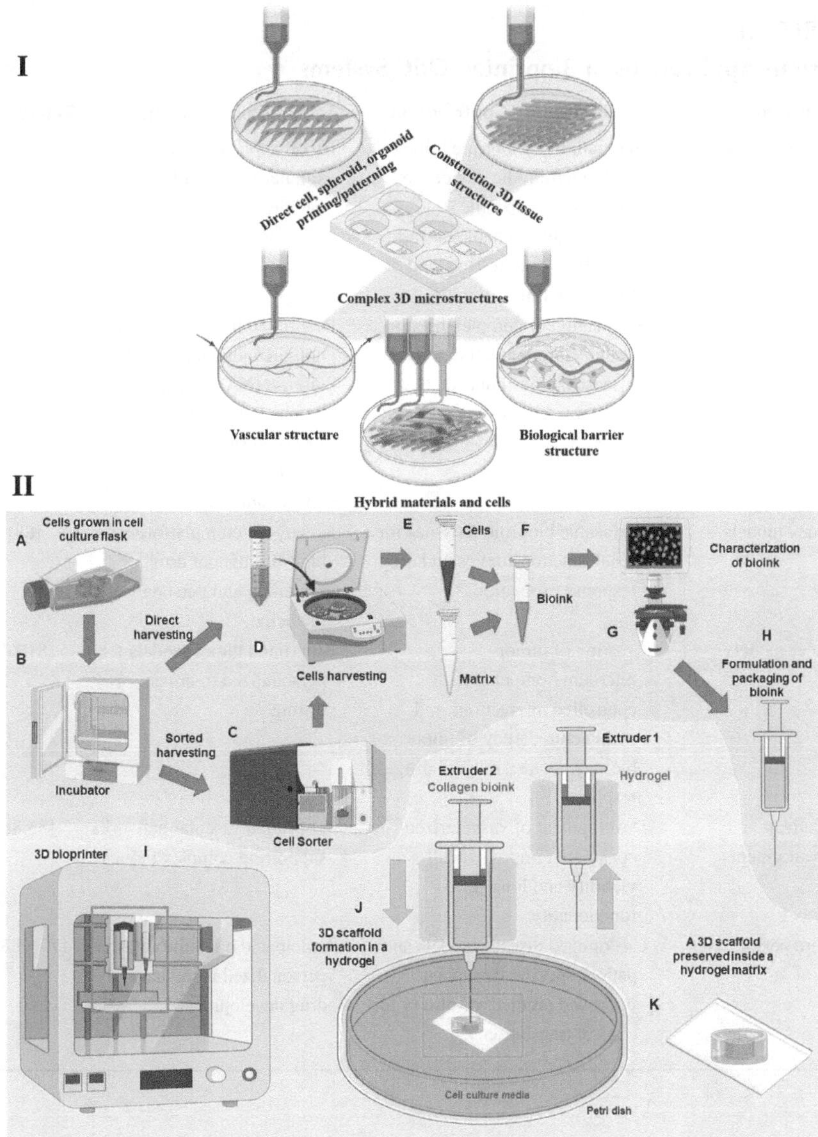

FIGURE 8.4 Overview of 3D bioprinting workflow and its integration with organ-on-chip systems which can be used for drug screening and toxicology. (I) The bioprinting process involves culturing and harvesting cells, preparing and characterizing bioinks, and fabricating 3D scaffolds within hydrogels using a bioprinter. (Figure is recreated under a Creative Commons Attribution (CC BY 4.0) Wiley license [4].) (II) Integration with OoC platforms enables the construction of complex biomimetic structures, including cell/organoid patterns, 3D tissues, vascular structures, biological barriers, and hybrid material–cell assemblies, advancing the development of physiologically relevant *in vitro* models. (Figure is recreated under a Creative Commons Attribution American Chemical Society licensed CC-BY-NC-ND 4.0 [77].)

TABLE 8.1
Various Applications of Bioprinted OoC Systems

Application Area	Bioprinting Contribution	Examples/Evidence	References
General OoC systems	Integration of bioprinted tissues with microfluidic devices to mimic organ-specific environments; enable disease modeling, drug testing, and therapy optimization.	Broad applications in simulating physiology and pathology across organ systems.	[11,78, 79]
Liver models	Replication of complex hepatic architecture; modeling liver diseases; drug-induced hepatotoxicity testing.	Bioprinted liver tissues for non-alcoholic fatty liver disease (NAFLD) studies; human induced pluripotent stem cell (hiPSC)-derived liver tissues mimicking *in vivo* conditions.	[80–82]
Kidney models	Perfusable bioprinted tissues for renal function studies and drug response evaluation.	Kidney-on-chip platforms for high-throughput drug screening and personalized medicine.	[83]
Cancer models	Creation of tumor microenvironments with controlled interactions and architecture; study of tumor biology, metastasis, and drug responses.	Bioprinted tumor models for personalized treatment testing.	[81,84]
Technical advancements	Development of vascularized constructs; improved cell viability and long-term functionality.	3D-printed vascular networks supporting complex tissues.	[85,86]
Future perspectives	Customized disease models and patient-specific therapies; improved predictive validity for clinical translation.	Anticipated breakthroughs in personalized medicine and drug development.	[79,87,88]

over traditional two-dimensional cultures and animal models. As summarized in Table 8.1, applications span multiple organ systems: liver-on-chip systems have been developed to study nonalcoholic fatty liver disease and drug-induced hepatotoxicity, while kidney models allow investigations of renal function and drug responses in perfusable chips. Cancer research has particularly benefited from bioprinted tumor models, where the TME and cellular interactions can be precisely controlled to study tumor progression, metastasis, and drug resistance. Technical innovations such as vascularized constructs and self-healing hydrogels have further enhanced the fidelity and functionality of bioprinted tissues, ensuring long-term viability and mimicking *in vivo* repair mechanisms. Collectively, these advances underscore the transformative role of bioprinting in OoC systems, paving the way for patient-specific disease models, personalized drug testing, and more accurate therapeutic predictions.

8.5.3 Personalized Medicine through Patient-Specific Bioprinting

The field of personalized medicine has been significantly enhanced by advances in bioprinting technology, facilitating the development of patient-specific models for disease modeling, drug testing, and therapeutic interventions. Bioprinting allows for the precise construction of biomimetic tissues and organs tailored to the genetic and phenotypic characteristics of individual patients, thereby addressing the limitations of traditional one-size-fits-all treatment approaches. Study on cancer modeling and treatment is one of the main areas of personalized medicine where bioprinting is being used. Therefore, 3D bioprinted cancer models using patient-derived tumor cells provide more accurate predictions of the disease and therapy efficacy. These models have shown promise in illuminating medication response, tumor behavior, and potential resistance pathways by mimicking the complex TME. The potential of bioprinted models to inform treatment plans based on unique tumor characteristics has been shown by research highlights like patient-derived breast cancer spheroids; however, issues with reproducibility and material sourcing still exist [89,90]. Likewise, the combination of 3D bioprinting and high-throughput screening methods has expedited the development and evaluation of customized anticancer medications [91]. Additionally, using induced pluripotent stem cells in bioprinting provides a revolutionary way to produce disease models tailored to individual patients. Because iPSC-derived tissues are customized, it is possible to simulate particular genetic mutations linked to distinct patient profiles. This is especially important for diseases like neuroblastoma, where patient-specific bioprinted models can help clarify how drugs work and improve treatment strategies [92,93]. By enabling improved cell survival and more complex interactions within the TME, the use of cutting-edge hydrogels in bioprinting also improves the functional characteristics of these tissues [72,94]. Bioprinting has advanced tissue engineering and regenerative medicine in addition to cancer applications. More and more, customized bioprinted tissues are being created to meet each patient's specific anatomical and biological needs, such as vascular constructs or bone grafts. In addition to restoring function in injured tissues, this customization improves integration and lowers rejection rates. Complex tissue architecture is required for therapeutic applications, and the bioprinting of vascularized tissues has been emphasized as essential for preserving tissue viability [95–97]. Optimizing bioinks and printing techniques is a major obstacle to the development of bioprinting technology for personalized medicine. To guarantee the functionality of the printed constructs, effective bioinks must promote cell viability, ease the transport of nutrients, and resemble the ECM found in nature.

8.5.4 Cancer-on-Chip and Tumor Microenvironment Replication

There is great potential for improving therapeutic approaches and expanding our knowledge of tumor biology through the incorporation of cancer-on-chip technology. Researchers can replicate the intricate TME, which is essential to the development of cancer and its response to therapy, by using microfluidics and 3D bioprinting. This technical advancement offers a platform for high-throughput drug testing, personalized therapy, and more accurate cancer modeling. The capacity of cancer-on-chip systems to closely resemble the biochemical and physical characteristics of human tumors, such as vascular networks, ECM structure, and cell composition, is one of its main advantages [98,99]. Given that the TME is known to affect tumor behavior, the probability of spread, and the response to treatment, this is crucial. OoC platforms, for example, can be made to mimic several TME features, such as immune cell interactions, cancer cell–stromal cell communication, and the dynamic nature of waste and nutrient exchange through perfusable channels [99,100]. According to recent research, cancer-on-chip models can accurately mimic processes like angiogenesis and extravasation, enabling scientists to study important mechanisms like tumor metastasis [101,102]. For instance, models that mimic how tumor cells and platelets interact in the setting of ovarian cancer have provided crucial information about the mechanisms underlying metastasis [101]. Additionally, these chips enable customized studies of distinct tumor responses to different anticancer treatments by integrating patient-derived cells and organoids, possibly opening the door for precision medicine approaches [97,100]. Research on breast and colorectal cancer has demonstrated that these systems are useful for a variety of cancer types. To assess the effectiveness of medications and pinpoint possible resistance mechanisms in specific patients, tumor-on-chip models have been created [102,103]. Furthermore, developments in multi-organ systems can be used to model the systematic spread of metastases and how they affect treatment, providing a thorough understanding of tumor biology that is frequently not possible with conventional *in vitro* or *in vivo* models [104,105]. Additionally, cancer-on-chip technology offers a dynamic setting for evaluating the toxicity and effectiveness of novel therapeutic agents. For instance, microfluidic designs enhance nutrition delivery and offer continuous flow that closely mimics physiological environments [106]. Researchers can now more precisely forecast and understand how a patient's tumor will react to a therapy, which has enormous implications for drug testing [107]. By utilizing platforms that allow for real-time monitoring and assessment of cellular behaviors under various treatment regimens, the predictive capabilities of preclinical models can be significantly improved [108,109]. In summary, the advances in cancer-on-chip systems signify a transformative approach to cancer research, offering more precise, relevant, and reproducible models that can lead to a better understanding of tumor dynamics and therapeutic efficacy. As technology evolves, the potential to integrate more sophisticated biomimetic components will further enhance these platforms, contributing to the ultimate goal of improved patient outcomes through personalized treatment strategies [110,111].

8.6 CHALLENGES AND FUTURE DIRECTIONS

Although bioprinting integrated with OoC platforms has demonstrated significant potential, several challenges must be overcome to ensure widespread adoption and translational impact. Ethical considerations will move beyond basic informed consent toward comprehensive governance models for the responsible use of patient-derived cells and organoids. The prospect of bioprinting human organs and tissues, including the concept of "growing your own organs," raises profound ethical questions regarding identity, bodily integrity, and consent, while from a broader socio-ethical perspective, concerns about equitable access, commercialization, and the potential exacerbation of healthcare inequalities remain central to the discourse [112]. Issues such as confidentiality in personalized organ modeling, usage and sources of biological material, security of all types of medical informatics, and equal access to patient-specific disease models will become increasingly important as precision medicine becomes widespread [113]. On the regulatory front, current evaluation frameworks remain fragmented, with limited harmonization across regions. In the near future, agencies such as the FDA and European Medicines Agency (EMA) are expected to propose specific guidelines for validating bioprinted OoC systems, potentially recognizing them as partial replacements for preclinical animal/human studies in disease modeling and efficacy testing [114].

Standardization is equally critical. At present, there is significant variability in bioink formulations, chip and material architecture, and analytical readouts, which hinders reproducibility and comparability across laboratories [115]. Establishing consensus standards for rheological properties of bioinks, cell viability assessment, microfluidic perfusion regimes, and tissue functionality metrics will be essential for scalability and industrial translation. On the technological side, AI and machine learning are emerging as powerful enablers that can accelerate bioink formulation, guide the rational design of complex tissue architectures, optimize printing parameters in real time, and extract hidden patterns from high-dimensional OoC datasets. AI-driven generative design tools may accelerate the development of vascularized, multicellular constructs [116], while machine learning models could optimize printing parameters, predict cell–material interactions, and automate adaptive control of chip performance. In addition, computational approaches will be vital for interpreting the vast, multidimensional datasets produced by multiplexed OoC platforms, enabling deeper biological insights [117].

In the realistic near-term, advances may include semiautomated bioprinting workflows, standardized chip platforms for specific tissues, and regulatory-recognized benchmarks for safety and performance [118]. By aligning ethical responsibility, regulatory clarity, and computational intelligence, bioprinting with OoC technology is positioned to deliver robust, predictive, and clinically relevant models that will reshape drug discovery, biomolecular testing, disease modeling, and personalized healthcare [119].

8.7 CONCLUSION

A revolutionary development in biomedical engineering is the combination of 3D bioprinting with OoC technology, which successfully closes the crucial gap between traditional preclinical models and human physiology. The accurate, automated creation of intricate, 3D, and physiologically significant human tissue models *in vitro* is made possible by this potent combination. Researchers can now form living tissues with complex cellular hierarchies and perfusable vascular networks by utilizing cutting-edge bioprinting techniques, including VP, ME, and MJ. The necessary biochemical and biomechanical cues to direct cell destiny and guarantee long-term functionality are provided by the concurrent formation of complex bioinks. Since these platforms can provide more predictive, human-relevant results, they have the potential to completely transform drug screening, toxicological evaluation, and disease modeling, decreasing the need for animal testing and speeding up the discovery of new treatments.

Notwithstanding notable advancements, resolving important obstacles is necessary to realize the full translational potential of bioprinted OoCs. To ensure reproducibility and dependability, these include setting uniform standards for materials and fabrication, attaining robust vascularization, and sustaining long-term tissue maturation. Additionally, proactive measures must be taken to handle the changing ethical and regulatory environment. AI and machine learning are inextricably related to the field's future because they can come close to tissue architecture design, optimize bioink compositions, and decipher complicated data outputs. The ultimate objective is the development of high-throughput, automated systems for customized medicine, in which a patient's own bioprinted tissues can be used to test treatments. Bioprinted OoC technology has the potential to transform drug development, disease modeling, and the future of healthcare by tackling these issues through interdisciplinary innovation.

ACKNOWLEDGMENTS

This study was supported by the Scientific and Technological Research Council of Türkiye (TÜBİTAK) 1004 under grant numbers 20AG003, 20AG031, and TÜBİTAK-1005 with the grant number of 123E013, as well as TÜBİTAK 3501 under grant number 222M468. This work has also been supported by the Health Institutes of Türkiye (TUSEB-32056) and Eskisehir Osmangazi University Scientific Research Projects Coordination Unit under grant numbers TOA-2022–2307, FOA-2025–3201, TDK-2024–3000 with FYL-2025–3442, FYL-2025–3450, FYL-2025–3402, and FYL-2025–3430.

REFERENCES

1. Carvalho V, Goncalves I, Lage T, Rodrigues RO, Minas G, Teixeira SF, et al. 3D printing techniques and their applications to organ-on-a-chip platforms: a systematic review. *Sensors*. 2021;21(9):3304.
2. Schöneberg J, De Lorenzi F, Theek B, Blaeser A, Rommel D, Kuehne AJ, et al. Engineering biofunctional in vitro vessel models using a multilayer bioprinting technique. *Scientific Reports*. 2018;8(1):10430.
3. Fetah K, Tebon P, Goudie MJ, Eichenbaum J, Ren L, Barros N, et al. The emergence of 3D bioprinting in organ-on-chip systems. *Progress in Biomedical Engineering*. 2019;1(1):012001.
4. Tabatabaei Rezaei N, Kumar H, Liu H, Lee SS, Park SS, Kim K. Recent advances in organ-on-chips integrated with bioprinting technologies for drug screening. *Advanced Healthcare Materials*. 2023;12(20):2203172.
5. D'Orazio M, Filippi J, Antonelli G, Curci G, Casti P, Mencattini A, et al. Cells in the 3D biomatrix on-chip: better mimicking the real micro-physiological system. *Next Materials*. 2024;5:100229.

6. Wu Z, Liu R, Shao N, Zhao Y. Developing 3D bioprinting for organs-on-chips. *Lab on a Chip.* 2025;25(5):1081–96.
7. Wu X, Shi W, Liu X, Gu Z. Recent advances in 3D-printing-based organ-on-a-chip. *EngMedicine.* 2024;1(1):100003.
8. Ortiz-Cárdenas JE, Zatorski JM, Arneja A, Montalbine AN, Munson JM, Luckey CJ, Pompano RR. Towards spatially-organized organs-on-chip: photopatterning cell-laden thiol-ene and methacryloyl hydrogels in a microfluidic device. *Organs-on-a-Chip.* 202 2;4:100018.
9. Ferrari E, Nebuloni F, Rasponi M, Occhetta P. Photo and soft lithography for organ-on-chip applications. *Organ-on-a-Chip: Methods and Protocols*, ed. M Rasponi: Springer; 2021. pp. 1–19.
10. Díaz Lantada A, Pfleging W, Besser H, Guttmann M, Wissmann M, Plewa K, et al. Research on the methods for the mass production of multi-scale organs-on-chips. *Polymers.* 2018;10(11):1238.
11. Thakare K, Jerpseth L, Pei Z, Elwany A, Quek F, Qin H. Bioprinting of organ-on-chip systems: a literature review from a manufacturing perspective. *Journal of Manufacturing and Materials Processing.* 2021;5(3):91.
12. Yang Q, Lian Q, Xu F. Perspective: fabrication of integrated organ-on-a-chip via bioprinting. *Biomicrofluidics.* 2017;11(3): 031301.
13. Mehrotra S, Moses JC, Bandyopadhyay A, Mandal BB. 3D printing/bioprinting based tailoring of in vitro tissue models: recent advances and challenges. *ACS Applied Bio Materials.* 2019;2(4):1385–405.
14. Jain A, Mathur T, Pandian NK, Selahi A. Organ-on-a-chip and 3D printing as preclinical models for medical research and practice. *Precision Medicine for Investigators, Practitioners and Providers*, eds. J Faintuch, S. Faintuch: Elsevier; 2020. pp. 83–95.
15. Xiang Y, Miller K, Guan J, Kiratitanaporn W, Tang M, Chen S. 3D bioprinting of complex tissues in vitro: state-of-the-art and future perspectives. *Archives of Toxicology.* 2022;96(3):691–710.
16. Yu F, Choudhury D. Microfluidic bioprinting for organ-on-a-chip models. *Drug Discovery Today.* 2019;24(6):1248–57.
17. De Spirito M, Palmieri V, Perini G, Papi M. Bridging the gap: integrating 3D bioprinting and microfluidics for advanced multi-organ models in biomedical research. *Bioengineering.* 2024;11(7):664.
18. Rodrigues RO, Sousa PC, Gaspar J, Bañobre-López M, Lima R, Minas G. Organ-on-a-chip: a preclinical microfluidic platform for the progress of nanomedicine. *Small.* 2020;16(51):2003517.
19. Leung CM, De Haan P, Ronaldson-Bouchard K, Kim G-A, Ko J, Rho HS, et al. A guide to the organ-on-a-chip. *Nature Reviews Methods Primers.* 2022;2(1):33.
20. Tan LJ, Zhu W, Zhou K. Recent progress on polymer materials for additive manufacturing. *Advanced Functional Materials.* 2020;30(43):2003062.
21. Pranzo D, Larizza P, Filippini D, Percoco G. Extrusion-based 3D printing of microfluidic devices for chemical and biomedical applications: a topical review. *Micromachines.* 2018;9(8):374.
22. Mandt D, Gruber P, Markovic M, Tromayer M, Rothbauer M, Kratz SRA, et al. Fabrication of biomimetic placental barrier structures within a microfluidic device utilizing two-photon polymerization. *International Journal of Bioprinting.* 2018;4(2):144.
23. Dahlberg T, Stangner T, Zhang H, Wiklund K, Lundberg P, Edman L, Andersson M. 3D printed water-soluble scaffolds for rapid production of PDMS micro-fluidic flow chambers. *Scientific Reports.* 2018;8(1):1–10.
24. Zuchowska A, Skorupska S. Multi-organ-on-chip approach in cancer research. *Organs-on-a-Chip.* 2022;4:100014.

25. Mehta V, Rath SN. 3D printed microfluidic devices: a review focused on four fundamental manufacturing approaches and implications on the field of healthcare. *Bio-Design and Manufacturing*. 2021;4(2):311–43.
26. Gonzalez G, Roppolo I, Pirri CF, Chiappone A. Current and emerging trends in polymeric 3D printed microfluidic devices. *Additive Manufacturing*. 2022;55:102867.
27. Ebrahimi A, Ghorbanpoor H, Apaydın E, Cevizlidere BD, Özel C, Tüfekçioğlu E, et al. Convenient rapid prototyping microphysiological niche for mimicking liver native basement membrane: liver sinusoid on a chip. *Colloids and Surfaces B: Biointerfaces*. 2025;245:114292.
28. Warr C, Valdoz JC, Bickham BP, Knight CJ, Franks NA, Chartrand N, et al. Biocompatible PEGDA resin for 3D printing. *ACS Applied Bio Materials*. 2020;3(4):2239–44.
29. Mehta V, Vilikkathala Sudhakaran S, Rath SN. Facile route for 3D printing of transparent PETg-based hybrid biomicrofluidic devices promoting cell adhesion. *ACS Biomaterials Science & Engineering*. 2021;7(8):3947–63.
30. Bressan LP, Adamo CB, Quero RF, de Jesus DP, da Silva JA. A simple procedure to produce FDM-based 3D-printed microfluidic devices with an integrated PMMA optical window. *Analytical Methods*. 2019;11(8):1014–20.
31. Donderwinkel I, Van Hest JC, Cameron NR. Bio-inks for 3D bioprinting: recent advances and future prospects. *Polymer Chemistry*. 2017;8(31):4451–71.
32. Panwar A, Tan LP. Current status of bioinks for micro-extrusion-based 3D bioprinting. *Molecules*. 2016;21(6):685.
33. Ji S, Guvendiren M. Recent advances in bioink design for 3D bioprinting of tissues and organs. *Frontiers in Bioengineering and Biotechnology*. 2017;5:23.
34. Choi Y-J, Park H, Ha D-H, Yun H-S, Yi H-G, Lee H. 3D bioprinting of in vitro models using hydrogel-based bioinks. *Polymers*. 2021;13(3):366.
35. Habib A, Khoda B. Development of clay based novel hybrid bio-ink for 3D bio-printing process. *Journal of Manufacturing Processes*. 2019;38:76–87.
36. Zhang W, Du A, Liu S, Lv M, Chen S. Research progress in decellularized extracellular matrix-derived hydrogels. *Regenerative Therapy*. 2021;18:88–96.
37. Gong J, Schuurmans CC, Genderen AMv, Cao X, Li W, Cheng F, et al. Complexation-induced resolution enhancement of 3D-printed hydrogel constructs. *Nature Communications*. 2020;11(1):1267.
38. Kutluk H, Bastounis EE, Constantinou I. Integration of extracellular matrices into organ-on-chip systems. *Advanced Healthcare Materials*. 2023;12(20):2203256.
39. Ma J, Wang Y, Liu J. Bioprinting of 3D tissues/organs combined with microfluidics. *RSC Advances*. 2018;8(39):21712–27.
40. Ribeiro S, Watigny A, Bayon Y, Biggs M, Zeugolis DI. It takes two to tango: controlling human mesenchymal stromal cell response via substrate stiffness and surface topography. *Advanced NanoBiomed Research*. 2024;4(1):2300042.
41. Yan Z, Qian Y, Fan C. Biomimicry in 3D printing design: implications for peripheral nerve regeneration. *Regenerative Medicine*. 2021;16(7):683–701.
42. Janani G, Priya S, Dey S, Mandal BB. Mimicking native liver lobule microarchitecture in vitro with parenchymal and non-parenchymal cells using 3D bioprinting for drug toxicity and drug screening applications. *ACS Applied Materials & Interfaces*. 2022;14(8):10167–86.
43. Loukelis K, Jammalamadaka U, Mikos AG. 3D printing-enabled spatial patterning of biomimetic signals for bone tissue engineering. *Advanced Drug Delivery Reviews*. 2025:115656.
44. Cheng Y, Luo X, Payne GF, Rubloff GW. Biofabrication: programmable assembly of polysaccharide hydrogels in microfluidics as biocompatible scaffolds. *Journal of Materials Chemistry*. 2012;22(16):7659–66.

45. Yu T, Yang Q, Peng B, Gu Z, Zhu D. Vascularized organoid-on-a-chip: design, imaging, and analysis. *Angiogenesis*. 2024;27(2):147–72.
46. Kong Z, Wang X. Bioprinting technologies and bioinks for vascular model establishment. *International Journal of Molecular Sciences*. 2023;24(1):891.
47. Liu S, Wang T, Li S, Wang X. Application status of sacrificial biomaterials in 3D bioprinting. *Polymers*. 2022;14(11):2182.
48. Budharaju H, Sundaramurthi D, Sethuraman S. Embedded 3D bioprinting – an emerging strategy to fabricate biomimetic & large vascularized tissue constructs. *Bioactive Materials*. 2024;32:356–84.
49. Kim W, Kim G. Intestinal villi model with blood capillaries fabricated using collagen-based bioink and dual-cell-printing process. *ACS Applied Materials & Interfaces*. 2018;10(48):41185–96.
50. Fang Z, Wu MC, Lim KS, Ju LA. Integrating microfluidics, hydrogels, and 3D bioprinting for personalized vessel-on-a-chip platforms. *Biomaterials Science*. 2025;13(5):1131–60.
51. Shrestha S, Lekkala VKR, Acharya P, Siddhpura D, Lee M-Y. Recent advances in microarray 3D bioprinting for high-throughput spheroid and tissue culture and analysis. *Essays in biochemistry*. 2021;65(3):481–9.
52. Janssen R, Benito-Zarza L, Cleijpool P, Valverde MG, Mihăilă SM, Bastiaan-Net S, et al. Biofabrication directions in recapitulating the immune system-on-a-chip. *Advanced healthcare materials*. 2025;14(5):2304569.
53. Shah KR, Garriga-Cerda L, Pappalardo A, Sorrells L, Jeong HJ, Lee CH, Abaci HE. A biopsy-sized 3D skin model with a perifollicular vascular plexus enables studying immune cell trafficking in the skin. *Biofabrication*. 2024;16(4):045006.
54. Vesperini D, Montalvo G, Qu B, Lautenschläger F. Characterization of immune cell migration using microfabrication. *Biophysical Reviews*. 2021;13(2):185–202.
55. Antill-O'Brien N, Bourke J, O'Connell CD. Layer-by-layer: the case for 3D bioprinting neurons to create patient-specific epilepsy models. *Materials*. 2019;12(19):3218.
56. Park W, Choi MJ, Lee JS, Ahn M, Han W, Gao G, et al. Embedded 3D-coaxial bioprinting of stenotic brain vessels with a mechanically enhanced extracellular matrix bioink for investigating hemodynamic force-induced endothelial responses. *Advanced Functional Materials*. 2025:e04276.
57. Jain N, Shashi Bhushan B, Natarajan M, Mehta R, Saini DK, Chatterjee K. Advanced 3D in vitro lung fibrosis models: contemporary status, clinical uptake, and prospective outlooks. *ACS Biomaterials Science & Engineering*. 2024;10(3):1235–61.
58. Sırma Tarım B, Tamburacı S, Uysal B, Top A. Integration of leu-asp-val cell attachment motif into self-assembling peptide sequences for nanofibrillar hydrogel formation in wound healing. *ACS Applied Nano Materials*. 2025;8(11):5302–14.
59. Zhang Y, Liu Y, Shu C, Shen Y, Li M, Ma N, Zhao J. 3D bioprinting of the airways and lungs for applications in tissue engineering and in vitro models. *Journal of Tissue Engineering*. 2024;15:20417314241309183.
60. Moutinho S. *Researchers and Regulators Plan for a Future without Lab Animals*: Nature Publishing Group US New York; 2023.
61. Halldorsson S, Lucumi E, Gómez-Sjöberg R, Fleming RM. Advantages and challenges of microfluidic cell culture in polydimethylsiloxane devices. *Biosensors and Bioelectronics*. 2015;63:218–31.
62. Miri AK, Mostafavi E, Khorsandi D, Hu S-K, Malpica M, Khademhosseini A. Bioprinters for organs-on-chips. *Biofabrication*. 2019;11(4):042002.
63. Ashammakhi N, Ahadian S, Xu C, Montazerian H, Ko H, Nasiri R, et al. Bioinks and bioprinting technologies to make heterogeneous and biomimetic tissue constructs. *Materials Today Bio*. 2019;1:100008.

64. Fritschen A, Lindner N, Scholpp S, Richthof P, Dietz J, Linke P, et al. High-scale 3D-bioprinting platform for the automated production of vascularized organs-on-a-chip. *Advanced Healthcare Materials.* 2024;13(17):2304028.
65. Zhang YS, Aleman J, Shin SR, Kilic T, Kim D, Mousavi Shaegh SA, et al. Multisensor-integrated organs-on-chips platform for automated and continual in situ monitoring of organoid behaviors. *Proceedings of the National Academy of Sciences of the United States of America.* 2017;114(12):E2293–302.
66. Kilic T, Navaee F, Stradolini F, Renaud P, Carrara S. Organs-on-chip monitoring: sensors and other strategies. *Microphysiological Systems.* 2018;2. doi: 10.21037/mps.2018.01.01
67. Zhang X, Wang T, Wang P, Hu N. High-throughput assessment of drug cardiac safety using a high-speed impedance detection technology-based heart-on-a-chip. *Micromachines.* 2016;7(7):122.
68. Azizgolshani H, Coppeta J, Vedula E, Marr E, Cain B, Luu R, et al. High-throughput organ-on-chip platform with integrated programmable fluid flow and real-time sensing for complex tissue models in drug development workflows. *Lab on a Chip.* 2021;21(8):1454–74.
69. Meneses J, Conceição F, Van Der Meer A, de Wit S, Moreira Teixeira L. Guiding organs-on-chips towards applications: a balancing act between integration of advanced technologies and standardization. *Frontiers in Lab on a Chip Technologies.* 2024;3:1376964.
70. Chliara MA, Elezoglou S, Zergioti I. Bioprinting on organ-on-chip: development and applications. *Biosensors.* 2022;12(12):1135.
71. Kim MH, Singh YP, Celik N, Yeo M, Rizk E, Hayes DJ, Ozbolat IT. High-throughput bioprinting of spheroids for scalable tissue fabrication. *Nature Communications.* 2024;15(1):10083.
72. Fonseca AC, Melchels FP, Ferreira MJ, Moxon SR, Potjewyd G, Dargaville TR, et al. Emulating human tissues and organs: a bioprinting perspective toward personalized medicine. *Chemical Reviews.* 2020;120(19):11093–139.
73. Ye C, Han X, Wang Y, Chen Z, Lu Y, Liu T, et al. Drug toxicity evaluation based on organ-on-a-chip technology: a review. *Micromachines.* 2020;11(4):381.
74. Lee H, Chae S, Kim JY, Han W, Kim J, Choi YJ, Cho DW. Cell-printed 3D liver-on-a-chip possessing a liver microenvironment and biliary system. *Biofabrication.* 2019;11(2):025001.
75. Wang Y, Wang P, Qin J. Microfluidic organs-on-a-chip for modeling human infectious diseases. *Accounts of Chemical Research.* 2021;54(18):3550–62.
76. Paek K, Kim S, Tak S, Kim MK, Park J, Chung S, et al. A high-throughput biomimetic bone-on-a-chip platform with artificial intelligence-assisted image analysis for osteoporosis drug testing. *Bioengineering & Translational Medicine.* 2022;8(1).
77. Verma S, Khanna V, Kumar S, Kumar S. The art of building living tissues: exploring the frontiers of biofabrication with 3D bioprinting. *ACS Omega.* 2023;8(50):47322–39.
78. Bhardwaj N, Dey S, Bhar B, Mandal BB. Bioprinted in vitro tissue models: an emerging platform for developing therapeutic interventions and disease modelling. *Progress in Biomedical Engineering.* 2023;6(1):012003.
79. Ma X, Liu J, Zhu W, Tang M, Lawrence N, Yu C, et al. 3D bioprinting of functional tissue models for personalized drug screening and in vitro disease modeling. *Advanced Drug Delivery Reviews.* 2018;132:235–51.
80. Ming Z, Tang X, Liu J, Ruan BF. Advancements in research on constructing physiological and pathological liver models and their applications utilizing bioprinting technology. *Molecules.* 2023;28(9):3683.
81. Mao S, Pang Y, Liu T, Shao Y, He J, Yang H, et al. Bioprinting of *in vitro* tumor models for personalized cancer treatment: a review. *Biofabrication.* 2020;12(4):042001.

82. He J, Wang J, Pang Y, Yu H, Qin X, Su K, et al. Bioprinting of a hepatic tissue model using humaninduced pluripotent stem cell-derived hepatocytes for drug-induced hepatotoxicity evaluation. *International Journal of Bioprinting.* 2022;8(3):581.
83. Homan KA, Kolesky DB, Skylar-Scott MA, Herrmann JE, Obuobi H, Moisan A, Lewis JA. Bioprinting of 3D convoluted renal proximal tubules on perfusable chips. *Scientific Reports.* 2016;6(1).
84. Briones YL, Pascua BPG, Tiangco NMJ, Crisostomo IC, Casiguran SL, Remenyi R. Assessing the landscape of clinical trials involving bioprinting: a scoping review. *3D Printing in Medicine.* 2024;11(1):5.
85. Demir E, Metli SN, Tutum BE, Gökyer Ş, Oto Ç, Huri PY. Hand-held bioprinters assisting *in situ* bioprinting. *Biomedical Materials.* 2025;20(2):022012.
86. Ayan B, Heo DN, Zhang Z, Dey M, Povilianskas A, Drapaca CS, Özbolat İT. Aspiration-assisted bioprinting for precise positioning of biologics. *Science Advances.* 2020;6(10).
87. Veeravalli RS, Vejandla B, Savani S, Nelluri A, Peddi NC. Three-dimensional bioprinting in medicine: a comprehensive overview of current progress and challenges faced. *Cureus.* 2023.
88. Cui H, Miao S, Esworthy T, Zhou X, Lee SJ, Liu C, et al. 3D bioprinting for cardiovascular regeneration and pharmacology. *Advanced Drug Delivery Reviews.* 2018;132:252–69.
89. Augustine R, Kalva SN, Ahmad R, Zahid AA, Hasan S, Nayeem A, et al. 3D bioprinted cancer models: revolutionizing personalized cancer therapy. *Translational Oncology.* 2021;14(4):101015.
90. Joshi P, Nascimento HSd, Kang SY, Lee M, Vanga MG, Lee SH, et al. Dynamic culture of bioprinted liver tumor spheroids in a pillar/perfusion plate for predictive screening of anticancer drugs. *Biotechnology and Bioengineering.* 2025;122(4):995–1009.
91. Jeong MH, Kim I-H, Park K, Ku B, Lee DW, Park KR, et al. An automated high-throughput screening (HTS) spotter for 3D tumor spheroid formation. *International Journal of Molecular Sciences.* 2023;24(2):1006.
92. Ning L, Shim J, Tomov ML, Liu R, Mehta R, Mingee A, et al. A 3D bioprinted in vitro model of neuroblastoma recapitulates dynamic tumor-endothelial cell interactions contributing to solid tumor aggressive behavior. *Advanced Science.* 2022;9(23):e2200244.
93. Nothdurfter D, Ploner C, Coraça-Huber DC, Wilflingseder D, Müller T, Hermann M, et al. 3D bioprinted, vascularized neuroblastoma tumor environment in fluidic chip devices for precision medicine drug testing. *Biofabrication.* 2022;14(3):035002.
94. Lee KK, Go K, Lee EB, Kim H, Kim S, Kim J, et al. Multifunctional hydrogels for advanced cancer treatment: diagnostic imaging and therapeutic modalities. *Gels.* 2025;11(6):426.
95. Arrigoni C, Gilardi M, Bersini S, Candrian C, Moretti M. Bioprinting and organ-on-chip applications towards personalized medicine for bone diseases. *Stem Cell Reviews and Reports.* 2017;13(3):407–17.
96. Gentile C, Lim KS, Vozzi G. Editorial: 3D bioprinting of vascularized tissues for in vitro and in vivo applications. *Frontiers in Bioengineering and Biotechnology.* 2021;9:754124.
97. Zhai X, Ma Y, Hou C, Gao F, Zhang Y, Ruan C, et al. 3D-printed high strength bioactive supramolecular polymer/clay nanocomposite hydrogel scaffold for bone regeneration. *ACS Biomaterials Science & Engineering.* 2017;3(6):1109–18.
98. Kronemberger GS, Guilherme ASCM, Tavares RSN, Montenegro BM, Kopke Úd A, Baptista LS. Recapitulating tumorigenesis in vitro: opportunities and challenges of 3D bioprinting. *Frontiers in Bioengineering and Biotechnology.* 2021;9:682498.
99. Nolan J, Pearce OM, Screen HRC, Knight MM, Verbruggen SW. Organ-on-a-chip and microfluidic platforms for oncology in the UK. *Cancers.* 2023;15(3):635.

100. Strelez C, Chilakala S, Ghaffarian K, Lau R, Spiller E, Ung N, et al. Human colorectal cancer-on-chip model to study the microenvironmental influence on early metastatic spread. *Iscience.* 2021;24(5):102509.
101. Saha B, Mathur T, Handley KF, Hu W, Afshar-Kharghan V, Sood AK, Jain A. OvCa-chip microsystem recreates vascular endothelium–mediated platelet extravasation in ovarian cancer. *Blood Advances.* 2020;4(14):3329–42.
102. Komen J, van Neerven SM, van den Berg A, Vermeulen L, van der Meer AD. Mimicking and surpassing the xenograft model with cancer-on-chip technology. *Ebiomedicine.* 2021;66:103303.
103. Neagu A-N, Whitham D, Bruno P, Versaci N, Biggers P, Darie CC. Tumor-on-chip platforms for breast cancer continuum concept modeling. *Frontiers in Bioengineering and Biotechnology.* 2024;12:1436393.
104. Xu H, Jia Z, Liu F, Li J, Huang Y, Jiang Y, et al. Biomarkers and experimental models for cancer immunology investigation. *Medcomm.* 2023;4(6):e437.
105. Aleman J, Skardal A. A multi-site metastasis-on-a-chip microphysiological system for assessing metastatic preference of cancer cells. *Biotechnology and Bioengineering.* 2018;116(4):936–44.
106. Regmi S, Poudel C, Adhikari R, Luo KQ. Applications of microfluidics and organ-on-a-chip in cancer research. *Biosensors.* 2022;12(7):459.
107. Kasendra M, Tovaglieri A, Sontheimer-Phelps A, Jalili-Firoozinezhad S, Bein A, Chalkiadaki A, et al. Development of a primary human small intestine-on-a-chip using biopsy-derived organoids. *Scientific Reports.* 2018;8(1):2871.
108. Zhang YS, Zhang Y-N, Zhang W. Cancer-on-a-chip systems at the frontier of nanomedicine. *Drug Discovery Today.* 2017;22(9):1392–9.
109. Wang Y, Wu D, Wu G, Wu J, Lu S, Lo J, et al. Metastasis-on-a-chip mimicking the progression of kidney cancer in the liver for predicting treatment efficacy. *Theranostics.* 2020;10(1):300–11.
110. Sun C, Li H, Chen H, Shi M, Liu Q, Pan ZQ, et al. Decreased expression of CHIP leads to increased angiogenesis via VEGF-VEGFR2 pathway and poor prognosis in human renal cell carcinoma. *Scientific Reports.* 2015;5(1):9774.
111. Meng X, Yan M, Zhang J, Xu Q, Chen W. Carboxy-terminus Hsc70 interacting protein exerts a tumor inhibition function in head and neck cancer. *Oncology Reports.* 2017;38(3):1629–36.
112. Vermeulen N, Haddow G, Seymour T, Faulkner-Jones A, Shu W. 3D bioprint me: a socioethical view of bioprinting human organs and tissues. *Journal of Medical Ethics.* 2017;43(9):618–24.
113. Goddard E, Dodds S. Ethics and policy for bioprinting. *3D Bioprinting: Principles and Protocols*, ed. JM Crook: Springer; 2020. pp. 43–64.
114. Bonaccorsi S. Organ-on-a-chip technology roadmap: regulatory framework, industry adoption, key players, technology transfer, validation, and ethical considerations. *Lab-on-a-Chip Devices for Advanced Biomedicines*, eds. A Parihar, PP Mehta: Royal Society of Chemistry; 2024. pp. 461–504.
115. Ricci G, Gibelli F, Sirignano A. Three-dimensional bioprinting of human organs and tissues: bioethical and medico-legal implications examined through a scoping review. *Bioengineering.* 2023;10(9):1052.
116. Zhou C, Liu C, Liao Z, Pang Y, Sun W. AI for biofabrication. *Biofabrication.* 2024;17(1):012004.
117. Lee H. Engineering in vitro models: bioprinting of organoids with artificial intelligence. *Cyborg and Bionic Systems.* 2023;4:0018.
118. Lin Y, Liu Z. *Future of Intelligent Biomaterials. Intelligent Biomaterials: Fundamentals, Principles and Applications*: Springer; 2025. pp. 511–24.
119. Gangadevi E, Shri ML, Dhanaraj RK, Balusamy B. *Computational Intelligence in Bioprinting: Challenges and Future Directions*: John Wiley & Sons; 2024.

9 *In Vivo* Studies of Bioprinted Tissues and Organs

Jiaxuan Fan and Zeyu Luo

9.1 INTRODUCTION

3D bioprinting is an innovative biofabrication technology that employs a computer-assisted transfer process to pattern and assemble both biological and non-biological materials into a predetermined three-dimensional structure, enabling the creation of bioengineered constructs [1]. This technology offers significant advantages in areas such as 3D cell culture, organoid development, and regenerative medicine. Among these applications, 3D bioprinted scaffolds are increasingly recognized for their exceptional bioactivity and functionality, making them a focal point in the fabrication of biomimetic organs and the replacement of diseased tissues [2]. The functional characterization of 3D bioprinted scaffolds is typically validated through *in vivo* studies, which are considered the most accurate means of assessing how these printed scaffolds perform within a biological environment.

In vivo studies involve the implantation of fabricated scaffolds into experimental animals, followed by the observation of *in vivo* changes at predetermined time points. For the *in vivo* evaluation of 3D bioprinted scaffolds, it is essential to first establish appropriate animal disease models, after which the scaffolds are implanted and monitored for biological responses. Common validation methods include imaging, histological analysis, and behavioral-functional assessments, with the goal of achieving structures and functions that closely mimic those of natural tissues [3]. Currently, 3D bioprinted scaffolds have been extensively studied across a range of tissue and organ disease models, demonstrating their potential for diverse therapeutic applications.

9.2 BONE

Bone is the hardest tissue in the human body and exhibits remarkable regenerative capacity. Minor defects resulting from trauma or disease can typically self-heal and restore their mechanical properties [4]. However, large bone defects are difficult to heal naturally and often require surgical intervention for repair [5]. Currently, autologous bone grafting is considered the gold standard for the clinical treatment of bone defects; however, issues such as nonhealing, infection, and surgical trauma limit its broader clinical application [6]. Consequently, the development of bioactive scaffolds for bone regeneration through 3D bioprinting has emerged as a promising strategy for repairing bone defects.

DOI: 10.1201/9781032638164-9

The functional validation of bone regeneration scaffolds *in vivo* is primarily conducted using bone defect animal models, in which defects are surgically induced and the prepared scaffolds are implanted into the defects. Common bone defect models include cranial defects, femoral condyloid defects, and segmental bone defects [7–9]. (Figure 9.1a) At designated time points, scaffolds are harvested for evaluation. Gross observation provides insight into the rate of bone repair, [10] while micro-CT scanning allows for the assessment of bone growth and the integration of newly formed bone tissue with surrounding natural bone [11,12]. Histological staining techniques, such as those for osteopontin and osteocalcin, are used to assess new bone formation, and functional outcomes are evaluated based on the amount of new bone and the inflammatory response [13,14] (Figure 9.1b).

Unlike cranial bone defect models, segmental bone defects occur in load-bearing or locomotor bones, necessitating scaffolds with high mechanical strength [15]. Following the implantation of 3D bioprinted scaffolds, support and fixation with steel plates are typically required [16] (Figure 9.1c). The characterization process is similar to that of cranial defects. A more refined experimental design involves performing functional studies on animals after defect repair to assess the impact of the treatment on the locomotor abilities of the animals [17] (Figure 9.1d).

In addition to bone tissue defects, healing at the tendon-bone interface presents unique challenges, including the need to establish a strong bone-tendon interface and construct a natural gradient structure between tendon and bone, while also promoting bone tissue regeneration [18]. *In vivo* evaluations are typically conducted using animal models of rotator cuff injury. The deltoid muscle is incised to expose the supraspinatus muscle, which is then separated at the junction between the supraspinatus and the tibia. A tunnel is drilled through the greater tuberosity of the humerus, and the supraspinatus muscle is reattached to the greater tuberosity using a silk suture, with a bracket placed between the tendon and bone suture [19]. Following successful modeling, magnetic resonance imaging (MRI) and computed tomography (CT) imaging can be performed at predetermined time points. A well-healed tendon appears plump and tense on MRI, while CT imaging clearly demonstrates the regeneration of bone tissue [18] (Figure 9.1e). Histological analysis of the tendon-bone interface focuses on the establishment of healing and fibrocartilage growth, with common staining methods including Toluidine blue and Safranin-O. A large area of fibrocartilage with well-organized fibers indicates successful tendon-bone healing [20]. The degree of tendon-bone repair can also be evaluated using tissue maturity scores, and combined with load tests such as tensile strength assessments, provides a more comprehensive evaluation of tendon-bone healing [18] (Figure 9.1f).

9.3 CARTILAGE

Cartilage tissue is widely distributed throughout the human body, including in the ears, nose, joints, trachea, and thorax [21]. As a tissue with distinct mechanical properties, cartilage primarily functions to provide support, lubrication, and cushioning. Articular cartilage, for example, is organized into several distinct zones: the superficial, intermediate, deep, and calcified regions. This hierarchical structure significantly enhances the compressive capacity of the tissue. Therefore, the key

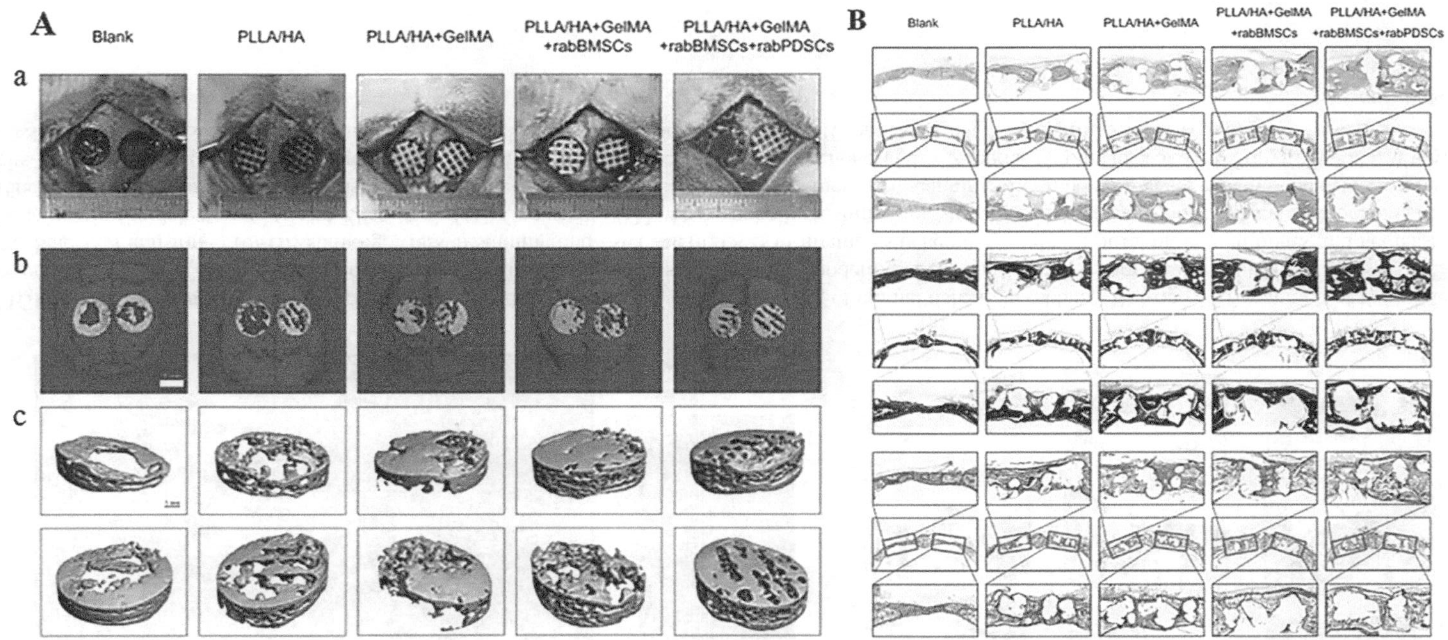

FIGURE 9.1 3D bioprinting in the field of bone tissue. (a) (A) Modeling of cranial defects in rabbits; (B) Micro-CT scanning of the model of cranial defects; (C) Three-dimensional reconstruction of micro-CT scanning after modeling of cranial defects. (From Zhao et al. [11]. Copyright 2023, AccScience Publishing.) (b) HE staining, Masson staining and osteocalcin (OCN) immunohistochemistry staining of rabbit cranial bones and neoplastic bone within the defect area. (From Zhao et al. [11]. Copyright 2023, AccScience Publishing.) (c) Modeling of segmental bone defects in rabbits. (From Pitacco et al. [17]. Copyright 2023, Elsevier.) (d) Three-dimensional reconstruction of micro-CT scanning after modeling of segmental bone defects in rabbits. (From Pitacco et al. [17]. Copyright 2023, Elsevier.) (e) Micro-CT scanning of osteochondral defect model. (From Du et al. [18]. Copyright 2023, Wiley.) (f) Safranin-O Fast Green, HE staining and Masson staining after osteochondral defect. (From Du et al. [18]. Copyright 2023, Wiley.)

(Continued)

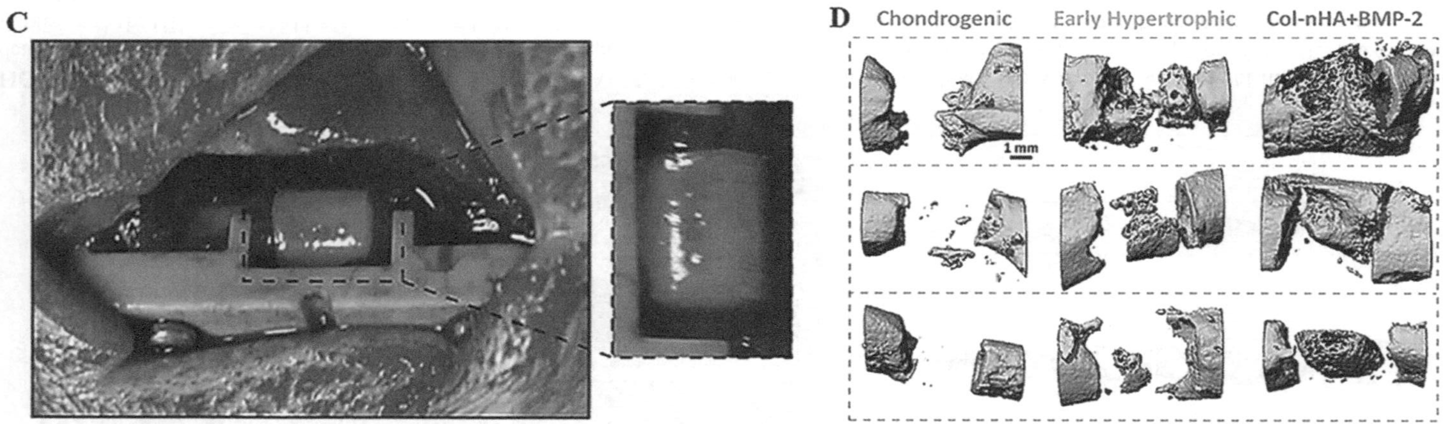

FIGURE 9.1 (*Continued*) 3D bioprinting in the field of bone tissue. (a) (A) Modeling of cranial defects in rabbits; (B) Micro-CT scanning of the model of cranial defects; (C) Three-dimensional reconstruction of micro-CT scanning after modeling of cranial defects. (From Zhao et al. [11]. Copyright 2023, AccScience Publishing.) (b) HE staining, Masson staining and osteocalcin (OCN) immunohistochemistry staining of rabbit cranial bones and neoplastic bone within the defect area. (From Zhao et al. [11]. Copyright 2023, AccScience Publishing.) (c) Modeling of segmental bone defects in rabbits. (From Pitacco et al. [17]. Copyright 2023, Elsevier.) (d) Three-dimensional reconstruction of micro-CT scanning after modeling of segmental bone defects in rabbits. (From Pitacco et al. [17]. Copyright 2023, Elsevier.) (e) Micro-CT scanning of osteochondral defect model. (From Du et al. [18]. Copyright 2023, Wiley.) (f) Safranin-O Fast Green, HE staining and Masson staining after osteochondral defect. (From Du et al. [18]. Copyright 2023, Wiley.)

(Continued)

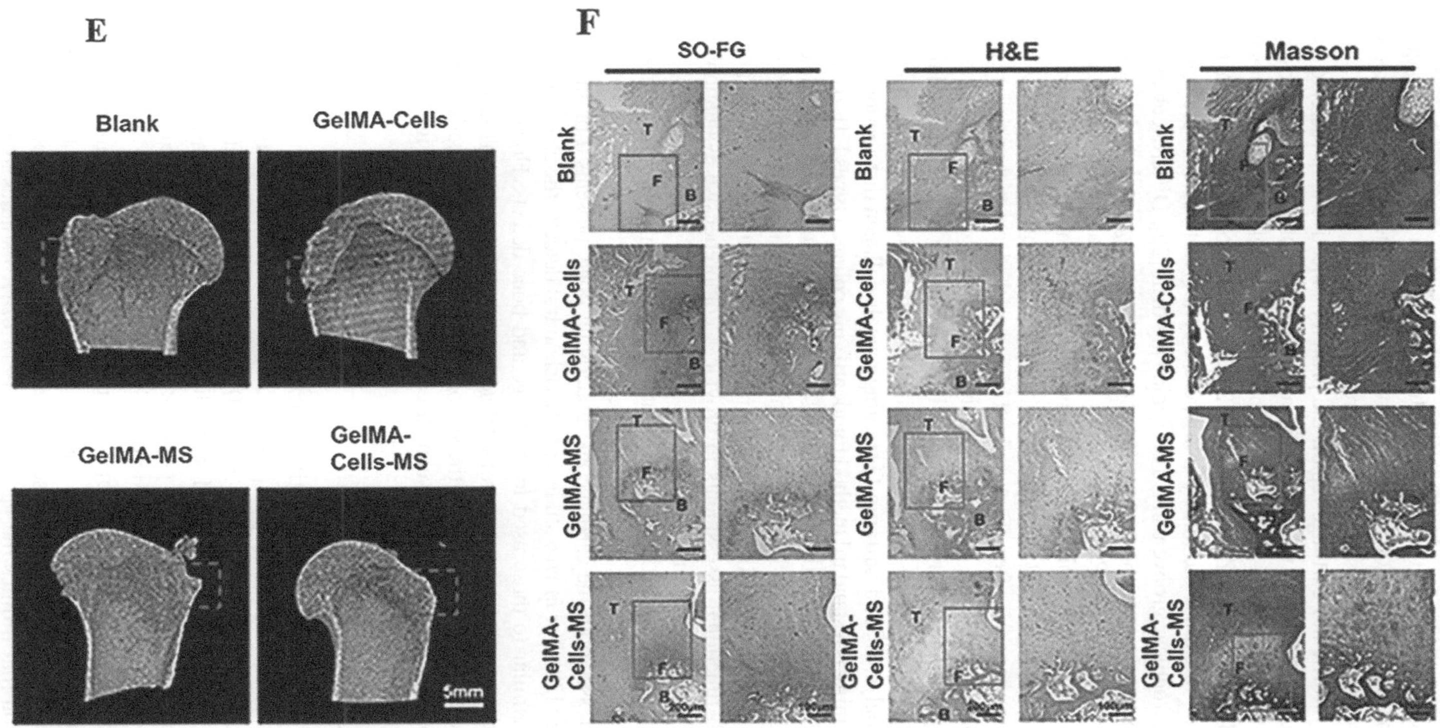

FIGURE 9.1 (*Continued*) 3D bioprinting in the field of bone tissue. (a) (A) Modeling of cranial defects in rabbits; (B) Micro-CT scanning of the model of cranial defects; (C) Three-dimensional reconstruction of micro-CT scanning after modeling of cranial defects. (From Zhao et al. [11]. Copyright 2023, AccScience Publishing.) (b) HE staining, Masson staining and osteocalcin (OCN) immunohistochemistry staining of rabbit cranial bones and neoplastic bone within the defect area. (From Zhao et al. [11]. Copyright 2023, AccScience Publishing.) (c) Modeling of segmental bone defects in rabbits. (From Pitacco et al. [17]. Copyright 2023, Elsevier.) (d) Three-dimensional reconstruction of micro-CT scanning after modeling of segmental bone defects in rabbits. (From Pitacco et al. [17]. Copyright 2023, Elsevier.) (e) Micro-CT scanning of osteochondral defect model. (From Du et al. [18]. Copyright 2023, Wiley.) (f) Safranin-O Fast Green, HE staining and Masson staining after osteochondral defect. (From Du et al. [18]. Copyright 2023, Wiley.)

to effectively repairing natural cartilage is to restore this layered architecture [22]. In contrast to articular cartilage, tissues such as the ear, nose, and trachea have unique morphological characteristics. For the repair of these tissues, the primary goal is to recreate their precise shape and structural features [23].

In the context of articular cartilage repair, the primary objective is to recreate the micro-layered structure and achieve compressive and lubricating properties that closely resemble those of natural cartilage. A common experimental model for cartilage defects involves the distal femur of New Zealand rabbits [24]. Briefly, following anesthesia, the patella is dislocated to expose the knee joint, where a cylindrical defect is created in the distal femoral trochlear groove using a coracoid ring drill [25]. Differences in the rate of repair can be observed between different experimental groups during gross examination [26] (Figure 9.2a). Radiographic imaging is essential for evaluating cartilage repair, with micro-CT typically used to assess the restoration of subchondral bone, while MRI provides insight into the thickness of the cartilage [26] (Figure 9.2c). Suboptimal cartilage repair is often characterized by reduced edema and a thicker cartilage layer. Histological analysis, including staining for collagen distribution and gradient, is critical for assessing the repair process. Hematoxylin and Eosin (HE) staining is commonly used for routine tissue analysis, while Toluidine blue staining highlights regenerated proteoglycans, and Safranin-O staining reveals collagen distribution [25]. Picrosirius red staining is a standard method for identifying collagen types I, II, III, and X [26] (Figure 9.2b). The International Cartilage Repair Society score and the Mankin score are widely utilized scoring systems to evaluate cartilage damage [22]. For cartilage defects in osteoarthritis models, it is recommended that histological evaluations be combined with functional assessments to provide a comprehensive evaluation of cartilage repair and disease treatment [27].

In cases of severe articular cartilage injuries that also involve damage to the subchondral bone, repair of the cartilage alone is insufficient. In these instances, osteochondral repair, which addresses both the cartilage and underlying bone, presents a promising therapeutic strategy [28]. For *in vivo* studies of osteochondral defects, the characterization methods are similar to those used for cartilage and bone defects. However, it is important to note that an ideal osteochondral scaffold must ensure that the cartilage layer and bone layer are properly aligned with the surrounding tissues. Additionally, a subchondral bone layer should be present between the cartilage and bone [24] (Figure 9.2d).

9.4 MENISCUS

The meniscus is a crescent-shaped cartilage structure located between the distal femur and the proximal tibial condyle, playing a crucial role in maintaining joint stability and absorbing mechanical forces [29,30]. The meniscus exhibits complex anisotropy, with its outer edge enriched with blood vessels that facilitate nutrient delivery, while the inner side is densely populated with collagen fibers and glycosaminoglycans to withstand pressure within the joint.

3D bioprinting offers significant advantages in the fabrication of meniscal scaffolds. This technique not only enables the precise replication of the meniscus's unique crescent-shaped structure but also facilitates the creation of an anisotropic internal distribution that mimics the natural tissue. In *in vivo* studies assessing the

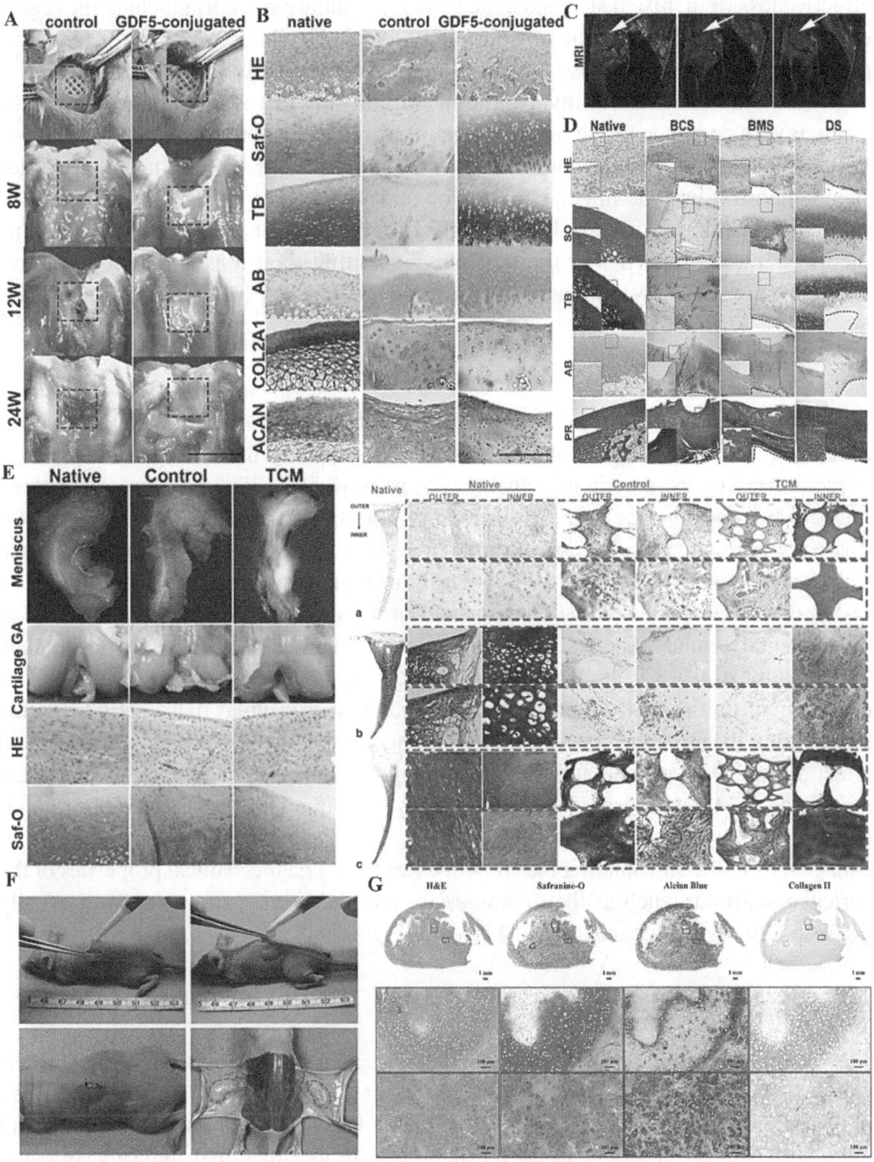

FIGURE 9.2 3D bioprinting in the field of cartilage tissue. (a) Modeling of cartilage defects and gross observations. (From Sun et al. [22]. Copyright 2019, Ivyspring International Publisher.) (b) Histological analysis of cartilage defect staining: HE Safranin-O, Toluidine blue, Alcian blue, ACAN and type II collagen. (From Sun et al. [22]. Copyright 2019, Ivyspring International Publisher.) (c) MRI scanning for repair of cartilage defects. (From Sun et al. [26]. Copyright 2020, AAAS Publisher.) (d) Histological staining of osteochondral defect repair. (From Sun et al. [26]. Copyright 2020, AAAS Publisher.) (e) Gross observation and histological staining of the meniscus. (From Sun et al. [31]. Copyright 2019, Ivyspring International Publisher.) (f) The process of subcutaneous implantation in the auricle of nude mice and gross observation. (From Xie et al. [35]. Copyright 2022, Wiley.) (g) HE, Safranin-O, Alcian blue, and type II collagen staining of regenerated auricular cartilage after 24 weeks of *in vivo* culture results.

effectiveness of meniscal scaffolds, the primary evaluation criteria include the regeneration of cartilage tissue, the anisotropic vascular distribution, and the mechanical properties that resemble those of natural meniscus tissue [31] (Figure 9.2e).

In vivo studies typically involve the in situ grafting of the medial meniscus. The evaluation of cartilage tissue regeneration in the meniscus follows standard protocols for cartilage characterization and can also be monitored by implanting the scaffolds subcutaneously in nude mice. The development of anisotropic structures within the scaffolds is primarily assessed through the distribution of neovascularization, while the mechanical properties of the scaffolds, including their tensile and compressive strengths, are routinely evaluated to ensure their suitability for meniscal repair [31].

9.5 EAR

Microtia is a common congenital maxillofacial deformity that affects both the appearance and certain aspects of auditory function. Consequently, there is significant interest in reconstructing the auricle for patients with microtia [32]. 3D bioprinting technology offers distinct advantages in the fabrication of bioactive scaffolds with specific shapes. These scaffolds can be tailored to the individual characteristics of the patient, and animal studies are essential to evaluate the biological functionality of auricular scaffolds [33].

For *in vivo* evaluation of tissue-engineered auricles, nude mice are commonly used as experimental animals. The scaffolds are typically implanted subcutaneously to simulate the conditions of in situ transplantation [34]. After subcutaneous implantation, chondrocytes within the scaffold proliferate and secrete extracellular matrix (ECM) while maintaining the structural integrity of the printed shape, thereby achieving the desired effect of the 3D bioprinted auricle. HE staining and Safranin-O staining are routinely used to assess tissue morphology. Additionally, immunofluorescence staining for collagen helps to visualize the presence of cartilage lacunae and the formation of abundant collagenous tissue surrounding the chondrocytes [35]. The mechanical properties of the auricular scaffolds, such as their compressive and indentation strengths, are typically evaluated through mechanical testing [36,37] (Figure 9.2f).

9.6 TRACHEA

The natural trachea possesses a complex heterogeneous structure, consisting of alternating C-shaped cartilage rings connected by vascularized fibrous tissue and lined with intraluminal epithelial layers [38]. Additionally, the cellular distribution and microstructure of the trachea play a crucial role in its functional integrity. In cases where diseases affect the trachea and severely impair tracheal ventilation, surgical treatment typically involves tracheal transplantation, where either autologous tissue or artificial trachea is used to replace the diseased segment [39]. However, existing artificial scaffolds often struggle to maintain long-term functionality, and tracheal stenosis may lead to graft failure. 3D bioprinting offers significant advantages in the construction of artificial trachea, enabling the fabrication of hollow, tubular structures that mimic the trachea's microstructure and appearance through advanced printing techniques. This approach holds great potential for creating tracheal substitutes that closely resemble the native tissue [40].

In vivo studies of 3D bioprinted tracheal scaffolds typically involve replacing diseased tracheal segments with the 3D bioprinted alternatives and observing both structural changes and functional outcomes [41]. The animal model for tracheal transplantation often involves excising four rings from the cervical trachea through a median cervical spinal incision, followed by the implantation of the artificial scaffold with proximal and distal end-to-end anastomoses [42]. Postimplantation, gross observations, and tracheoscopy are used to assess the integration of the scaffold with the surrounding natural trachea. X-ray and CT scanning are also employed to evaluate whether the artificial trachea is properly connected to the adjacent tissue and to identify any formation of granulation or scar tissue, which can be visualized through animal tracheoscopy [43]. Histological staining techniques are utilized to characterize the cartilage and fibrous tissue within the scaffold. The cartilage region typically displays distinct indentation and ECM deposition, while angiogenesis can be observed in the fibrous tissue. CD31 staining is commonly used to examine blood vessel distribution [44]. It is essential that the cartilage and fibrous tissue regions are tightly integrated. Furthermore, reconstructing the luminal surface features of the trachea is crucial for restoring its physiological function. Positive keratin staining of epithelial cells is indicative of successful epithelial regeneration, which plays a critical role in restoring normal tracheal function [40]. Additionally, the inflammatory response at the graft site should be carefully monitored as part of the evaluation of the biological function of the artificial trachea [45].

9.7 SKELETAL MUSCLE

Skeletal muscle constitutes a significant portion of the human body and is primarily responsible for contraction and movement in response to nervous system stimulation. Although skeletal muscle has the ability to regenerate after injury [46,47], the process of self-regeneration becomes increasingly difficult when extensive muscle damage occurs, leading to muscle dysfunction. Volumetric muscle loss (VML), which results from severe trauma, tumor excision, or muscular dystrophy, significantly reduces the muscle's endogenous healing capacity and causes loss of muscle function [48]. One common treatment approach for this condition is the use of autologous localized muscle flaps [49]. This technique enhances blood supply and promotes muscle growth by covering the damaged area with surrounding muscle tissue; however, it does not address the root cause of muscle tissue loss.

In contrast, the primary approach to repairing VML using 3D bioprinted scaffolds is to fill the muscle defect and guide muscle regeneration [47]. Animal models typically involve rats, where the middle third of the tibialis anterior muscle is excised to create the VML, while the extensor digitorum longus and extensor hallucis longus muscles are also removed to prevent compensatory hypertrophy during muscle regeneration (Figure 9.3a). After successful modeling, the 3D bioprinted constructs are implanted into the muscle defects and covered with fascia [50]. Functionally, electromyography and muscle strength testing are the most commonly used techniques to evaluate muscle function [51]. The regenerative status of muscle tissue can also be assessed by measuring the mass of the muscle tissue post-surgery and comparing the changes in mass. Histological evaluations are primarily conducted

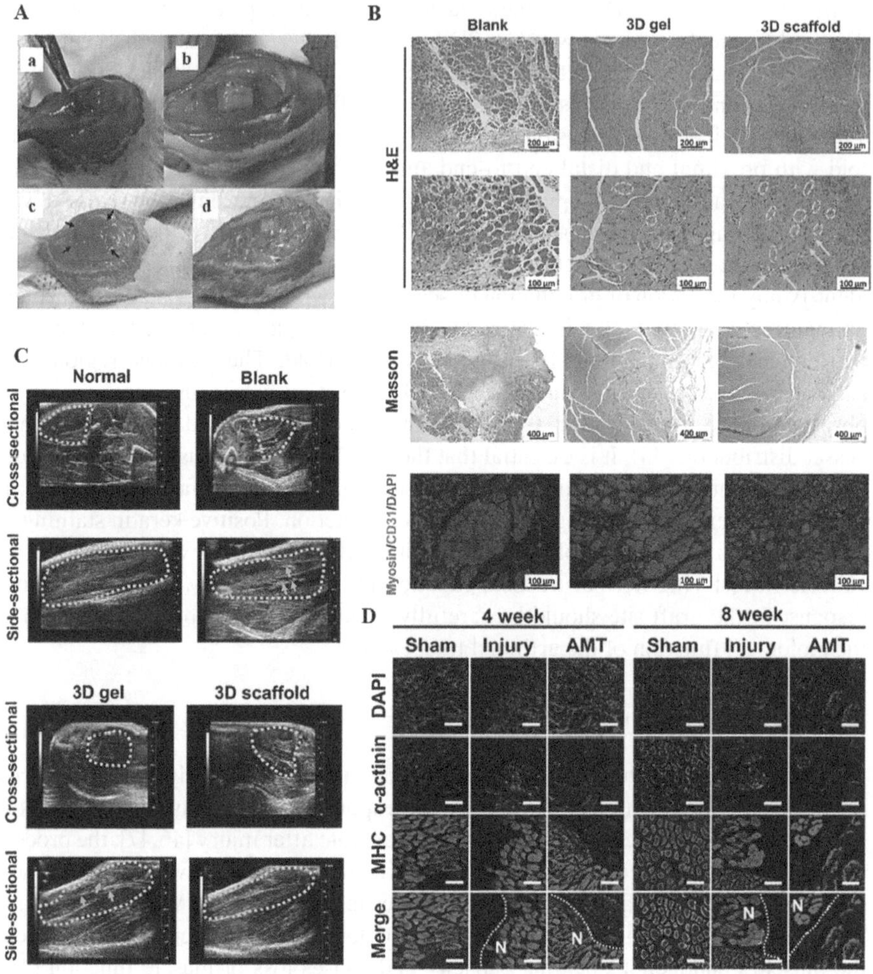

FIGURE 9.3 3D bioprinting for repair of volumetric muscle loss (VML) models. (a) After VML modeling, the 3D bioprinted scaffold was implanted and secured. (From Christensen et al. [53]. Copyright 2021, Wiley.) (b) HE, Masson staining and immunofluorescence staining of regenerated muscle at 14 days postoperatively. (From Li et al. [52]. Copyright 2023, Elsevier.) (c) Ultrasound Images of 3D bioprinted repair VML models. (From Li et al. [52]. Copyright 2023, Elsevier.) (d) Immunofluorescence of α-actinin, MHC, and DAPI in repaired muscle. (From Lee et al. [51]. Copyright 2022, Wiley.)

using tissue staining methods. Standard tissue staining allows for the observation of muscle fiber arrangement and the extent of neovascularization, with minimal fibrosis being the desired outcome of the repair (Figure 9.3b). Additionally, ultrasonography can be employed to visualize the recovery of muscle tissue *in vivo* [52] (Figure 9.3c). Immunofluorescence staining is used to assess the number and distribution of regenerating muscle fibers, with myosin heavy chain (MHC) being the most commonly used marker [52] (Figure 9.3d). An ideal muscle repair results in well-aligned muscle fibers, with small blood vessels distributed within the fibers. The new muscle tissue should be closely integrated with the surrounding natural muscle and capable of contracting in synchrony with nerve stimulation.

9.8 PERIPHERAL NERVE

Peripheral nerves serve as a crucial link between the central nervous system and the motor system, enabling various motor functions of the human body [54]. However, peripheral nerves are delicate and can be damaged by trauma or surgical procedures [55]. Natural recovery from peripheral nerve damage is difficult, necessitating surgical intervention for repair [55]. Nerve repair conduit technology offers a promising solution by facilitating nerve regeneration through the creation of artificial nerve conduits with biological functions, providing an optimal microenvironment for repair [2,56]. Recent studies have focused on the use of cell-free conduits for nerve repair, with the combination of specialized structural designs and nerve repair additives accelerating the healing of nerve injuries and minimizing scar formation. While cell-free scaffolds primarily promote nerve healing by directing cell migration, 3D bioprinting allows for the design of nerve repair conduits that include cells.

Functional evaluation of 3D bioprinted nerve conduits is typically conducted using animal models of peripheral nerve injury [57]. Under general anesthesia, the animal is positioned prone, and a longitudinal skin incision is made in the posterior thigh. The sciatic nerve is exposed via a gluteal muscle separation approach, and a sharp incision is made at the mid-thigh to create a nerve defect (Figure 9.4a). Nerve repair can then be assessed through both histological and functional recovery measures. Kinematic analysis is used to evaluate the movement of muscle groups innervated by the nerve [57,58], while gait analysis assesses the recovery of nerve function post-repair [59]. Sensory recovery is evaluated using the needle prick test, with results categorized into a score of 0–3 according to Siemionow et al. [60]: grade 0, no response to stimulation; grade 1, withdrawal response induced by heel stimulation; grade 2, withdrawal response from dorsal stimulation; and grade 3, withdrawal response from toe stimulation. Motor recovery is evaluated through the paw extension test, where toe spreading is graded from 0 to 3: grade 0, no toe spreading; grade 1, any sign of toe movement; grade 2, toe abduction; and grade 3, toe abduction and stretching [60].

The number of axons in the nerve tissue, the thickness of the myelin sheath, and the degree of axonal alignment serve as key indicators of nerve repair. Special staining techniques can be employed to determine the number of sensory and motor neurons, with a higher number of neurons suggesting better repair outcomes [53,61] (Figure 9.4b and d). The degree of muscle atrophy in the innervated muscles, such as the gastrocnemius muscle innervated by the sciatic nerve, can also provide insight into nerve regeneration. Sections of the gastrocnemius muscle are routinely analyzed and compared with their wet weights, with reduced muscle atrophy and increased wet weight indicating improved nerve repair [62] (Figure 9.4c). Additionally, the activity and differentiation capacity of cells within the conduit are evaluated through in situ and subcutaneous grafts [63].

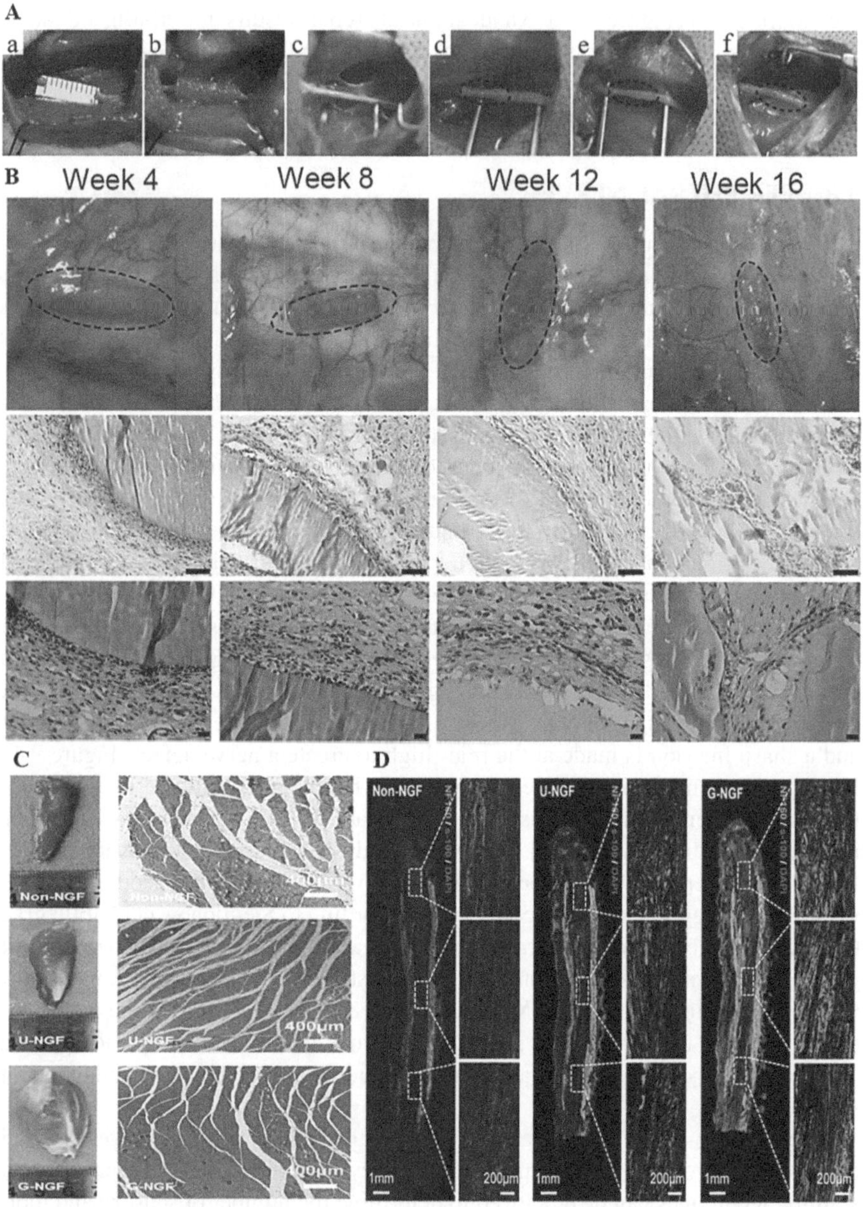

FIGURE 9.4 3D bioprinted conduit to repair peripheral nerves. (a) Modeling of peripheral nerve defect and implantation of a nerve repair conduit. (From Hu et al. [64]. Copyright 2016, Springer Nature.) (b) Gross observation, HE staining and anti-CD68 antibody staining at 4, 8, 12 and 16 weeks after implantation. (From Tao et al. [65]. Copyright 2019, Elsevier.) (c) Gastrocnemius muscle gross observation and Masson staining at 12 weeks postoperatively. (From Wang et al. [62]. Copyright 2023, Wiley.) (d) Immunofluorescence staining of nerve cross sections at 12 weeks postoperatively. (From Wang et al. [62]. Copyright 2023, Wiley.)

9.9 SPINAL CORD

The spinal cord, part of the central nervous system, is responsible for the bidirectional conduction of signals. Spinal cord injury (SCI) is a severe and traumatic condition characterized by partial or complete loss of sensory and motor functions below the injured segment [66]. This condition is often accompanied by processes such as the loss of nerve cells, axonal disruption, and demyelination [66]. To promote recovery from SCI, researchers aim to replace damaged spinal cord tissue with bioengineered scaffolds that mimic the function of the natural spinal cord, fill the injured area, and encourage spinal cord regeneration.

Implanting a 3D bioprinted spinal cord scaffold into the injury site and assessing its integration and functionality are a widely used approach for evaluating spinal cord scaffolds [67]. The rat model is commonly employed in these studies. After anesthetizing the rat, a 2 cm incision is made along the back to expose the T7–T10 vertebrae. A dorsal transverse laminectomy is performed at T7–T10, exposing the spinal cord at T8–T9, which is then transected to create a 4 mm injury [67]. Successful establishment of the model is indicated by symptoms such as bilateral hind limb twitching, hindfoot stretching, muscle weakness, and flaccidity [68,69].

Evaluation of spinal cord scaffolds involves both functional and histological assessments after a specific recovery period. Functional assessments commonly include the Basso–Beattie–Bresnahan motor score [70] and inclined plane tests [71]. Postoperative electrophysiological testing is performed to evaluate nerve healing by inserting stimulating electrodes into the motor projection areas and recording electrodes into hindlimb muscle groups [68]. MRI is used to monitor the healing of spinal cord lesions, with reduced edema and scarring at the junction being desirable outcomes. Histological evaluation is performed through tissue staining methods. HE staining and immunohistochemical staining are used to assess the formation of new tissue on the surface and within the scaffold. Key factors include the alignment of nerve fibers inside the scaffold and the extent of scar proliferation in the healing area [68]. Electron microscopy is another tool for assessing axonal growth, providing insights into the potential for functional recovery after nerve regeneration [72].

9.10 VESSEL

In the design of artificial blood vessels, commonly used arterial models include the femoral arteries and aorta [73], while venous models typically involve the vena cava and popliteal vein [74,75]. Following the implantation of artificial blood vessels, precise anastomosis of the ports and strict infection prevention are critical to avoid animal mortality. Postimplantation deaths are often associated with thromboembolism caused by the implant, with thrombosis being the primary cause of implantation failure [73]. After the procedure, it is essential to evaluate whether integration occurs between the artificial conduit and the natural blood vessel, as well as whether the layers within the artificial conduit differentiate appropriately.

Microvascular tissue, which plays a crucial role in nourishing surrounding tissues and facilitating material exchange, is frequently co-constructed with other target tissues to enhance viability. Unlike traditional tubular structures, pure microvascular networks are often fabricated as mesh-like scaffolds [73]. *In vivo* studies of microvascular networks focus primarily on the biocompatibility of the scaffolds, ensuring their survival and functionality postimplantation. These scaffolds must differentiate into network structures, establish connections with peripheral vascular networks, and form a localized artificial vascular system capable of nutrient delivery. Additionally, minimizing the inflammatory response is crucial [76]. Common *in vivo* studies involve subcutaneous implantation of the scaffolds in rats. Postimplantation evaluation is typically conducted through histological staining after tissue sampling. A key indicator of successful vascularization is the observation of smooth muscle tissue and endothelial tissue, along with the formation of small hollow channels within the scaffolds [77].

9.11 SKIN

The skin is the largest organ in the human body, accounting for approximately 15% of an adult's body weight [78,79]. It has a layered structure comprising three main layers: the epidermis, dermis, and subcutaneous tissue. The epidermis, the outermost layer, consists of keratin-producing cells; the dermis, the middle layer, contains collagen cells and fibroblasts; and the subcutaneous tissue, the innermost layer, is composed of adipocytes and collagen [80]. While the skin can naturally heal from minor trauma or surgical interventions, severe trauma, burns, infections, or tumors can result in significant skin defects that are difficult to heal without intervention. Such defects may lead to extensive scarring, necessitating external measures for proper recovery. The primary goal of skin tissue repair using artificial scaffolds is not only to repair the defective area but also to restore the skin's structure and function [81].

For *in vivo* studies of skin defects, the standard approach involves creating a skin defect model in experimental animals (Figure 9.5a). Following the implantation of artificial scaffolds into the defect, gross observation is used to assess the recovery rate of the damaged area (Figure 9.5b). HE staining can evaluate the repair of skin tissues, and keratin staining is necessary for characterizing the layered structure of new skin and neovascularization [82] (Figure 9.5c). Additionally, other stains, such as those for sebaceous glands or collagen, may be employed depending on the specific study design to demonstrate the functional restoration of skin tissues [83].

In cases where skin defects are accompanied by other conditions, such as diabetes mellitus, disease modeling requires modifications. To create diabetic skin models, experimental animals are first induced into a diabetic state via intraperitoneal injections of streptozotocin, and their blood glucose levels are monitored using glucose meters. Rats are considered successfully induced into a diabetic model when non-fasting blood glucose levels exceed 20×10^{-3} M, accompanied by symptoms such as polydipsia, polyuria, and weight loss. Once diabetes is established, skin defects are created, and diabetic-specific husbandry, including a controlled diet, is maintained [84]. For infected skin defect models, the procedure is similar to conventional skin defect modeling but includes the injection of representative bacteria into the wound to simulate infection [84] (Figure 9.5d).

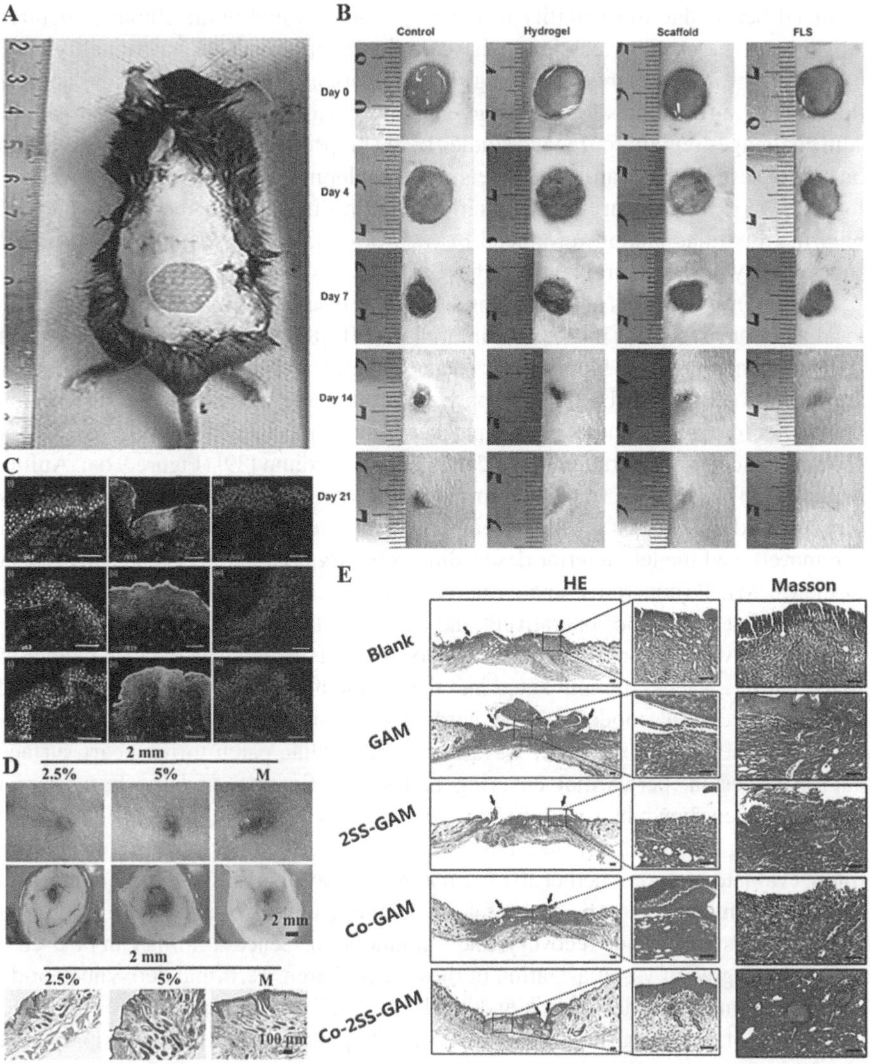

FIGURE 9.5 3D bioprinted scaffolds for skin defect repair. (a) Mouse skin defect model. (From Ma et al. [84]. Copyright 2021, Wiley.) (b) Gross observation of healing of skin defects. (From Zhou et al. [82]. Copyright 2020, Elsevier.) (c) P63 (white), K19 (black) and Ki67 (gray) staining demonstrates the layered structure of skin and scaffolds. (From Kim et al. [85]. Copyright 2018, Wiley.) (d) HE staining, Masson staining, and collagen fiber deposition (dotted black) in a diabetic skin defect model. (From Ma et al. [84]. Copyright 2021, Wiley.) (e) HE staining, Masson staining, and collagen fiber deposition in a diabetic skin defect model.

9.12 HEART

The ultimate goal of cardiac bioprinting technology is to fabricate functional cardiac organs *in vitro* and maintain their proper function after transplantation into the body [86]. 3D bioprinting has emerged as a promising technology for constructing artificial hearts due to its ability to fabricate complex and multicellular structures. Advances in bioprinting technology have gradually improved the functionality of 3D bioprinted heart structures, including the conduction of neural signals and applications as organ substitutes for pathology and pharmacology studies. However, significant challenges remain for *in vivo* studies of 3D bioprinted cardiac structures. On the one hand, establishing animal models and developing mature surgical procedures for partial or whole-heart transplantation remain difficult. On the other hand, 3D bioprinted cardiac analogs produced *in vitro* often fall short of replicating the full functionality of the natural heart [30].

Current *in vivo* studies of bioprinting for cardiac diseases primarily focus on treating localized lesions, such as myocardial infarction (MI) [87]. A commonly used approach is the implantation of 3D bioprinted cardiac patches, which are applied to the infarcted area to restore myocardial blood supply and contractile function while minimizing scar tissue formation. These cardiac patches provide mechanical support [87,88] and promote vascular regeneration in the damaged myocardium [89] (Figure 9.6a). Animal models of MI have well-established surgical procedures. Briefly, the animals are anesthetized, and the chest is opened left at the fourth intercostal space. The pericardium is removed, and the left anterior descending coronary artery was permanently ligated to induce MI. Postoperative analgesia and anti-infection are given [87]. Baseline is established at 2 days postoperatively and subsequent patch implantation procedures are initiated, with rats anesthetized and left open chest dissection at the fifth intercostal space, cardiac patches are implanted into the region of the infarcted myocardium [90].

After successful modeling, the cardiac patch is implanted into the animal. Currently, there are three main ways to fix the cardiac patch to the heart surface: natural adhesion, pericardial covering and suture fixation, and the best fixation effect has been shown by suture fixation in a study by Bejleri et al. [91] (Figure 9.6b). In evaluating the biological function of the patch, staining of tissue sections is routinely evaluated to see whether the cardiac patch plays a positive role in controlling ventricular thickness, scar tissue area, and infarct area. Collagen staining can be used to assess local tissue recovery, and immunofluorescence staining can be used to assess the degree of vascularization of the diseased area. Terminal deoxynucleotidyl transferase -mediated dUTP nick end labeling (TUNEL) staining is one of the effective means of assessing the level of myocardial apoptosis, and ideally, implantation of a 3D bioprinted cardiac patch would reduce the level of myocardial apoptosis [87]. Cardiac function is further assessed through echocardiography, which measures key parameters such as left ventricular ejection fraction, left ventricular shortening fraction, left ventricular systolic internal diameter, and left ventricular diastolic internal diameter. These measurements provide a comprehensive evaluation of cardiac pathology and function. Advanced imaging techniques, such as CMRI and PET-CT, have been employed to evaluate structural changes and the extent of MI, providing enhanced characterization of the *in vivo* performance of cardiac patches [90].

Two main experimental methods are used to assess the biocompatibility of 3D bioprinted cardiac patches *in vivo*. The first involves subcutaneous implantation of the sterilized patch into the backs of rats, followed by histological analysis. HE staining is used to examine tissue response, while CD68 and CCR7 immunostaining assess macrophage infiltration at the implantation site. The formation of neovascular

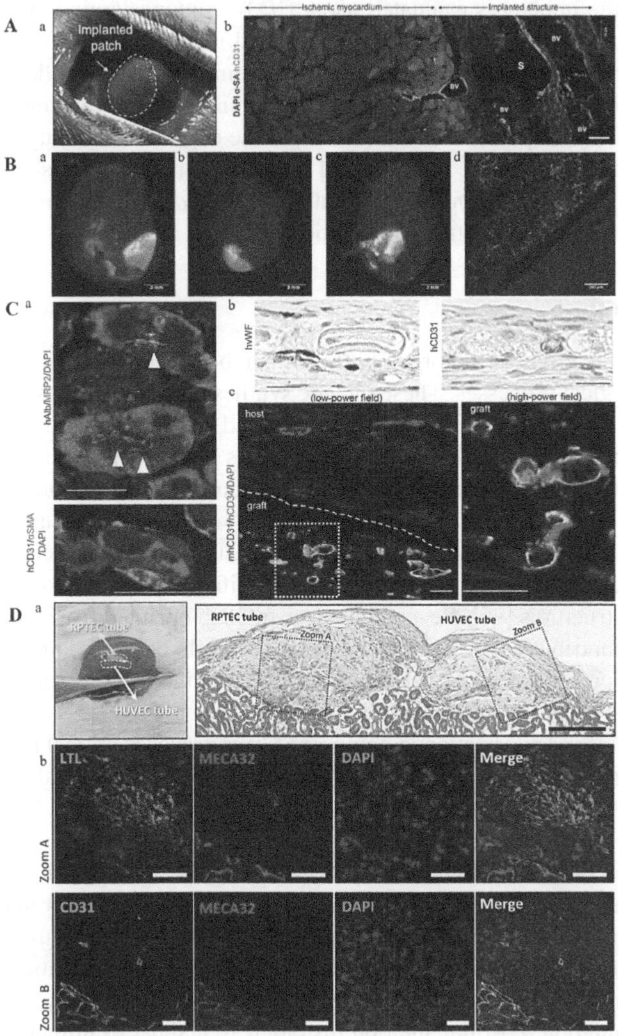

FIGURE 9.6 3D bioprinting for heart, liver and kidney organ repair. (a) (A) 3D bioprinted heart patch implanted on the surface of the heart in myocardial infarction; (B) Neovascularization within the patch and migration to the injured myocardium. (From Cui et al. [105]. Copyright 2018, Elsevier.) (b) (A) Suture method; (B) pericardial folding method; (C) postimplantation suture method; (D) immunohistological analysis of angiogenesis (black) and cells (grey) after 14 days *in vivo*. (From Bejleri et al. [91]. Copyright 2018, Wiley.) (c) Histological analysis of blood vessels in pre-vascularized liver tissue. (A) MRP2-positive bile duct-like structures (black) are located in the middle of the hepatocyte mass, suggestive of bile duct formation. (B) Human-specific CD31 antibody, human-specific vWF antibody demonstrating blood vessels. (C) MHCd31-positive and HCd34-negative tubules (white) are present suggestive of mouse capillaries. (From Sasaki et al. [99]. Copyright 2018, Elsevier.) (d) (A) Transplantation of kidney-like tissue into the subperitoneum of the kidney; (B) Histological staining after transplantation; (C) Angiogenesis after transplantation. (From Singh et al. [104]. Copyright 2020, Elsevier.)

tissue near the implant is evaluated using CD31 immunostaining, with quantitative analysis of neovascularization [92]. The second method involves applying the cardiac patch to the surface of a normal heart. Specimens are then collected, fixed, and sectioned for histological analysis to detect immune responses and quantify the presence of CD3+ and CD68+ cells. To evaluate the degradation ability of the patch, it is subcutaneously implanted in rats, and the patch is removed, washed, lyophilized, and weighed at predetermined time points. The *in vivo* degradation rate is calculated based on weight changes after implantation [93].

9.13 LIVER

The liver is the largest solid organ in the human body, playing a vital role in numerous physiological processes. These include synthesizing compounds essential for the coagulation cascade, metabolizing nutrients and toxins, regulating blood glucose levels, and producing bile to emulsify dietary fats [94]. The liver's ability to perform such diverse functions is attributed to its complex anatomy, characterized by a hierarchical and compartmentalized network of blood vessels and bile ducts that facilitate efficient and orderly biological processes [95]. 3D bioprinting technology has significant potential to enable the fabrication of artificial livers due to its customizable bioink and structures [96]. Recent advances in 3D bioprinted liver tissue have made significant contributions to drug metabolism research, catalysis studies, and disease modeling. For *in vivo* characterization of liver organoids, key parameters include survivability, vascularization, and biological functionality [97].

The level of vascularization in engineered liver tissues is critical for their survival and functionality *in vivo*. To evaluate angiogenic capacity, artificial liver tissues are often implanted subcutaneously in animal models. Immunohistochemical staining of the samples reveals fluorescently labeled vascular structures within the tissues. The presence of abundant and widely distributed vascular networks is foundational for subsequent liver tissue functionality [98] (Figure 9.6c). Another major important ductal system within liver tissue is the bile duct system, and immunohistochemical staining shows MRP2+ duct-like structures, indicating the formation of bile ducts [99]. The functionality of artificial liver tissues can be assessed following subcutaneous implantation. Postimplantation histological analysis examines morphological changes, including the formation of large tissue clusters and their prolonged survival *in vivo*, which indicate functional activity of the 3D bioprinted liver tissues [100].

A more physiologically relevant method involves transplanting 3D bioprinted liver tissues into the abdominal cavity of experimental animals. After implantation, the metabolic capacity of the artificial liver tissue is evaluated through blood analysis. Key biochemical markers include albumin, total protein, bilirubin, alanine aminotransferase, aspartate aminotransferase, lactate dehydrogenase, γ-glutamyl transpeptidase, alkaline phosphatase, and the albumin-to-globulin ratio. The presence and levels of these markers provide insight into the liver's metabolic and synthetic activity. Additionally, the drug-metabolizing capability of the 3D bioprinted tissues is assessed by administering drugs to experimental animals and analyzing the resulting metabolites in the blood. Combining these metabolic indices with histological analysis offers a comprehensive evaluation of the effectiveness of 3D bioprinted liver tissues [98].

9.14 KIDNEY

The kidney is a highly vascularized vital organ responsible for filtering molecules and regulating physiological states such as fluid balance and blood pressure [101,102]. The artificial construction of kidney-related tissues or whole kidney organs offers a promising platform for *in vitro* applications, including drug nephrotoxicity prediction, drug screening, and disease modeling. Moreover, for patients with end-stage renal disease, the development of physiologically functional artificial kidneys presents a potential solution to the shortage of donor organs. Advances in bioprinting technology, with its unique capabilities in multicellular distribution, microstructure fabrication, and shape replication, make it possible to construct transplantable, functionalized kidneys [103]. The kidney's complex structure and diverse functions present significant challenges for artificial kidney construction. In vivo studies are essential for advancing this field, focusing not only on reproducing the histological structure of natural kidneys but also on assessing renal function through animal experiments.

Currently, there are limited *in vivo* studies involving transplantable renal tissues, with most research centered on disease models such as the unilateral ureteral obstruction (UUO) model. In this model, the ureter is accessed through a dorsal incision in rats and blocked mid-ureter with a two-point silk ligation to induce kidney injury. Singh et al. employed coaxial 3D cell printing technology to fabricate tubular and vascularized renal parenchyma using renal tubular epithelial and endothelial cells, respectively. These 3D bioprinted tubular tissues were transplanted beneath the renal peritoneum in rats with UUO-induced kidney injury. After an 8-week period, the 3D bioprinted tissues were retrieved for evaluation. Observations revealed that the grafts retained their original structure, and host blood vessels had grown around the vascularized grafts (Figure 9.6d). Additionally, premature maturation of proximal tubular structures was observed near the bionic renal tissue grafts, demonstrating their therapeutic potential in chronic renal disease models [104].

9.15 CONCLUSION AND PERSPECTIVE

The results of *in vivo* studies serve as a crucial foundation for transforming 3D bioprinted constructs into viable products and are essential for advancing 3D bioprinting for human applications. With the continuous advancement of tissue staining and imaging technologies, the functionality of 3D bioprinted scaffolds in animals has been more accurately characterized, particularly for tissues and organs such as bone, cartilage, muscle, and skin. For these tissues, *in vivo* characterization has significantly improved. However, for parenchymal organs such as the heart, liver, and kidneys, the available animal models for *in vivo* studies remain limited. Furthermore, due to the complex cellular composition and intricate structure of parenchymal organs, current 3D bioprinting technologies have not yet reached the capability to fully replicate their architecture and functions. As a result, *in vivo* studies involving 3D bioprinted scaffolds for these organs continue to present significant challenges.

Additionally, the biosafety of 3D bioprinted scaffolds cannot be overlooked. Inflammatory responses at the implantation site, as well as systemic immune reactions, may compromise scaffold functionality and even the health of the experimental animals. Evaluating the long-term functionality of the implants is also essential. Structural and functional changes over time, following the implant's long-term presence, are important indicators for assessing the safety of these implants within the body.

REFERENCES

1. Moroni, L., et al., Biofabrication strategies for 3D in vitro models and regenerative medicine. *Nat Rev Mater*, 2018. **3**(5): p. 21–37.
2. Murphy, S.V., P. De Coppi, and A. Atala, Opportunities and challenges of translational 3D bioprinting. *Nat Biomed Eng*, 2020. **4**(4): p. 370–380.
3. Chimene, D., R. Kaunas, and A.K. Gaharwar, Hydrogel bioink reinforcement for additive manufacturing: a focused review of emerging strategies. *Adv Mater*, 2020. **32**(1): p. e1902026.
4. Chen, Z., et al., A stone-cottage-inspired printing strategy to build microsphere patterned scaffolds for accelerated bone regeneration. *Adv Funct Mater*, 2025. **35**(14): p. 2417836.
5. Roddy, E., et al., Treatment of critical-sized bone defects: clinical and tissue engineering perspectives. *Eur J Orthop Surg Traumatol*, 2018. **28**(3): p. 351–362.
6. Enneking, W.F., J.L. Eady, and H. Burchardt, Autogenous cortical bone grafts in the reconstruction of segmental skeletal defects. *J Bone Joint Surg Am*, 1980. **62**(7): p. 1039–1058.
7. Li, G., et al., ECM-mimicking composite hydrogel for accelerated vascularized bone regeneration. *Bioact Mater*, 2024. **42**: p. 241–256.
8. Wang, J., et al., Engineering large-scale self-mineralizing bone organoids with bone matrix-inspired hydroxyapatite hybrid bioinks. *Adv Mater*, 2024. **36**(30): p. e2309875.
9. Liu, Y., et al., Cellular scale curvature in bioceramic scaffolds enhanced bone regeneration by regulating skeletal stem cells and vascularization. *Adv Healthc Mater*, 2024. **13**(29): p. e2401667.
10. Liu, B., et al., 3D-bioprinted functional and biomimetic hydrogel scaffolds incorporated with nanosilicates to promote bone healing in rat calvarial defect model. *Mater Sci Eng C Mater Biol Appl*, 2020. **112**: p. 110905.
11. Zhao, D., et al., Co-culture bioprinting of tissue-engineered bone-periosteum biphasic complex for repairing critical-sized skull defects in rabbits. *Int J Bioprint*, 2023. **9**(3): p. 698.
12. Kim, J., et al., Thermo-responsive nanocomposite bioink with growth-factor holding and its application to bone regeneration. *Small*, 2023. **19**(9): p. e2203464.
13. Kim, W., C.H. Jang, and G. Kim, Bone tissue engineering supported by bioprinted cell constructs with endothelial cell spheroids. *Theranostics*, 2022. **12**(12): p. 5404–5417.
14. Moncal, K.K., et al., Controlled co-delivery of pPDGF-B and pBMP-2 from intraoperatively bioprinted bone constructs improves the repair of calvarial defects in rats. *Biomaterials*, 2022. **281**: p. 121333.
15. Zheng, C., et al., 3D-printed HA15-loaded β-tricalcium phosphate/poly (lactic-co-glycolic acid) bone tissue scaffold promotes bone regeneration in rabbit radial defects. *Int J Bioprint*, 2021. **7**(1): p. 317.
16. Daly, A.C., et al., 3D printed microchannel networks to direct vascularisation during endochondral bone repair. *Biomaterials*, 2018. **162**: p. 34–46.
17. Pitacco, P., et al., 3D bioprinting of cartilaginous templates for large bone defect healing. *Acta Biomater*, 2023. **156**: p. 61–74.
18. Du, L., et al., Multicellular bioprinting of biomimetic inks for tendon-to-bone regeneration. *Adv Sci (Weinh)*, 2023. **10**(21): p. e2301309.
19. Yang, R., et al., Gradient bimetallic ion-based hydrogels for tissue microstructure reconstruction of tendon-to-bone insertion. *Sci Adv*, 2021. **7**(26): p. eabg3816.

20. Zhang, X., et al., Three-dimensional bioprinting of a structure-, composition-, and mechanics-graded biomimetic scaffold coated with specific decellularized extracellular matrix to improve the tendon-to-bone healing. *ACS Appl Mater Interfaces*, 2023. **15**(24): p. 28964–28980.
21. Visscher, D.O., et al., A photo-crosslinkable cartilage-derived extracellular matrix bioink for auricular cartilage tissue engineering. *Acta Biomater*, 2021. **121**: p. 193–203.
22. Sun, Y., et al., 3D-bioprinting a genetically inspired cartilage scaffold with GDF5-conjugated BMSC-laden hydrogel and polymer for cartilage repair. *Theranostics*, 2019. **9**(23): p. 6949–6961.
23. Luo, Z., et al., 3D assembly of cryo(bio)printed modular units for shelf-ready scalable tissue fabrication. *Adv Funct Mater*, 2024. **34**(4): p. 2309173.
24. Shim, J.H., et al., Three-dimensional bioprinting of multilayered constructs containing human mesenchymal stromal cells for osteochondral tissue regeneration in the rabbit knee joint. *Biofabrication*, 2016. **8**(1): p. 014102.
25. Pei, Z., et al., Experimental study on repair of cartilage defects in the rabbits with GelMA-MSCs scaffold prepared by three-dimensional bioprinting. *Int J Bioprint*, 2023. **9**(2): p. 662.
26. Sun, Y., et al., 3D bioprinting dual-factor releasing and gradient-structured constructs ready to implant for anisotropic cartilage regeneration. *Sci Adv*, 2020. **6**(37).
27. Liu, Y., et al., 3D-bioprinted BMSC-laden biomimetic multiphasic scaffolds for efficient repair of osteochondral defects in an osteoarthritic rat model. *Biomaterials*, 2021. **279**: p. 121216.
28. Zhang, X., et al., 3D bioprinting of biomimetic bilayered scaffold consisting of decellularized extracellular matrix and silk fibroin for osteochondral repair. *Int J Bioprint*, 2021. **7**(4): p. 401.
29. Katz, J.N., et al., Surgery versus physical therapy for a meniscal tear and osteoarthritis. *N Engl J Med*, 2013. **368**(18): p. 1675–1684.
30. Lian, L., et al., Rapid volumetric bioprinting of decellularized extracellular matrix bioinks. *Adv Mater*, 2024. **36**: p. e2304846.
31. Sun, Y., et al., 3D-bioprinting ready-to-implant anisotropic menisci recapitulate healthy meniscus phenotype and prevent secondary joint degeneration. *Theranostics*, 2021. **11**(11): p. 5160–5173.
32. Yamada, A., Autologous rib microtia construction: nagata technique. *Facial Plast Surg Clin North Am*, 2018. **26**(1): p. 41–55.
33. Bly, R.A., et al., Microtia reconstruction. *Facial Plast Surg Clin North Am*, 2016. **24**(4): p. 577–591.
34. Jia, L., et al., Bioprinting and regeneration of auricular cartilage using a bioactive bioink based on microporous photocrosslinkable acellular cartilage matrix. *Bioact Mater*, 2022. **16**: p. 66–81.
35. Xie, X., et al., Microtissue-based bioink as a chondrocyte microshelter for DLP bioprinting. *Adv Healthc Mater*, 2022. **11**(22): p. e2201877.
36. Zielinska, D., et al., Combining bioengineered human skin with bioprinted cartilage for ear reconstruction. *Sci Adv*, 2023. **9**(40): p. eadh1890.
37. Chae, S., et al., 3D cell-printing of biocompatible and functional meniscus constructs using meniscus-derived bioink. *Biomaterials*, 2021. **267**: p. 120466.
38. Furlow, P.W. and D.J. Mathisen, Surgical anatomy of the trachea. *Ann Cardiothorac Surg*, 2018. **7**(2): p. 255–260.
39. Li, D., et al., Regeneration of trachea graft with cartilage support, vascularization, and epithelization. *Acta Biomater*, 2019. **89**: p. 206–216.
40. Huo, Y., et al., Functional trachea reconstruction using 3D-bioprinted native-like tissue architecture based on designable tissue-specific bioinks. *Adv Sci (Weinh)*, 2022. **9**(29): p. e2202181.

41. Jungebluth, P., et al., Tracheal tissue engineering in rats. *Nat Protoc*, 2014. **9**(9): p. 2164–2179.
42. Sun, Y., et al., Instant trachea reconstruction using 3D-bioprinted C-shape biomimetic trachea based on tissue-specific matrix hydrogels. *Bioact Mater*, 2024. **32**: p. 52–65.
43. Bae, S.W., et al., 3D bioprinted artificial trachea with epithelial cells and chondrogenic-differentiated bone marrow-derived mesenchymal stem cells. *Int J Mol Sci*, 2018. **19**(6), 1624.
44. Park, J.H., et al., 3D bioprinting of a trachea-mimetic cellular construct of a clinically relevant size. *Biomaterials*, 2021. **279**: p. 121246.
45. Liu, Y., et al., A cell-free tissue-engineered tracheal substitute with sequential cytokine release maintained airway opening in a rabbit tracheal full circumferential defect model. *Biomaterials*, 2023. **300**: p. 122208.
46. Jana, S., S.K. Levengood, and M. Zhang, Anisotropic materials for skeletal-muscle-tissue engineering. *Adv Mater*, 2016. **28**(48): p. 10588–10612.
47. Luo, Z., et al., Vertical extrusion cryo(bio)printing for anisotropic tissue manufacturing. *Adv Mater*, 2022. **34**(12): p. 2108931.
48. Agrawal, G., A. Aung, and S. Varghese, Skeletal muscle-on-a-chip: an in vitro model to evaluate tissue formation and injury. *Lab Chip*, 2017. **17**(20): p. 3447–3461.
49. Quarta, M., et al., Bioengineered constructs combined with exercise enhance stem cell-mediated treatment of volumetric muscle loss. *Nat Commun*, 2017. **8**: p. 15613.
50. Kim, J.H., et al., Neural cell integration into 3D bioprinted skeletal muscle constructs accelerates restoration of muscle function. *Nat Commun*, 2020. **11**(1): p. 1025.
51. Lee, H., et al., Functional skeletal muscle regeneration using muscle mimetic tissue fabricated by microvalve-assisted coaxial 3D bioprinting. *Adv Healthc Mater*, 2023. **12**(7): p. e2202664.
52. Li, T., et al., Bioprinted anisotropic scaffolds with fast stress relaxation bioink for engineering 3D skeletal muscle and repairing volumetric muscle loss. *Acta Biomater*, 2023. **156**: p. 21–36.
53. Christensen, K.W., et al., Assembled cell-decorated collagen (AC-DC) fiber bioprinted implants with musculoskeletal tissue properties promote functional recovery in volumetric muscle loss. *Adv Healthc Mater*, 2022. **11**(3): p. e2101357.
54. Pfister, B.J., et al., Biomedical engineering strategies for peripheral nerve repair: surgical applications, state of the art, and future challenges. *Crit Rev Biomed Eng*, 2011. **39**(2): p. 81–124.
55. Panagopoulos, G.N., P.D. Megaloikonomos, and A.F. Mavrogenis, The present and future for peripheral nerve regeneration. *Orthopedics*, 2017. **40**(1): p. e141–e156.
56. Adams, A.M., et al., Scaffoldless tissue-engineered nerve conduit promotes peripheral nerve regeneration and functional recovery after tibial nerve injury in rats. *Neural Regen Res*, 2017. **12**(9): p. 1529–1537.
57. Yurie, H., et al., The efficacy of a scaffold-free Bio 3D conduit developed from human fibroblasts on peripheral nerve regeneration in a rat sciatic nerve model. *PLoS One*, 2017. **12**(2): p. e0171448.
58. Tajino, J., et al., Three-dimensional motion analysis for comprehensive understanding of gait characteristics after sciatic nerve lesion in rodents. *Sci Rep*, 2018. **8**(1): p. 13585.
59. Bain, J.R., S.E. Mackinnon, and D.A. Hunter, Functional evaluation of complete sciatic, peroneal, and posterior tibial nerve lesions in the rat. *Plast Reconstr Surg*, 1989. **83**(1): p. 129–138.
60. Siemionow, M., et al., Peripheral nerve defect repair with epineural tubes supported with bone marrow stromal cells: a preliminary report. *Ann Plast Surg*, 2011. **67**(1): p. 73–84.
61. Hwangbo, H., et al., Bio-printing of aligned GelMa-based cell-laden structure for muscle tissue regeneration. *Bioact Mater*, 2022. **8**: p. 57–70.

62. Wang, H., et al., Quantitative biofabrication platform for collagen-based peripheral nerve grafts with structural and chemical guidance. *Adv Healthc Mater*, 2024. **13**(9): p. e2303505.
63. Mitsuzawa, S., et al., Pro-angiogenic scaffold-free Bio three-dimensional conduit developed from human induced pluripotent stem cell-derived mesenchymal stem cells promotes peripheral nerve regeneration. *Sci Rep*, 2020. **10**(1): p. 12034.
64. Hu, Y., et al., 3D-engineering of cellularized conduits for peripheral nerve regeneration. *Sci Rep*, 2016. **6**: p. 32184.
65. Tao, J., et al., Rapid 3D printing of functional nanoparticle-enhanced conduits for effective nerve repair. *Acta Biomater*, 2019. **90**: p. 49–59.
66. Hsieh, F.Y. and S.H. Hsu, 3D bioprinting: a new insight into the therapeutic strategy of neural tissue regeneration. *Organogenesis*, 2015. **11**(4): p. 153–158.
67. Liu, X., et al., 3D bioprinted neural tissue constructs for spinal cord injury repair. *Biomaterials*, 2021. **272**: p. 120771.
68. Jiang, J.P., et al., Three-dimensional bioprinting collagen/silk fibroin scaffold combined with neural stem cells promotes nerve regeneration after spinal cord injury. *Neural Regen Res*, 2020. **15**(5): p. 959–968.
69. Liu, X., et al., Release of O-GlcNAc transferase inhibitor promotes neuronal differentiation of neural stem cells in 3D bioprinted supramolecular hydrogel scaffold for spinal cord injury repair. *Acta Biomater*, 2022. **151**: p. 148–162.
70. Du, X.J., et al., Neural stem cell transplantation inhibits glial cell proliferation and P2X receptor-mediated neuropathic pain in spinal cord injury rats. *Neural Regen Res*, 2019. **14**(5): p. 876–885.
71. Zhang, C., et al., Early electrical field stimulation prevents the loss of spinal cord anterior horn motoneurons and muscle atrophy following spinal cord injury. *Neural Regen Res*, 2018. **13**(5): p. 869–876.
72. Koffler, J., et al., Biomimetic 3D-printed scaffolds for spinal cord injury repair. *Nat Med*, 2019. **25**(2): p. 263–269.
73. Szklanny, A.A., et al., 3D bioprinting of engineered tissue flaps with hierarchical vessel networks (vesselnet) for direct host-to-implant perfusion. *Adv Mater*, 2021. **33**(42): p. e2102661.
74. Wang, D., et al., Microfluidic bioprinting of tough hydrogel-based vascular conduits for functional blood vessels. *Sci Adv*, 2022. **8**(43): p. eabq6900.
75. Tang, G., et al., Liquid-embedded (bio)printing of alginate-free, standalone, ultrafine, and ultrathin-walled cannular structures. *Proc Natl Acad Sci USA*, 2023. **120**(7): p. e2206762120.
76. Son, J., et al., Bioprinting of pre-vascularized constructs for enhancedin vivoneo-vascularization. *Biofabrication*, 2023. **15**(3).
77. Cui, H., et al., In vitro and in vivo evaluation of 3D bioprinted small-diameter vasculature with smooth muscle and endothelium. *Biofabrication*, 2019. **12**(1): p. 015004.
78. Dashnyam, K., et al., Promoting angiogenesis with mesoporous microcarriers through a synergistic action of delivered silicon ion and VEGF. *Biomaterials*, 2017. 116: p. 145–157.
79. Kechichian, E. and K. Ezzedine, Vitamin D and the skin: an update for dermatologists. *Am J Clin Dermatol*, 2018. **19**(2): p. 223–235.
80. Weng, T., et al., 3D bioprinting for skin tissue engineering: current status and perspectives. *J Tissue Eng*, 2021. **12**: p. 20417314211028574.
81. Jin, R., et al., Three-dimensional bioprinting of a full-thickness functional skin model using acellular dermal matrix and gelatin methacrylamide bioink. *Acta Biomater*, 2021. **131**: p. 248–261.
82. Zhou, F., et al., Rapid printing of bio-inspired 3D tissue constructs for skin regeneration. *Biomaterials*, 2020. **258**: p. 120287.

83. Chen, H., et al., Robot-assisted in situ bioprinting of gelatin methacrylate hydrogels with stem cells induces hair follicle-inclusive skin regeneration. *Biomed Pharmacother*, 2023. **158**: p. 114140.
84. Ma, J., et al., 3D printing of strontium silicate microcylinder-containing multicellular biomaterial inks for vascularized skin regeneration. *Adv Healthc Mater*, 2021. **10**(16): p. e2100523.
85. Kim, B.S., et al., 3D cell printing of perfusable vascularized human skin equivalent composed of epidermis, dermis, and hypodermis for better structural recapitulation of native skin. *Adv Healthc Mater*, 2019. **8**(7): p. e1801019.
86. Zimmermann, W.H., Tissue engineering: polymers flex their muscles. *Nat Mater*, 2008. **7**(12): p. 932–933.
87. Yang, Y., et al., Elastic 3D-printed hybrid polymeric scaffold improves cardiac remodeling after myocardial infarction. *Adv Healthc Mater*, 2019. **8**(10): p. e1900065.
88. Zimmermann, W.H., et al., Engineered heart tissue grafts improve systolic and diastolic function in infarcted rat hearts. *Nat Med*, 2006. **12**(4): p. 452–458.
89. Sun, X., W. Altalhi, and S.S. Nunes, Vascularization strategies of engineered tissues and their application in cardiac regeneration. *Adv Drug Deliv Rev*, 2016. **96**: p. 183–194.
90. Huang, S., et al., A perfusable, multifunctional epicardial device improves cardiac function and tissue repair. *Nat Med*, 2021. **27**(3): p. 480–490.
91. Bejleri, D., et al., A bioprinted cardiac patch composed of cardiac-specific extracellular matrix and progenitor cells for heart repair. *Adv Healthc Mater*, 2018. **7**(23): p. e1800672.
92. Mehrotra, S., et al., Engineering microsphere-loaded non-mulberry silk-based 3D bioprinted vascularized cardiac patches with oxygen-releasing and immunomodulatory potential. *ACS Appl Mater Interfaces*, 2021. **13**(43): p. 50744–50759.
93. Annabi, N., et al., Engineering a highly elastic human protein-based sealant for surgical applications. *Sci Transl Med*, 2017. **9**(410).
94. Moon, A.M., A.G. Singal, and E.B. Tapper, Contemporary epidemiology of chronic liver disease and cirrhosis. *Clin Gastroenterol Hepatol*, 2020. **18**(12): p. 2650–2666.
95. Cross-Najafi, A.A., et al., The long road to develop custom-built livers: current status of 3D liver bioprinting. *Transplantation*, 2024. **108**(2): p. 357–368.
96. da Silva Morais, A., et al., Advanced biomaterials and processing methods for liver regeneration: state-of-the-art and future trends. *Adv Healthc Mater*, 2020. **9**(5): p. e1901435.
97. Vijayavenkataraman, S., et al., 3D bioprinting of tissues and organs for regenerative medicine. *Adv Drug Deliv Rev*, 2018. **132**: p. 296–332.
98. Yang, H., et al., Three-dimensional bioprinted hepatorganoids prolong survival of mice with liver failure. *Gut*, 2021. **70**(3): p. 567–574.
99. Sasaki, K., et al., Construction of three-dimensional vascularized functional human liver tissue using a layer-by-layer cell coating technique. *Biomaterials*, 2017. **133**: p. 263–274.
100. Ohashi, K., et al., Engineering functional two- and three-dimensional liver systems in vivo using hepatic tissue sheets. *Nat Med*, 2007. **13**(7): p. 880–885.
101. Kim, S. and S. Takayama, Organ-on-a-chip and the kidney. *Kidney Res Clin Pract*, 2015. **34**(3): p. 165–169.
102. Sochol, R.D., N.R. Gupta, and J.V. Bonventre, A role for 3D printing in kidney-on-a-chip platforms. *Curr Transplant Rep*, 2016. **3**(1): p. 82–92.
103. Ibi, Y. and R. Nishinakamura, Kidney bioengineering for transplantation. *Transplantation*, 2023. **107**(9): p. 1883–1894.
104. Singh, N.K., et al., Three-dimensional cell-printing of advanced renal tubular tissue analogue. *Biomaterials*, 2020. **232**: p. 119734.
105. Cui, H., et al., 3D bioprinting for cardiovascular regeneration and pharmacology. *Adv Drug Deliv Rev*, 2018. **132**: p. 252–269.

10 Future Directions and Emerging Trends in 3D Bioprinting

Chuyue Cui and Thomas J. Webster

10.1 INTRODUCTION

Three-dimensional (3D) printing, also known as additive manufacturing, is an advanced rapid prototyping technology. Its core principle involves the precise construction of 3D objects based on digital model files through layer-by-layer printing and incremental fabrication (Wu et al., 2023, Fang et al., 2023). As an emerging subfield, 3D bioprinting combines 3D printing techniques with biological materials. It uses active molecules and living cells as fundamental building blocks and assembles them under the control of digital 3D models to produce biomimetic structures, tissues, and even organs, with wide applications in the biomedical field. This technology represents an interdisciplinary integration of manufacturing science, materials science, biology, informatics, and medicine. It has successfully enabled the fabrication of various biomedical materials and shows great promise for both research and clinical applications (Schneider et al., 2023). At present, 3D bioprinting is widely applied in producing complex and otherwise hard-to-replicate anatomical structures for surgical planning, intraoperative navigation, postoperative repair, surgical training, patient education, and patient-specific treatments. In addition, it allows for the precise deposition of biomaterials and living cells and can be combined with biotechnology to facilitate new drug development. It is considered a key enabler in advancing and accelerating the field of regenerative medicine.

10.2 EMERGING TRENDS IN 3D BIOPRINTING

10.2.1 4D Bioprinting and Smart Materials

3D bioprinting is a rapidly evolving technology that utilizes functional bioinks to fabricate complex, cell-laden 3D tissue constructs designed to replicate the architecture and function of native biological tissues. This technique has shown promising applications in engineering soft tissues such as cartilage, bone, and skin (Di Marzio et al., 2020, Mohammed et al., 2020, Midha et al., 2019). Common bioprinting methods include extrusion-based, inkjet, and laser-assisted approaches (Ghilan et al., 2020, Daly et al., 2015, Khorsandi et al., 2021). Building upon these capabilities, the emerging concept of four-dimensional (4D) bioprinting introduces "time" as an additional dimension (Wan et al., 2020). By integrating smart, stimuli-responsive biomaterials,

DOI: 10.1201/9781032638164-10

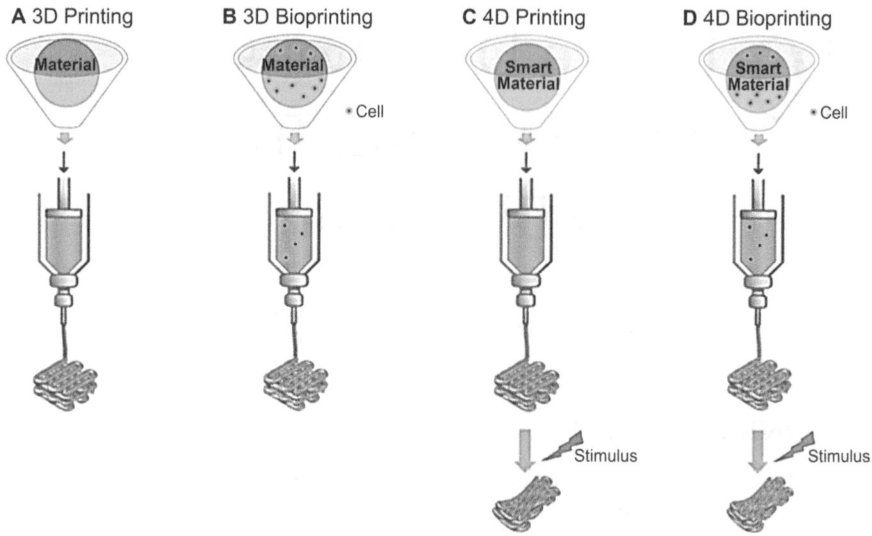

FIGURE 10.1 This schematic compares 3D and 4D printing technologies, including their bioprinting variants. While bioprinting incorporates living cells, 4D bioprinting involves cell-laden constructs that can change over time in response to external stimuli or internal cellular forces.

4D bioprinting enables printed constructs to dynamically transform their shape or functionality in response to external cues, offering new possibilities for fabricating adaptive, functional tissue architectures (Figure 10.1) (Zheng et al., 2022).

4D bioprinting encompasses a range of programmable technologies capable of self-assembly, self-folding, or structural adaptation over time (An et al., 2016). It is characterized by three key elements: (1) a human-designed, programmable structure rather than one derived from nature; (2) the use of 2D or 3D bioprinting techniques for fabrication; and (3) a post-printing evolution process, in which the printed constructs undergo dynamic changes driven by embedded cells or biomaterials in response to external stimuli.

Figure 10.2 illustrates three representative strategies currently adopted in 4D bioprinting, each based on a different mechanism. The first strategy is rooted in the original concept proposed by the Massachusetts Institute of Technology (MIT), where a smart material such as a responsive hydrogel serves as the structural base. Upon exposure to specific stimuli, the substrate transforms into a preprogrammed 3D shape, while the encapsulated cells or tissues adapt passively to this transformation, resulting in a desired spatial configuration (Mironov, 2014). The second strategy can be considered a form of "in vivo 4D bioprinting." Here, a bioresorbable 3D-printed implant is placed into the body and acts as a temporary scaffold to guide tissue regeneration. Over time, as the biological tissue grows and strengthens, the implanted device gradually degrades and is absorbed, with tissue development itself acting as the driving stimulus (Morrison et al., 2015). The third strategy centers on active self-assembly. In this case, cells are printed in specific microscale

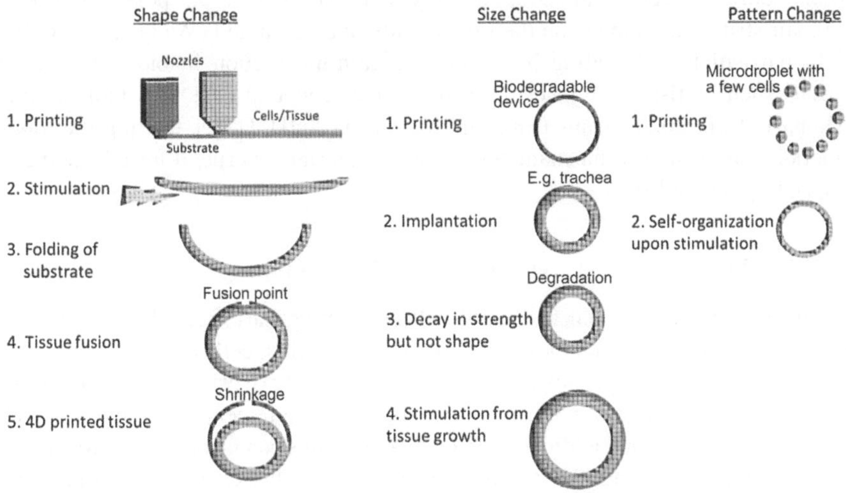

FIGURE 10.2 Three approaches in 4D bioprinting.

arrangements, and subsequent structural changes arise autonomously through intercellular signaling and collective behavior. Although self-organization is encouraged, the exact triggers for pattern evolution remain unclear (Agarwal et al., 2023). Given the limited research available for each approach, it is premature to determine which is most effective. However, all three strategies present novel possibilities and merit further investigation in future studies (Figure 10.2).

Stimuli-responsive materials (SMs), widely used in 4D bioprinting, can generally be categorized into two main groups: shape-changing materials (SCMs) and shape-memory materials (SMMs), along with those that exhibit variations in stiffness or phase transitions (Zhao et al., 2022, Su et al., 2018, Haleem et al., 2021). SCMs react to environmental changes by altering their shape and then returning to their original configuration once the external stimulus is withdrawn, indicating that their deformation pathways are inherently predefined (McLellan et al., 2022, Mani et al., 2022). In contrast, SMMs require a programming phase during which they are "trained" to transform into complex forms upon stimulation. These are further divided into shape-memory alloys (SMAs) and shape-memory polymers (SMPs) (Shie et al., 2019, Palmara et al., 2021).

Various smart materials, including SMAs, SMPs, SMP composites, hydrogels, elastomers, and SCMs—have been adapted for use in 4D bioprinting systems (Heidarian et al., 2021, Heidarian et al., 2020, Bom et al., 2022). These materials are capable of exhibiting five core intelligent behaviors: shape memory, self-assembly, self-actuation, self-sensing, and self-healing (Wang and Li, 2021). Specifically, SMMs can switch into preconfigured shapes under external triggers (Arif et al., 2021), while self-assembly relies on stimuli to induce folding or alignment into intended forms (Zhao et al., 2018). Self-actuating systems respond autonomously to stimuli, whereas self-sensing materials detect and assess changes in their surroundings (Pingale et al.,

2023, Piedrahita-Bello et al., 2020). Finally, self-healing materials possess the ability to repair structural damage on their own, without external aid (Wang et al., 2020).

In particular, self-healing hydrogels are gaining traction in biomedical applications such as tissue engineering, drug delivery, wound care, and biofabrication (Manjari et al., 2020, Amukarimi and Mozafari, 2021). Understanding the unique functions and response mechanisms of these materials is crucial for advancing 4D bioprinting technologies.

10.2.2 Multi-Material and Multi-Cell Bioprinting

Advances in multi-material and multi-cell bioprinting have been driven largely by the development of tailored bioinks that can carry distinct cell types while providing local biochemical and mechanical cues. Recent surveys of extrusion-compatible bioinks emphasize strategies for blending natural and synthetic polymers, decellularized-ECM fractions, and functional additives so that different inks can be optimized for specific cell phenotypes (e.g., endothelial, stromal, cardiomyocytes, etc.) without compromising printability or viability (Tarassoli et al., 2021, Kim et al., 2022). Multichannel and coaxial printheads enable simultaneous deposition of heterogeneous inks (allowing core–shell or Janus filaments that spatially segregate cell populations and permit sacrificial materials for later perfusable channel formation) which is an approach that has been used to produce vascularized cardiac constructs and other multicellular architectures (Mohan et al., 2022, Maiullari et al., 2018). To better mimic native tissue complexity, contemporary strategies combine: (1) gradient or layered deposition of compositionally distinct bioinks to recreate extracellular matrix (ECM) and mechanical heterogeneity, (2) incorporation of instructive biochemical cues (growth factors, ECM fragments, etc.) to guide cell fate and self-organization, and (3) the use of dynamic or sacrificial components to generate microvascular networks and interstitial spaces that permit mass transport (Ravanbakhsh et al., 2021, Hwang et al., 2021). Together, these material- and process-level advances are enabling increasingly biomimetic, multicellular constructs that approach the structural and functional hallmarks of native tissues (Zhang, 2022).

10.2.3 Artificial intelligence (AI) and Machine Learning in Bioprinting

The integration of artificial intelligence and machine learning (ML) into bioprinting workflows is transforming how print parameters and bioink formulations are optimized. Data-driven algorithms can rapidly correlate rheological, mechanical, and biological datasets with deposition fidelity, enabling an automated adjustment of extrusion pressure, nozzle speed, and temperature to maintain print resolution and cell viability across diverse bioink compositions (Ruberu et al., 2021). In addition, multi-objective optimization frameworks have been applied to fine-tune composite bioinks (balancing viscosity, crosslinking kinetics, and biochemical content) thereby reducing the need for extensive trial-and-error experimentation (Freeman et al., 2022).

Beyond process optimization, predictive modeling powered by ML is increasingly used to forecast cell behavior and tissue maturation within printed constructs.

Models trained on time-lapse imaging, gene expression profiles, and biomechanical data can anticipate proliferation, differentiation, and ECM deposition patterns, offering early indicators of tissue functionality (Boehm et al., 2022, Li, 2021). Such predictive tools support the rational design of dynamic culture regimes and adaptive bioprinting strategies, ultimately improving the reproducibility and clinical readiness of engineered tissues (Ramesh et al., 2024).

10.3 FUTURE DIRECTIONS IN 3D BIOPRINTING

10.3.1 Personalized Medicine and Patient-Specific Bioprinting

The concept of personalized medicine is transforming healthcare from a model of standardized treatment toward one that accounts for the genetic, anatomical, and physiological differences between individuals. In bioprinting, this approach has manifested in the development of patient-specific implants, grafts, and tissues, which are fabricated based on each patient's own anatomical data and, in many cases, their own cells. The integration of medical imaging techniques such as computed tomography and magnetic resonance imaging with computer-aided design allows for the creation of highly detailed 3D digital models of defects or organs. These models are then translated into printer instructions, enabling the precise deposition of biomaterials to match patient-specific geometries with remarkable fidelity (Kennedy et al., 2025).

Personalized bioprinting goes beyond geometry. Biological compatibility is also optimized by incorporating autologous cells—stem cells or differentiated cells derived from the patient—into bioinks. This strategy mitigates the risk of immune rejection and improves integration with the surrounding tissue after implantation. Recent research has demonstrated the feasibility of fabricating cartilage constructs seeded with patient-derived chondrocytes for repairing joint defects, as well as cardiac patches embedded with a patient' s own induced pluripotent stem cells to promote myocardial regeneration (Shopova et al., 2023).

Emerging 4D bioprinting technologies—where printed constructs are designed to change shape, properties, or function in response to environmental stimuli—add an extra layer of personalization. For example, shape-memory polymers and stimuli-responsive hydrogels can adapt their mechanical stiffness to match the healing progression of surrounding tissues, or release therapeutic agents in response to changes in pH or temperature. This adaptability could allow implants to "co-evolve" with the patient's recovery process, aligning treatment with individual healing trajectories. The growing convergence of patient-specific digital design, cell sourcing, and smart material science thus represents a critical frontier in translating bioprinting from the laboratory to personalized clinical care.

10.3.2 Bioprinting for In Vitro Models and Drug Testing

Drug development is an expensive and time-consuming process, with a high rate of late-stage failures—often because traditional in vitro and in vivo models fail to accurately predict human responses. Bioprinted in vitro tissue models address this problem by replicating the 3D microenvironment of human tissues, capturing not only the spatial organization of cells but also their interactions with ECM components and mechanical cues (Budharaju et al., 2025).

For example, liver tissue models constructed from primary human hepatocytes and non-parenchymal cells have been printed into perfusable hydrogel matrices that sustain metabolic function for weeks. These models allow for more accurate predictions of drug clearance rates, metabolic pathways, and potential hepatotoxicity than conventional 2D monolayer cultures. In oncology, 3D bioprinted tumor models embedded within vascular-like channels mimic the nutrient and oxygen gradients of solid tumors, enabling the evaluation of drug penetration and efficacy under physiologically relevant conditions (Mallya et al., 2025).

A major advantage of bioprinted models is their reproducibility. Unlike patient-derived xenografts in animals, which vary due to interspecies differences and host physiology, printed models can be standardized to produce uniform testing platforms for high-throughput drug screening. This consistency is particularly valuable for toxicity testing in the cosmetics industry, which faces increasing restrictions on animal testing. Furthermore, combining these models with organ-on-a-chip systems allows dynamic fluid flow, further enhancing physiological relevance. The synergy between bioprinting and microfluidics is opening the door to multi-organ "human-on-a-chip" systems that could one day simulate systemic drug responses in vitro (Paradiso et al., 2023).

By improving predictive accuracy, bioprinted in vitro models not only accelerate preclinical research but also align with ethical imperatives to reduce animal testing. As these models become more sophisticated (integrating immune cells, vasculature, and even neural components) they may eventually replace certain categories of animal studies altogether.

10.3.3 Toward Fully Functional Organ Printing

The dream of fabricating fully functional, transplantable organs is one of the most ambitious goals in regenerative medicine. Significant progress has been made in printing small tissue constructs and organoids, yet scaling up to whole organs presents formidable scientific and engineering challenges. The most critical among these is vascularization—creating dense, hierarchical networks of blood vessels that can supply oxygen and nutrients to all regions of the tissue (Sexton et al., 2023). Without such networks, cell death occurs rapidly in thick constructs due to diffusion limits.

Recent strategies for overcoming this barrier include sacrificial-ink printing, in which fugitive materials are deposited during the printing process and later removed to leave behind perfusable channels. Another promising approach is coaxial extrusion bioprinting, which allows for the simultaneous deposition of vessel-like tubular structures lined with endothelial cells. Integration of microfluidic designs into bioprinting workflows enables precise control over channel geometry and interconnectivity, which is critical for achieving physiologically relevant perfusion.

Beyond vasculature, fully functional organ printing also requires the incorporation and coordination of multiple cell types (parenchymal, stromal, endothelial, and immune cells) in correct spatial arrangements. For instance, in printing kidney-like constructs, not only must the nephrons be replicated, but they must also connect functionally to the collecting ducts and vascular networks. Mechanical properties are equally important; printed heart tissue must withstand cyclic loading, while printed cartilage must endure compressive forces. Advanced biomaterials such as decellularized ECM bioinks are being investigated for their ability to provide tissue-specific biochemical cues that promote cell differentiation and maturation (Sun et al., 2024).

Finally, the long-term survival and function of printed organs depend on immune compatibility and integration with the host body. Gene editing tools such as CRISPR–Cas9 are being explored to modify donor-derived cells to reduce immunogenicity. These converging advances (vascularization strategies, multicellular organization, biomaterial innovation, and immunomodulation) suggest that while fully functional organ printing is not yet a clinical reality, the gap between possibility and practice is steadily narrowing.

10.3.4 Ethical and Regulatory Considerations

The bioprinting of human tissues and organs raises complex ethical, legal, and societal questions. At the heart of these concerns is the issue of ownership: if a patient's cells are used to create a bioprinted organ, does the organ belong to the patient, the healthcare provider, or the company that manufactured it? Current legal frameworks offer limited guidance, leading to uncertainty and potential disputes (Yaneva et al., 2023).

Another critical issue is informed consent. Donors must be made aware not only of the immediate use of their cells but also of any potential future applications, such as research, commercial products, or storage in biobanks. This is particularly important when cells are genetically modified or combined with other biological materials. The potential for misuse (such as the unregulated printing of tissues for enhancement purposes or nontherapeutic applications) has also prompted calls for strict biosecurity measures.

Regulatory pathways for bioprinted products are still evolving. In most jurisdictions, these products do not fit neatly into existing categories of medical devices or biologics. This ambiguity can slow the translation of laboratory advances into clinical therapies. Regulatory agencies are beginning to develop new classifications and guidelines, emphasizing quality control, safety testing, and postimplantation monitoring. Some have proposed adaptive regulatory frameworks that can evolve alongside the technology (Briones et al., 2025).

International cooperation will be essential to harmonize standards, especially as the global market for bioprinted products expands. Without coordinated efforts, disparities in regulatory requirements could lead to "medical tourism" for unapproved treatments, raising safety and ethical concerns. Ultimately, robust ethical oversight and clear regulatory guidelines are not obstacles to innovation, but enablers that can ensure public trust and responsible clinical translation.

10.3.5 Commercialized 3D-Printed Materials

Although the field of bioprinting is often associated with experimental research, several categories of 3D-printed materials have already reached the commercial stage. In orthopedics, patient-specific titanium alloy implants manufactured via powder bed fusion are now routinely used for complex joint reconstructions and spinal surgeries. In dentistry, custom ceramic crowns and bridges fabricated by 3D printing offer both aesthetic and functional advantages over traditional manufacturing.

In the realm of biofabrication, companies like Organovo have pioneered the commercial production of bioprinted tissue models for pharmaceutical testing. Their human liver and cancer models provide more predictive data on drug metabolism and toxicity than conventional preclinical methods, allowing pharmaceutical companies to identify promising compounds earlier and reduce costly late-stage failures.

Beyond hard tissues, there is a growing market for bioinks—specialized printable materials that may contain cells, growth factors, or other bioactive agents. These are being sold for research purposes, enabling labs without in-house formulation capabilities to experiment with tissue printing. Hybrid constructs that combine biodegradable polymers with embedded drugs or electrical conductivity are emerging for applications in regenerative medicine, where they can support tissue growth while delivering therapeutic cues or enabling functional stimulation (Mirsky et al., 2024).

Regulatory approval for living, cell-laden products remains rare, but as safety and efficacy data accumulate, more complex constructs are likely to reach the clinic. The success of current commercial products demonstrates that the technological and economic foundations for the bioprinting industry are already in place, paving the way for increasingly sophisticated applications.

10.4 CONCLUSIONS

This chapter summarizes 3D bioprinting, an extension of additive manufacturing, and its integration with digital design and biomaterials and living cells to create functional biological structures for biomedical research and clinical applications. This chapter introduces the foundations of 3D and 4D (where the fourth dimension is time) bioprinting, highlighting the role of smart, stimuli-responsive materials such as shape-memory polymers and hydrogels in enabling dynamic, adaptive tissue constructs. Emerging advances in multi-material and multi-cell bioprinting are discussed, with emphasis on the development of tailored bioinks and strategies for vascularization and tissue complexity. The integration of artificial intelligence and ML is also examined as a means of optimizing printing parameters, predicting cell behavior, and accelerating tissue maturation. Future directions address the potential of personalized, patient-specific bioprinting, the creation of in vitro models for drug discovery, and progress toward fully functional organ printing. Ethical and regulatory considerations are reviewed alongside current commercial applications of 3D-printed materials. Together, these developments illustrate the transformative potential of bioprinting to advance regenerative medicine and reshape healthcare.

REFERENCES

Agarwal, K., Srinivasan, V., Lather, V., Pandita, D. & Vasanthan, K. S. 2023. Insights of 3D bioprinting and focusing the paradigm shift towards 4D printing for biomedical applications. *Journal of Materials Research,* 38, 112–141.

Amukarimi, S. & Mozafari, M. 2021. 4D bioprinting of tissues and organs. *Bioprinting,* 23, e00161.

An, J., Chua, C. K. & Mironov, V. 2016. A perspective on 4D bioprinting. *International Journal of Bioprinting,* 2, 3–5.

Arif, M. M., Khan, S. M., Gull, N., Tabish, T. A., Zia, S., Khan, R. U., Awais, S. M. & Butt, M. A. 2021. Polymer-based biomaterials for chronic wound management: Promises and challenges. *International Journal of Pharmaceutics,* 598, 120270.

Boehm, K. M., Aherne, E. A., Ellenson, L., Nikolovski, I., Alghamdi, M., Vázquez-Garcí A, I., Zamarin, D., Roche, K. L., Liu, Y., Patel, D., Aukerman, A., Pasha, A., Rose, D., Selenica, P., Andrieu, P. I. C., Fong, C., Capanu, M., Reis, J. S., Vanguri, R., Veeraraghavan, H., Gangai, N., Sosa, R., Leung, S., Mcpherson, A., Gao, J. J., Lakhman, Y., Shah, S. H. P. & Consortium, M. M. 2022. Multimodal data integration using machine learning improves risk stratification of high-grade serous ovarian cancer. *Nature Cancer,* 3, 723.

Bom, S., Ribeiro, R., Ribeiro, H. M., Santos, C. & Marto, J. 2022. On the progress of hydrogel-based 3D printing: Correlating rheological properties with printing behaviour. *International Journal of Pharmaceutics,* 615, 121506.

Briones, Y., Pascua, B., Tiangco, N., Crisostomo, I., Casiguran, S. & Remenyi, R. 2025. Assessing the landscape of clinical and observational trials involving bioprinting: A scoping review. *3D Printing in Medicine,* 11, 5.

Budharaju, H., Singh, R. K. & Kim, H.-W. 2025. Bioprinting for drug screening: A path toward reducing animal testing or redefining preclinical research? *Bioactive Materials,* 51, 993–1017.

Daly, R., Harrington, T. S., Martin, G. D. & Hutchings, I. M. 2015. Inkjet printing for pharmaceutics–a review of research and manufacturing. *International Journal of Pharmaceutics,* 494, 554–567.

Di Marzio, N., Eglin, D., Serra, T. & Moroni, L. 2020. Bio-fabrication: convergence of 3D bioprinting and nano-biomaterials in tissue engineering and regenerative medicine. *Frontiers in Bioengineering and Biotechnology,* 8, 326.

Fang, Y., Chen, F., Wu, H. & Chen, B. 2023. Progress in the application of 3D printing technology in ophthalmology. *Graefe's Archive for Clinical and Experimental Ophthalmology,* 261, 903–912.

Freeman, S., Calabro, S., Williams, R., Jin, S. & Ye, K. M. 2022. Bioink formulation and machine learning-empowered bioprinting optimization. *Frontiers in Bioengineering and Biotechnology,* 10, 913579.

Ghilan, A., Chiriac, A. P., Nita, L. E., Rusu, A. G., Neamtu, I. & Chiriac, V. M. 2020. Trends in 3D printing processes for biomedical field: Opportunities and challenges. *Journal of Polymers and the Environment,* 28, 1345–1367.

Haleem, A., Javaid, M., Singh, R. P. & Suman, R. 2021. Significant roles of 4D printing using smart materials in the field of manufacturing. *Advanced Industrial and Engineering Polymer Research,* 4, 301–311.

Heidarian, P., Kaynak, A., Paulino, M., Zolfagharian, A., Varley, R. J. & Kouzani, A. Z. 2021. Dynamic nanocellulose hydrogels: Recent advancements and future outlook. *Carbohydrate Polymers,* 270, 118357.

Heidarian, P., Kouzani, A. Z., Kaynak, A., Paulino, M., Nasri-Nasrabadi, B., Zolfagharian, A. & Varley, R. 2020. Dynamic plant-derived polysaccharide-based hydrogels. *Carbohydrate Polymers,* 231, 115743.

Hwang, D. G., Choi, Y. M. & Jang, J. 2021. 3D bioprinting-based vascularized tissue models mimicking tissue-specific architecture and pathophysiology for *in vitro* studies. *Frontiers in Bioengineering and Biotechnology,* 9, 685507.

Kennedy, S. M., Sekar, M., Vasanthanathan, A. & Amudhan, K. 2025. 4D bioprinting for personalized medicine, innovations in implant fabrication and regenerative therapies. *Polymer-Plastics Technology and Materials,* 64, 1–26.

Khorsandi, D., Fahimipour, A., Abasian, P., Saber, S. S., Seyedi, M., Ghanavati, S., Ahmad, A., De Stephanis, A. A., Taghavinezhaddilami, F. & Leonova, A. 2021. 3D and 4D printing in dentistry and maxillofacial surgery: Printing techniques, materials, and applications. *Acta Biomaterialia,* 122, 26–49.

Kim, D., Kim, M., Lee, J. & Jang, J. 2022. Review on multicomponent hydrogel bioinks based on natural biomaterials for bioprinting 3D liver tissues. *Frontiers in Bioengineering and Biotechnology,* 10, 764682.

Li, Z. Y. 2021. Predicting bone regeneration from machine learning. *Nature Computational Science,* 1, 509–510.

Maiullari, F., Costantini, M., Milan, M., Pace, V., Chirivì, M., Maiullari, S., Rainer, A., Baci, D., Marei, H. E., Seliktar, D., Gargioli, C., Bearzi, C. & Rizzi, R. 2018. A multi-cellular 3D bioprinting approach for vascularized heart tissue engineering based on HUVECs and iPSC-derived cardiomyocytes. *Scientific Reports,* 8, 13532.

Mallya, D., Gadre, M. A., Varadharajan, S. & Vasanthan, K. S. 2025. 3D bioprinting for the construction of drug testing models-development strategies and regulatory concerns. *Frontiers in Bioengineering and Biotechnology,* 13, 1457872.

Mani, M. P., Sadia, M., Jaganathan, S. K., Khudzari, A. Z., Supriyanto, E., Saidin, S., Ramakrishna, S., Ismail, A. F. & Faudzi, A. A. M. 2022. A review on 3D printing in tissue engineering applications. *Journal of Polymer Engineering,* 42, 243–265.

Manjari, M. S., Aaron, K. P., Muralidharan, C. & Rose, C. 2020. Highly biocompatible novel polyphenol cross-linked collagen scaffold for potential tissue engineering applications. *Reactive & Functional Polymers,* 153, 104630.

Mclellan, K., Sun, Y. C. & Naguib, H. E. 2022. A review of 4D printing: Materials, structures, and designs towards the printing of biomedical wearable devices. *Bioprinting*, 27, e00217.

Midha, S., Dalela, M., Sybil, D., Patra, P. & Mohanty, S. 2019. Advances in three-dimensional bioprinting of bone: Progress and challenges. *Journal of Tissue Engineering and Regenerative Medicine,* 13, 925–945.

Mironov, V. 4D bioprinting: Biofabrication of rod-like and tubular tissue engineered constructs using programmable self-folding bioprinted biomaterials. *International Bioprinting Congress*, 2014, 24–25.

Mirsky, N. A., Ehlen, Q. T., Greenfield, J. A., Antonietti, M., Slavin, B. V., Nayak, V. V., Pelaez, D., Tse, D. T., Witek, L., Daunert, S. & Coelho, P. G. 2024. Three-dimensional bioprinting: A comprehensive review for applications in tissue engineering and regenerative medicine. *Bioengineering,* 11, 777.

Mohammed, A., Elshaer, A., Sareh, P., Elsayed, M. & Hassanin, H. 2020. Additive manufacturing technologies for drug delivery applications. *International Journal of Pharmaceutics,* 580.

Mohan, T. S., Datta, P., Nesaei, S., Ozbolat, V. & Ozbolat, I. T. 2022. 3D coaxial bioprinting: Process mechanisms, bioinks and applications. *Progress in Biomedical Engineering,* 4, 022003.

Morrison, R. J., Hollister, S. J., Niedner, M. F., Mahani, M. G., Park, A. H., Mehta, D. K., Ohye, R. G. & Green, G. E. 2015. Mitigation of tracheobronchomalacia with 3D-printed personalized medical devices in pediatric patients. *Science Translational Medicine,* 7, 285ra64.

Palmara, G., Frascella, F., Roppolo, I., Chiappone, A. & Chiadò, A. 2021. Functional 3D printing: Approaches and bioapplications. *Biosensors & Bioelectronics,* 175, 112849.

Paradiso, A., Volpi, M., Rinoldi, C., Celikkin, N., Negrini, N. C., Bilgen, M., Dallera, G., Pierini, F., Costantini, M., Swieszkowski, W. & Farè, S. 2023. *In vitro* functional models for human liver diseases and drug screening: beyond animal testing. *Biomaterials Science,* 11, 2988–3015.

Piedrahita-Bello, M., Angulo-Cervera, J. E., Courson, R., Molná R, G., Malaquin, L., Thibault, C., Tondu, B., Salmon, L. & Bousseksou, A. 2020. 4D printing with spin-crossover polymer composites. *Journal of Materials Chemistry C,* 8, 6001–6005.

Pingale, P., Dawre, S., Dhapte-Pawar, V., Dhas, N. & Rajput, A. 2023. Advances in 4D printing: From stimulation to simulation. *Drug Delivery and Translational Research,* 13, 164–188.

Ramesh, S., Deep, A., Tamayol, A., Kamaraj, A., Mahajan, C. & Madihally, S. 2024. Advancing 3D bioprinting through machine learning and artificial intelligence. *Bioprinting,* 38, e00331.

Ravanbakhsh, H., Karamzadeh, V., Bao, G. Y., Mongeau, L., Juncker, D. & Zhang, Y. S. 2021. Emerging technologies in multi-material bioprinting. *Advanced Materials,* 33, e2104730.

Ruberu, K., Senadeera, M., Rana, S., Gupta, S., Chung, J., Yue, Z. L., Venkatesh, S. & Wallace, G. 2021. Coupling machine learning with 3D bioprinting to fast track optimisation of extrusion printing. *Applied Materials Today,* 22, 100914.

Schneider, K. H., Oberoi, G., Unger, E., Janjic, K., Rohringer, S., Heber, S., Agis, H., Schedle, A., Kiss, H. & Podesser, B. K. 2023. Medical 3D printing with polyjet technology: Effect of material type and printing orientation on printability, surface structure and cytotoxicity. *3D Printing in Medicine,* 9, 27.

Sexton, Z. A., Hudson, A. R., Herrmann, J. E., Shiwarski, D. J., Pham, J., Szafron, J. M., Wu, S. M., Skylar-Scott, M., Feinberg, A. W. & Marsden, A. 2023. Rapid model-guided design of organ-scale synthetic vasculature for biomanufacturing. *ArXiv,* arXiv:2308.07586v1.

Shie, M. Y., Shen, Y. F., Astuti, S. D., Lee, A. K. X., Lin, S. H., Dwijaksara, N. L. B. & Chen, Y. W. 2019. Review of polymeric materials in 4D printing biomedical applications. *Polymers,* 11, 1864.

Shopova, D., Yaneva, A., Bakova, D., Mihaylova, A., Kasnakova, P., Hristozova, M., Sbirkov, Y., Sarafian, V. & SEMERDZHIEVA, M. 2023. (Bio)printing in personalized medicine-opportunities and potential benefits. *Bioengineering,* 10, 287.

Su, J.-W., Tao, X., Deng, H., Zhang, C., Jiang, S., Lin, Y. & Lin, J. 2018. 4D printing of a self-morphing polymer driven by a swellable guest medium. *Soft Matter,* 14, 765–772.

Sun, X. M., Ren, W., Xie, L. Y., Ren, Q. Q., Zhu, Z. J., Jia, Q. F., Jiang, W. S., Jin, Z. & Yu, Y. 2024. Recent advances in 3D bioprinting of tissues and organs for transplantation and drug screening. *Virtual and Physical Prototyping,* 19, e2384662.

Tarassoli, S. P., Jessop, Z. M., Jovic, T., Hawkins, K. & Whitaker, I. S. 2021. Candidate bioinks for extrusion 3D bioprinting–a systematic review of the literature. *Frontiers in Bioengineering and Biotechnology,* 9, 616753.

Wan, Z., Zhang, P., Liu, Y., Lv, L. & Zhou, Y. 2020. Four-dimensional bioprinting: Current developments and applications in bone tissue engineering. *Acta Biomaterialia,* 101, 26–42.

Wang, F. F., Yuan, C., Wang, D., Rosen, D. W. & Ge, Q. 2020. A phase evolution based constitutive model for shape memory polymer and its application in 4D printing. *Smart Materials and Structures,* 29, 055016.

Wang, Y. N. & Li, X. 2021. 4D-printed bi-material composite laminate for manufacturing reversible shape-change structures. *Composites Part B-Engineering,* 219, 108918.

Wu, W., Sabharwal, S., Bunker, M. & Sabharwal, S. 2023. 3D printing technology in pediatric orthopedics: A primer for the clinician. *Current Reviews in Musculoskeletal Medicine,* 16, 398–409.

Yaneva, A., Shopova, D., Bakova, D., Mihaylova, A., Kasnakova, P., Hristozova, M. & Semerdjieva, M. 2023. The progress in bioprinting and its potential impact on health-related quality of life. *Bioengineering,* 10, 910.

Zhang, W. J. 2022. Recent progress in bioprinting: From bioink design to applications. *Bioengineering,* 9, 785.

Zhao, D., Pang, B., Zhu, Y., Cheng, W., Cao, K., Ye, D., Si, C., Xu, G., Chen, C. & Yu, H. 2022. A stiffness-switchable, biomimetic smart material enabled by supramolecular reconfiguration.*Advanced Materials,* 34, 2107857.

Zhao, T. T., Yu, R., Li, X. P., Cheng, B., Zhang, Y., YANG, X., Zhao, X. J., Zhao, Y. L. & Huang, W. 2018. 4D printing of shape memory polyurethane via stereolithography. *European Polymer Journal,* 101, 120–126.

Zheng, Z. R., Patel, M. & Patel, R. 2022. Hyaluronic acid-based materials for bone regeneration: A review. *Reactive & Functional Polymers,* 171, 105151.

Index

V

W

X

Y

Z

For Product Safety Concerns and Information please contact our EU representative GPSR@taylorandfrancis.com Taylor & Francis Verlag GmbH, Kaufingerstraße 24, 80331 München, Germany